Carcinogen Risk Assessment

CONTEMPORARY ISSUES IN RISK ANALYSIS

Sponsored by the Society for Risk Analysis

Carcinogen Risk Assessment

Edited by

Curtis C. Travis

Oak Ridge National Laboratory
Oak Ridge, Tennessee

Plenum Press • *New York and London*

Library of Congress Cataloging in Publication Data

Carcinogen risk assessment / edited by Curtis C. Travis.
    p.   cm. — (Contemporary issues in risk analysis; v. 3)
    Includes bibliographical references and index.
    ISBN-13: 978-1-4684-5486-4   **e-ISBN-13: 978-1-4684-5484-0**
    DOI: 10.1007/ 978-1-4684-5484-0
    1. Carcinogenicity testing. 2. Health risk assessment. 3. Cancer — Prevention. I.
Travis, C. C. II. Series.
RC268.65.C365   1988
616.99′4071 — dc19   87-37403
                                                                  CIP

© 1988 Plenum Press, New York
Softcover reprint of the hardcover 1st edition 1988
A Division of Plenum Publishing Corporation
233 Spring Street, New York, N.Y. 10013

Contributors

Elizabeth L. Anderson   Clement Associates, Inc., Fairfax, Virginia 22031.

Edward J. Calabrese   Environmental Science Program, School of Public Health, University of Massachusetts, Amherst, Massachusetts 01003

Gail Charnley   Clement Associates, Inc., Fairfax, Virginia 22031

Vincent T. Covello   Risk Assessment Program, National Science Foundation, Washington, D.C. 20550

E. A. C. Crouch   Energy and Environmental Policy Center, Harvard University, and Meta-systems, Cambridge, Massachusetts 02138

W. Gary Flamm   Office of Toxicological Sciences, Center for Food Safety and Applied Nutrition, Food and Drug Administration, Washington, D.C. 20204

Ronald W. Hart   National Center for Toxicological Research, Food and Drug Administration, Jefferson, Arkansas 72079

Holly A. Hattemer-Frey   Office of Risk Analysis, Health and Safety Research Division, Oak Ridge National Laboratory, Oak Ridge, Tennessee 37831-6109

Lester B. Lave   Graduate School of Industrial Administration, Carnegie-Mellon University, Pittsburgh, Pennsylvania 15213

Donald Mackay   Institute for Environmental Studies, University of Toronto, Toronto M5S 1A4, Canada

Sally Paterson   Institute for Environmental Studies, University of Toronto, Toronto M5S 1A4, Canada

Frederica P. Perera   Division of Environmental Science, School of Public Health, Columbia University, New York, New York 10032

Robert J. Scheuplein   Office of Toxicological Sciences, Center for Food Safety and Applied Nutrition, Food and Drug Administration, Washington, D.C. 20204

Paul Slovic   Decision Research, Eugene, Oregon 97401

Todd W. Thorslund   Clement Associates, Inc., Fairfax, Virginia 22031

Curtis C. Travis   Office of Risk Analysis, Health and Safety Research Division, Oak Ridge National Laboratory, Oak Ridge, Tennessee 37831-6109

Angelo Turturro   National Center for Toxicological Research, Food and Drug Administration, Jefferson, Arkansas 72079

Elizabeth K. Weisburger   Division of Cancer Etiology, National Cancer Institute, Bethesda, Maryland 20892

Chris Whipple   Electric Power Research Institute, Palo Alto, California 94303

Richard Wilson   Department of Physics and the Energy and Environmental Policy Center, Harvard University, Cambridge, Massachusetts 02138

Detlof von Winterfeldt   Institute of Safety and System Management, University of Southern California, Los Angeles, California 90089

Contents

*Carcinogen
Risk Assessment*

I

Overview of Risk Assessment

1

The Risk Analysis Process

Elizabeth L. Anderson

RISK ASSESSMENT AND RISK MANAGEMENT

The process of risk assessment and risk management is widely recognized in the United States for making policy decisions to control the risk associated with toxic chemical exposures. This two-step process, to first evaluate risk and then decide what, if anything, should be done to reduce exposures, was first adopted by the Environmental Protection Agency (EPA) in 1976 in its announcement of guidelines for assessing cancer risk (EPA, 1976; Albert *et al.*, 1977). This approach was later endorsed by committees of the National Academy of Sciences (NAS) as the most appropriate process for informed public policy decisions to protect public health from toxic chemical exposures (NAS, 1982, 1983). Other United States federal interagency committees reviewed the basis for cancer risk assessment and published background documents that are largely consistent with the earlier and much briefer statement of risk assessment guidance published by the EPA in 1976 (IRLG, 1979; OSTP, 1984). The EPA has recently published updates of its cancer risk assessment guidelines and guidelines for other health effects that take into account its decade of experience in assessing cancer risks for hundreds of chemicals (EPA, 1984a–d, 1985a, 1986a–e).

Risk Assessment

Risk assessment is an organized approach to evaluating scientific data that involve considerable uncertainties. Risk assessment attempts to answer two questions: (1) How likely is an event to occur? and (2) If it does occur, how bad could it be in quantitative terms? This approach has long been used to estimate risks associated with a variety of activities, including economic forecasting, transportation safety, engineering safety (e.g.,

Elizabeth L. Anderson • Clement Associates Inc., Fairfax, Virginia 22031.

nuclear power plants), and radiation exposures. More recently, risk assessment approaches have been used to estimate risk associated with toxic chemical exposures (EPA, 1976; Albert *et al.*, 1977; NAS, 1982, 1983; IRLG, 1979; OSTP, 1984; EPA, 1984a–d, 1985a, 1986a–e).

Risk assessment of toxic chemical exposures may be defined as having four steps: (1) hazard identification, (2) dose–response modeling, (3) exposure assessment, and (4) risk characterization. The hazard identification step (or qualitative risk assessment) (EPA, 1976, 1984a–d, 1985a, 1986a–e) answers the first risk assessment question: How likely is a risk to occur? The next two steps, dose–response modeling and exposure assessment, are combined to quantify the risk associated with current and anticipated exposures. Finally, the risk characterization step presents both the qualitative likelihood of hazard and the quantitative estimates of risk.

Hazard identification for toxic chemicals is based on the evaluation of all available data (e.g., epidemiology, animal bioassay studies, and *in vivo* and *in vitro* studies) to characterize the strength of evidence indicating potential health effects which might occur in exposed human populations.

In the absence of human data to describe low-dose effects, two different approaches for dose–response characterization are most frequently used: one for "threshold" effects and the other for "nonthreshold" effects. The doses associated with human diseases that are thought to occur by a "threshold dose mechanism," i.e., no significant health risks are likely to occur until a certain dose is reached, are most frequently defined by applying safety factors to the no-observed-effect levels in animal bioassay studies. However, human data are used whenever possible. These so-called safe exposure levels are labeled acceptable daily intakes (ADIs) or reference doses. For nonthreshold effects (e.g., cancer), meaning that there may be some risks associated with any exposure, dose–response extrapolation models are used to estimate cancer risks associated with low-dose exposure based on observed incidence in humans and animals exposed at high doses. Since 1976, quantitative risk assessment has received widespread recognition and acceptance for describing health risks associated with toxic chemical exposure. The model most often relied upon for estimating cancer risk has been the linear nonthreshold model, which provides a plausible upper-bound cancer risk estimate (EPA, 1984a; IRLG, 1979; OSTP, 1984; Anderson, 1983). The conservative nature of the linear, nonthreshold approach, as well as its biological inflexibility, have stimulated scientists, regulators, and economists to search for methods that can incorporate a more biological understanding of the cancer process. A number of chemicals have been identified that most likely exert their carcinogenic effects in manners for which a linear nonthreshold relationship would be invalid at low doses. As a result of these concerns, scientists have sought to develop dose–response models that account for varying biological mechanisms.

For example, the biologically based dose–response relationship that results from clinical observations of human tumors has been described by Moolgavkar and Knudson in terms of two stages (Moolgavkar and Knudson, 1981). The two-stage model can account for the dose- and time-dependent effects of carcinogenic agents or mixtures of agents on various biological parameters. The model is valid for agents that exert their activity in a number of different ways, such as those that have genotoxic or nongenotoxic mechanisms, as well as cocarcinogens or inhibitors of carcinogenesis. It incorporates parameters that depend on mutation rates as well as cell proliferation rates, both of which play important roles in the process. As a result, it may be possible to estimate parameters in the model for a particular agent or mixture of agents using experimental information from bioassays other than chronic carcinogenicity tests, if the latter are unavailable. Furthermore, knowledge of differences in mutation or cell proliferation rates between species can be used to perform more meaningful interspecies extrapolations than the surface area or body weight adjustments currently used. In particular, the biologically based model is finding practical applications for chemicals thought to act primarily by mechanisms other than direct interaction with DNA (Thorslund, 1987; Thorslund and Charnley, in press; Thorslund et al., 1986, 1987a,b). This model is described in more detail in Chapter 8.

Other important efforts are attempting to model pharmacokinetic data that describe the pathway a toxic chemical follows through the body to deliver the effective carcinogen at the target organ that develops the cancer response. Earlier cancer models assumed that exposure or some adjustment of actual exposure according to uptake or absorption by skin, gastrointestinal tract, or the lungs constituted the effective dose. Current efforts have contributed to important progress toward describing the actual dose of the effective chemical carcinogen that is delivered to the target tissue (Andersen et al., 1980, 1984; Andersen, 1981a,b; Crump 1981, 1987). This topic is dealt with in more detail in Chapter 7.

Exposure assessment involves the characterization of populations exposed by various routes, such as ingestion, inhalation, or dermal absorption. Measured ambient levels of exposure are used whenever such data are available. Usually, it is necessary to use limited monitoring data in conjunction with estimates of exposure, often derived from various dispersion models, to estimate exposure levels. The best data come from directly monitored human data, but this information is rarely available or usable to estimate human dose. Wherever possible, it is most desirable to characterize the effective dose at the site of organ damage, but this information is even more difficult to measure or derive by modeling. The exposure assessment should include the number of people exposed, a profile of particularly sensitive individuals, and, wherever possible, information regarding the duration of exposure for different population subgroups.

Finally, risk characterization expresses the weight-of-evidence that different disease end points may be associated with exposure to the chemical under evaluation and combines the dose–response data with current and projected exposures to estimate the magnitude of potential risks.

Risk Management

Various studies have called for performing the risk assessment as a separate step from the risk management decision (EPA, 1976; NAS, 1982, 1983). This is to make sure that the assumptions necessary for dealing with scientific uncertainty in the risk assessment process are not biased by an eventual desired risk management outcome.

Factors considered in deciding how much health risk to accept inevitably include considerations of social benefits and costs, economic cost associated with control measures, and available technology for control. Various U.S. laws, however, call for somewhat different weighting of these factors in reaching a final risk management or policy decision to limit exposures. For example, the Clean Air Act calls for setting national ambient air quality standards (e.g., sulfur oxides, nitrogen oxides, and lead) based on health protection alone, without regard to social or economic considerations. The pesticide authorities in the United States call for balancing the risks of use versus the benefits, and the Drinking Water Act calls for basing final standards, maximum contaminant levels (MCLs), on the feasibility of control. The role of risk assessment in the risk management process, therefore, varies according to different legal constraints and practical circumstances.

APPLICATIONS OF RISK ASSESSMENT TO PUBLIC POLICY DECISIONS

The majority of experience with risk assessment approaches in public health protection has been in the areas of radiation and chemical carcinogenesis, though these approaches are not limited to these areas. The idea that is common to all risk assessments is to adopt an organized approach in the face of uncertainty and to make the most credible projections possible as a basis for management decisions. Most certainly, these same approaches are amenable to, and are being applied to, health effects data other than carcinogen data. For example, for acutely toxic effects that require rapid response in the case of an accidental release, risk assessment approaches may be used to identify the health effects of concern, the dose of concern, and, using physical and chemical parameters, estimate the area surrounding the release that may require evacuation (EPA, 1985b).

In the ecological area, consistent guidance for assessing risk is badly needed to achieve more organized approaches to evaluating these data to guide both national and international decision making for a host of problems, such as acid rain (NAS, 1986).

Applications with Emphasis on Carcinogens

Quantitative risk assessment, together with qualitative assessment of the biomedical evidence, has been used in five distinct situations in the U.S.: for deciding public policy to set priorities, to review residual risk after application of the best available technology to see if anything more should be done, to balance risks against benefits, to set standards and target levels of risk, and to provide information about the urgency of situations where population subgroups are inadvertently exposed to toxic agents, e.g., populations near uncontrolled waste sites. Several examples are discussed below.

Setting Priorities

Under provisions of the Clear Air Act, the EPA must list hazardous air pollutants and regulate sources of such air pollutants as necessary. In order to set priorities for reviewing hundreds of agents that may be potential air pollutants, the EPA's Office of Air Programs identified three groups of potentially toxic chemicals suspected of being present in the ambient air at levels of concern because of their use patterns (Tables 1 and 2). The highest priority for performing in-depth health evaluations was given to Group I, then to Group II, and finally to Group III. These priorities reflected judgments from the Office of Air Programs regarding those chemicals which, based on preliminary information for likely

Table 1. Chemicals Proposed by the EPA's Office of Air Programs for Unit Risk Assessment[a]

Group I	Group II
Acrylonitrile	Beryllium
Carbon tetrachloride	Cresols (ortho, meta, and para)
Chloroform	Formaldehyde
Ethylene dibromide	Maleic anhydride
Ethylene dichloride	Manganese
Nitrosamines (4)	Methylene chloride
Perchloroethylene	Nickel
Trichloroethylene	Nitrobenzene
Vinylidene chloride	Toluene
	Xylenes (ortho, meta, and para)

[a]Unit risk is the incremental excess lifetime risk associated with breathing 1 $\mu g/m^3$ of the chemical over a 70-year life span for a 70-kg person

exposure and possible toxicity, might present the greatest hazard to humans from air pollution. The Carcinogen Assessment Group (CAG), one of the health subgroups in the EPA's Office of Health and Environmental Assessment, provided a qualitative weight-of-evidence statement and an index of potency for chemicals selected from Groups I and II. The index of potency is expressed as an upper-bound unit risk estimate, with the unit risk estimate defined as the incremental excess lifetime risk for a 70-kg individual breathing air containing 1 $\mu g/m^3$ of the chemical of interest, for a 70-yr life span. The data is presented in Table 3. Notice that the potency index, expressed as unit risk, ranges a millionfold, and that chemicals having the strongest biomedical evidence for carcinogenicity based on responses in humans may have relatively low potencies. For example, vinyl chloride has a unit risk of 10^{-6} and benzene has a unit risk of 10^{-6}. Strong evidence of carcinogenicity need not also mean high potency. In the absence of information regarding potency, regulators are inclined to regulate human carcinogens more severely than animal

Table 2. Chemicals Proposed by the EPA's Office of Air Programs for Unit Risk Assessment[a]

Group III	
Acetaldehyde	Dioxane
Acetylene tetrachloride	Epichlorohydrin
Acrolein	Hexachlorocyclopentadiene
Allyl chloride	Methyl iodine
Benzyl chloride	Naphthylamine (1- and 2-)
Bischloromethyl ether (BCME)	2-Nitropropane
Chlorobenzene	Phenol
Chloromethylmethyl ether	Phosgene
Chloroprene	Polychlorinated biphenyls (PCBs)
Dichlorobenzene (ortho and para)	Propylene oxide

[a]Unit risk is incremental excess lifetime risk associated with breathing 1 $\mu g/m^3$ of the chemical over a 70-year life span for a 70-kg person.

Table 3. Upper-Bound Unit Calculations for
Suspected Carcinogenic Air Pollutants[a,b]

Chemical	Upper-bound unit risk estimates
Acrylonitrile	7×10^{-5}
Allyl chloride	5×10^{-8}
Arsenic	4×10^{-3}
Benzene	7×10^{-6}
Beryllium	6×10^{-4}
Diethylnitrosamine (DEN)	2×10^{-2}
Dimethylnitrosamine (DMN)	5×10^{-3}
Dioxin (2,3,7,8-tetrachloro-)[c]	1
Ethylene dibromide	6×10^{-5}
Ethylene dichloride	7×10^{-6}
Ethylene oxide	2×10^{-4}
Formaldehyde	5×10^{-5}
Manganese	4×10^{-4}
Nickel	6×10^{-4}
N-nitroso-N-ethylurea (NEU)	1×10^{-2}
N-nitroso-N-methylurea (NMU)	7×10^{-1}
Perchloroethylene	2×10^{-6}
Tricholoroethylene	3×10^{-6}
Vinyl chloride	4×10^{-6}
Vinylidene chloride	4×10^{-5}

[a]From EPA, Carcinogen Assessment Group Reports, 1976–1986. These
calculations are periodically revised as new data become available
[b]Unit risk is the incremental excess lifetime risk associated with breathing 1 $\mu g/m^3$ of the chemical over a 70-year life span for a 70-kg person.
[c]The potency of dioxin is estimated to be about 1600 times greater than
that of DEN at low exposure levels; therefore, for lifetime exposure to 1
$\mu g/m^3$ the upper-bound unit risk estimate is 100% chance of cancer
occurrence. The upper-bound estimate of the potency (slope) for dioxin
is 33 $\mu g/m^3$ or 3 3 $\times$ 10^{-2} ng/m^3.

carcinogens, even though some human carcinogens appear to be relatively much less potent than some chemicals whose carcinogenic effect has only been demonstrated in animal studies.

While there are many chemicals-of-concern, some pose a greater risk than others. The weight-of-evidence for carcinogenicity, the unit risk estimate as a measure of poten-cy, and information concerning exposure levels have all provided a basis for selecting the most hazardous air pollutants for further study and possible regulation, and for disre-garding others.

After an agent has been listed as a hazardous air pollutant, the EPA must decide which sources to regulate first, and indeed, whether or not regulation is warranted. Table 4 presents a comparison of data for different source categories contributing arsenic to the ambient air. The upper-bound risk estimates to population subgroups and the related upper-bound nationwide impacts always rely on estimates of exposures, which also have great uncertainties. Uncertainties must always be included in the exposure assessment and taken into account when using risk assessment information. For example, where estimates of exposure are highly uncertain it may be possible to present a range for the exposure. Risk estimates based on this range can be instructive, particularly in circumstances where

Table 4. Upper-Bound Lifetime Cancer Risk for Arsenic Exposures[a,b]

Source	Number exposed in highest two groups[c]	Highest two exposure levels ($\times 10^{-4}$ mg/kg per day)[d]	Associated lifetime upper-bound cancer risk	Upper-bound estimates/cases per year
Copper smelters	43,800	2.7–1.5	2–1 $\times 10^{-3}$	1.5–0.821
Lead smelters	3400	0.69–0.27	6–2 $\times 10^{-4}$	0.029–0.017
Zinc smelters	37,000	0.69–0.27	6–2 $\times 10^{-4}$	0.32–0.13
Cotton gins	32	15.4–6.9	13–6 $\times 10^{-3}$	0.0061–0.0027
Pesticide manufacturing	1480	0.026–0.014	2–1 $\times 10^{-5}$	0.0004–0.00025
Glass manufacturing	11,580	0.69–0.014	6–2 $\times 10^{-4}$	0.099–0.040

[a]From EPA, Carcinogen Assessment Group's Risk Assessment on Arsenic, May 2, 1980, National Technical Information Service, PB 81-20613

[b]The significant figures presented do not indicate precision or accuracy, rather they are included to make it easier to trace the derivation of these numbers through the various extrapolation and mathematical calculations.

[c]Population exposed to ambient levels of arsenic from the sources listed.

[d]For example, the highest exposure level for copper smelters is 2 7 $\times 10^{-4}$ mg/kg per day.

either the upper end of the range provides low estimates or, conversely, where the lower end of the range still suggests possible associated high risks.

Residual Risk

The next example of the use of Risk Management is in examining residual risk. Quantitative risk assessment was used to compare residual risk, after application of the best available technology to control ambient levels of vinyl chloride monomer, with the risk associated with other potentially hazardous air pollutants that had not yet been regulated (see Table 5). The risk assessment information indicated that reductions in risk had been considerable after regulation for vinyl chloride, and that the remaining risk was low relative to risks associated with the other air pollutants, namely, the individual risks for arsenic and benzene and the nationwide impacts for arsenic and benzene (Table 5). Relative individual risks and lifetime population risks (Table 5) are generally both considered in making regulatory decisions. Based on such analysis, the EPA's Office of Air Quality Programs allocated agency resources to consider other air pollutants and not to consider additional reductions in risks associated with vinyl chloride emissions. To date, vinyl chloride has not been further regulated. The agency has agreed, however, to periodically review the regulation of these emissions.

Balancing Risk and Benefits

Many decisions involving the balancing of risks and benefits under the EPA's pesticide registration authorities have relied on risk assessment. Table 6 presents the quantitative risk estimates associated with three examples for which registration decisions have been made. In the case of chlorobenzilate, a pesticide used on citrus fruit, the weight-of-evidence for carcinogenic potential is based on responses in the liver of both male and female mice; studies in rats were negative (EPA, 1978). There is considerable disagreement among some scientists regarding the appropriate weight to be given to such

Table 5. Comparison of Upper-Bound Risks Associated with Ambient Exposure to Carcinogenic Air Pollutants[a]

Chemical[b]	Upper-bound lifetime probability of cancer death due to maximum exposure near stationary sources[c]	Total number exposed[c,d]	Total number of cancer deaths/year at the upper bound in U.S. due to chemical in air[c]
Relative individual risks			
Arsenic	2×10^{-3}	44,000	1
Benzene	2×10^{-4}	55,000	0.1
Coke ovens	6×10^{-3}	1800	0.2
Vinyl chloride[e]			
Before regulation	4×10^{-3}	34,000	1.9
After regulation	2×10^{-4}	34,000	0.1
Lifetime population risks			
Arsenic	4×10^{-5}	25 million	16
Benzene	3×10^{-5}	220 million	78
Coke ovens	7×10^{-4}	15 million	150
Vinyl chloride[e]			
Before regulation	2×10^{-4}	5 million	20
After regulation	1×10^{-5}	5 million	1

[a]From EPA, Carcinogen Assessment Group Reports 1976–1981 These estimates may change as additional data become available.
[b]All risks are before regulations unless otherwise indicated
[c]The significant figures presented do not indicate precision or accuracy, rather they are included to make it easier to trace the derivation of these numbers through the various extrapolation and mathematical calculations.
[d]Population exposed to ambient levels of chemical listed. Exposure is from stationary air sources.
[e]If risks were based on the incidence of mammary tumors in the animal bioassay studies, the results would be four times higher.

responses. Nevertheless, based on the assumption that chlorobenzilate is a human carcinogen, quantitative risk estimates indicate that risk associated with exposure to the general population is relatively low—on the order of one chance in a million of increased risk—and the annual cancer rate on a nationwide basis is also relatively low. However, the risk to applicators of the pesticide was higher by two orders of magnitude. Since the pesticide act—The Federal Insecticide, Fungicide and Rodenticide Act (FIFRA)—requires the balancing of risks and benefits, the presence of increased risk to applicators was evaluated in view of the fact that no substitute exists for chlorobenzilate on citrus. The EPA decided that the risks did not outweigh the benefits and therefore retained the registration of chlorobenzilate for use on citrus. The agency added stringent requirements for the label on chlorobenzilate, urging applicators to take further protective measures.

The next example in Table 6 involved the application of risk assessment to the registration of the new pesticide BAAM for use on pears and apples. Only one carcinogenesis bioassay has been performed, and it provided very weak evidence of carcinogenic activity. In the absence of additional data but on the assumption that this one test reflected true biological activity, a quantitative risk assessment was performed. The calculated upper-bound risk estimates indicated on the order of one chance in a million of increased risk, a relatively low projected risk to the U.S. population as a whole. Balancing risks against benefits, the EPA made a decision to (1) permit a three-year temporary registration of BAAM for use on pears but not on apples, because substitutes were not available in the former case but were available in the latter; and (2) require submission of

Table 6. Upper-Bound Risk Estimates for Population Exposure to Suspected Carcinogenic Pesticides[a]

Pesticide	Population exposed	Upper-bound lifetime probability of cancer death due to exposure[b]	Number of expected cancer deaths/year at the upper bound
Chlorobenzilate	220 million–citrus consumption	2×10^{-6}	7
	–citrus applicators[c]	4×10^{-4}	—
		1×10^{-3}	
Amitraz (BAAM)	220 million–apple consumption	3×10^{-6}	8
	–pear consumption	2×10^{-6}	6
	1400 applicators–spraying apples	1×10^{-4}	0.002
	1550 applicators–spraying pears	6×10^{-5}	0.001
	1600 applicators–spraying pears	1×10^{-4}	0.003
Chlordane/heptachlor	220 million	2×10^{-4d}	500[b]
		5×10^{-5e}	150[d]

[a]From the EPA Carcinogen Assessment Group Reports 1976–1981 These estimates may change as addition data become available
[b]The significant figures presented do not indicate precision or accuracy; rather, they are included to make it easier to trace the derivation of these numbers through the various extrapolation and mathematical calculations
[c]The total number of applicators was not included in the study
[d]Based on total tumors
[e]Based on large carcinomas

more definitive data before granting a permanent registration for any uses. While the final results of these tests are not yet available, this example demonstrates how time and effort can be put to good use when guided by quantitative risk assessment.

In the third example in Table 6, risk assessment was used to balance risks and benefits for registered uses of chlordane/heptachlor. The biomedical evidence for the carcinogenicity of these chemicals is reasonably strong based on liver carcinomas in a series of bioassay studies in the mouse and rat. These chemicals bioaccumulate, and most humans carry a body burden of the chemicals in adipose tissue. Application of quantitative risk assessment indicated risks at least an order of magnitude higher than the previous two cases presented in Table 6; considerable potential nationwide impacts were also projected. The decision in this case was to cancel most uses of chlordane/heptachlor with the exception of underground applications for termite control, for which good substitutes were not available and potential exposures to humans were estimated to be less.

In the last example of the use of risk assessment to balance risks and benefits, data are presented in Table 7 for projected risks associated with the resumed manufacture of nitrilotriacetic acid (NTA) in the United States. The manufacture of NTA had been voluntarily suspended in the early 1970s because of the early indications of animal bioassay studies that NTA might be a carcinogen. This risk assessment was done because the manufacturer asked the EPA for guidance as to whether or not the EPA would regulate NTA if manufacturing resumed. NTA can be used in detergents to replace phosphates which contribute to the eutrophication of bodies of water. The benefits associated with using NTA would be a potential reduction of the concentration of phosphates in water. The risk estimates presented in Table 7 are based on monitoring data from Canada, where NTA has been in continuous use for a number of years. With the exception of private

Table 7. Upper-Bound Projected Lifetime Cancer Risk Based on One-Hit Model
from NTA Exposure–Response[a,b]

Type of exposure	Number exposed	Exposure levels in mg/kg per day[c]	Associated cancer risk at the upper bound	Cancer cases/year at the upper bound
Public drinking water	220 million	8×10^{-5}	4×10^{-7}	1
Range		7×10^{-4}	3×10^{-6}	10
Mean		4×10^{-5}	2×10^{-7}	1
Private wells	66 million	up to 0.1^{d}	4×10^{-4d}	370
Maximum[d]				
General consumers				
Laundry	125 million	2×10^{-4}	1×10^{-6}	2
Dishwashing	125 million	2×10^{-4}	1×10^{-6}	2
Residue on unrinsed dishes	2 million	0.01	6×10^{-5}	2
Workers	100	1×10^{-3}	6×10^{-6}	—
Manufacture		7×10^{-3}	3×10^{-5}	—
Formulations	1750	5×10^{-3}	2×10^{-5}	0.001
		5×10^{-2}	2×10^{-4}	

[a]From the EPA Office of Toxic Substances, Draft Report, 1979
[b]The significant figures presented do not indicate precision or accuracy, rather, they are included to make it easier to trace the derivation of these numbers through the various extrapolation and mathematical calculations
[c]Projected United States exposures based on Canadian monitoring data
[d]Insufficient data, based on only 21 samples of which only one was significantly contaminated

wells, where only 21 samples have been monitored, potential cancer risks from the Canadian data indicated low projected risks for populations in the United States. Although questions were raised about the applicability of the Canadian exposure data to projected exposures in the United States, the decision not to regulate the resumed manufacture of NTA cited these relatively low risk estimates as the reason.

Setting Target Levels of Risk

In this example (Table 8), the EPA was obligated to recommend nationwide water quality criteria for a large number of chemicals, including suspected carcinogens (EPA,

Table 8. Guidance for Water Quality Criteria
Upper-Bound Calculations With a Lower-Bound Approaching
Zero[a]

	Upper-bound slope B_H (mg/kg per day)$^{-1b}$	Water concentrations corresponding to a risk level of 10^{-5} (μg/liter) at the upper bound[b,c]
Acrylonitrile	0.6(2.0)	0.6(0.08)
Aldrin	11.4(6.3)	$7.4 \times 10^{-4}(5 \times 10^{-5})$
Arsenic[d]	14.0	0.02
Asbestos	—	300,000 (fibers/liter)(0.05)

Table 8. (*Continued*)

	Upper-bound slope B_H (mg/kg per day)$^{-1 b}$	Water concentrations corresponding to a risk level of 10^{-5} (µg/liter) at the upper bound[b,c]
Benzene[d]	0.1	7
Benzidine[d]	234.1	1×10^{-3}
Beryllium	4.9(3.4)	0.1(0.1)
Carbon tetrachloride	0.1(0.1)	4(3)
Chloroform	0.2(0.2)	2(2)
Chlordane	1.6(5.4)	$5 \times 10^{-3}(1 \times 10^{-3})$
Chloroalkyl ethers		
BCME	9300(13,600)	$4 \times 10^{-5}(2 \times 10^{-5})$
BCEE	1.1(0.7)	0.3(0.4)
Chlorinated benzenes		
HCB	1.7(2.5)	$7 \times 10^{-3}(1 \times 10^{-3})$
Chlorinated ethanes		
1,2-di-	0.04(0.05)	9(7)
1,1,2-tri-	0.1(0.1)	6(3)
1,1,2,2-tetra-	0.2(0.2)	2(2)
Hexa-	0.01(0.02)	19(6)
Dichlorobenzidine	2(2)	0.1(0.02)
DDT	8(18)	$2 \times 10^{-4}(4 \times 10^{-4})$
Dichloroethylenes		
1,1-dichloroethylene	1(0.3)	0.3(1)
Dieldrin	30(180)	$7 \times 10^{-4}(4 \times 10^{-4})$
Dinitroluene	0.3(0.4)	1(0.1)
Dioxins		
2,3,7,8-tetrachloro-	$4 \times 10^{-5}(1 \times 10^{-4})$	$2 \times 10^{-9}(5 \times 10^{-7})$
Diphenylhydrazine dioxin	0.8(0.7)	0.4(0.4)
Halomethanes	Same as chloroform	
Heptachlor	3 (30)	$3 \times 10^{-3}(2 \times 10^{-4})$
Hexachlorobutadiene	0.008(0.05)	5(1)
Hexachlorocyclohexane		
technical grade	5(2)	0.1(0.02)
alphaisomer	11(3)	0.02(0.02)
betaisomer	2(2)	0.1(0.03)
gammaisomer	1(1)	0.2(0.05)
Nitrosamines		
DMNA	26(13)	$1 \times 10^{-2}(3 \times 10^{-2})$
DENA	44(38)	$8 \times 10^{-3}(9 \times 10^{-3})$
DBNA	5(27)	0.1 (0.01)
N–N–P	2(4)	0.2(0.1)
PAH	12(28)	$3 \times 10^{-2}(10 \times 10^{-3})$
PCBs	4(3)	$8 \times 10^{-4}(3 \times 10^{-4})$
Tetrachloroethylene	0.04(0.1)	$8 \times (2.0)$
Trichloroethylene	0.01(0.01)	27(21)
Toxaphene	1(4)	$7 \times 10^{-3}(5 \times 10^{-4})$
Vinyl chloride[d]	0.02	20

[a]*Federal Register*, Vol 45, No 231, November 1980.
[b]The values in parentheses were calculated based on the one-hit model. Other values were calculated based on the multistage model.
[c]Assuming a lifetime daily consumption of 2 liters of water and 0.0065 kg fish Note that a daily consumption of 0.0187 kg fish was assumed in the calculation using the one-hit model, and some of the bioconcentration factors are different in the calculation using the multistage model
[d]Scope determined from epidemiological data

1980a). The statute under which these criteria were issued, the Federal Water Pollution Control Act, required that water quality criteria be published by the agency to protect the public health: no provisions were included in this section of the statute to incorporate social and economic factors in setting water quality criteria. Since threshold concentrations could not be established for suspected carcinogens, quantitative risk assessment was used to recommend concentrations in water associated with lifetime risks of 10^{-7} to 10^{-5}. Concentrations that would result in such risks were calculated by assuming an ingestion of two liters of drinking water per day and an average consumption of fish of 6.5 grams per day (edible portion). The upper bound slope of the dose-response curve for each chemical was calculated, as was the concentration in water for each chemical that would correspond to a cancer risk level of 10^{-5} at the upper bound. In calculating these data, an extrapolation must be used to estimate the dose of carcinogen needed to cause cancer. In the proposed criteria, the data were calculated using the one-hit model. In response to public comments, the agency reviewed alternative models and decided to adopt the Crump linearized, multistage model in order to make full use of all of the data points (EPA, 1980a; and see Armitage, 1985; Moolgavkar, 1986; Thorslund, 1987; Thorslund and Charnley, in press; and Thorslund *et al.*, 1987a,b for recent discussions of biological models of carcinogenesis). The upper-bound slope and the individual chemical concentrations are presented in Table 8 using the multistage model and one-hit model (EPA, 1979a–c). Both values have been included so that the relative slopes and concentrations can be compared. From these comparisons it is evident that the data derived from the one-hit model and from the multistage model are very close for most cases. The weight of the biomedical evidence varies enormously for the chemicals presented in Table 8, and this information should be taken into consideration in applying these target concentrations during the risk management process.

CONCLUSIONS AND FUTURE DIRECTIONS

These examples illustrate the applications of quantitative risk assessment in a variety of practical circumstances to provide information regarding risk as a basis for making public health policy decisions in the United States. These policy decisions did not hinge on any "acceptable level" of risk; each decision reflected achievability in some measure. Nevertheless, most risk management decisions regulated exposures so that individual lifetime cancer risks were near 10^{-5} at the upper bound. There were some circumstances in which this level of risk was not achievable, such as, in setting haloform standards for drinking water (EPA, 1978). Such decisions, in which risks higher than 10^{-5} were accepted, generally were justified on grounds of social and economic tradeoffs, such as the protective value of chlorination of the drinking water supply to prevent infection. Risks to the population as a whole that were lower than 10^{-5} were generally unregulated, as exemplified by the risk management decisions for NTA, vinyl chloride, and chlorobenzilate. Exceptions for risks lower than 10^{-5} include the voluntary cancellation of safrole as a dog repellent (risk of 10^{-7}) and the recommendation of water quality criteria associated with risks ranging from 10^{-7} to 10^{-5} (EPA, 1980). In a large sample of risk assessments for different chemicals in various exposure situations, the upper-bound risks fell into a relatively low risk range of 10^{-5} for about 80% to 90% of the cases studied.

Uncertainties in exposure estimates, and other uncertainties inherent in the extrapolation process, need to be taken into account on a case-by-case basis. Despite these deficiencies, the use of upper-bound estimates to identify those cases where the risks may be so low, even at the upper bound, as to fall into a low-priority category for regulatory consideration, has helped regulators to focus attention on more compelling public health problems.

The process of risk assessment is undergoing continual refinement and improvement. Considerable effort is now concentrated on improving the methods of dose and exposure assessment, centering on advances in molecular biology and our increasing ability to detect low levels of toxic chemicals and/or their metabolic products in human tissues and fluids.

Biologically motivated mathematical models are under development to reduce the uncertainty concerning the upper-bound cancer risk at low doses. Such efforts are necessary so that we do not "over regulate" chemicals where the true risks are significantly below the upper bound (Thorslund *et al.*, 1987a).

The risk analysis process begins with the generation of data on which to base the scientific analysis of health risk estimation, both in qualitative and quantitative terms. The management of these projected risks involves considerations of legal and general social and economic factors in deciding how to manage risk. Finally, risk communication and risk acceptance are essential concerns in the risk analysis process because the affected public is increasingly playing an active role in public health decisions. The complex area of risk communication is an interdisciplinary area that involves a spectrum of elements, including communication of scientific data, the effects of news communication, risk perceptions, risk and compensation tradeoffs, psychological factors of risk and control, and communication and arbitration processes. Historically these areas have been pursued by researchers working in the specialized areas mentioned above. New initiatives are needed to better integrate these disciplines to provide an improved basis for risk communication, an essential part of the risk analysis process. This issue is addressed in Chapter 12.

REFERENCES

Albert, R. E., Train, R. E., and Anderson, E. L., 1977, Rationale developed by the Environmental Protection Agency for the assessment of carcinogenic risks, *J. Natl. Cancer Inst.* **58**:1537–1541.

Andersen, M. E., Gargas, M. L., Jones, R. A., and Jenkins, L. J., Jr, 1980, Determination of the kinetic constants for metabolism of inhaled toxicants *in vivo* using gas uptake measurements, *Toxicol. Appl. Pharmacol.* **54**:100–116.

Andersen, M. E., 1981a, A physiologically based toxicokinetic description of the metabolism of inhaled gases and vapors. Analysis at steady state, *Toxicol. Appl. Pharmacol.* **60**:509–526.

Andersen, M. E., 1981b, Saturable metabolism and its relationship to toxicity, *CRC Crit. Rev. Toxicol.* **9**: 105–150.

Andersen, M. E., Gargas, M. L., and Ramsey, J. C., 1984, Inhalation pharmacokinetics: Evaluating systemic extraction, total *in vivo* metabolism, and the time course of enzyme induction for inhaled styrene in rats based on arterial blood: inhaled air concentration ratios, *Toxicol. Appl. Pharmacol.* **73**:176–187.

Anderson, E. L. and Carcinogen Assessment Group (CAG) of the Environmental Protection Agency, 1983, Quantitative approaches in use to assess cancer risk, *Risk Anal.* **3**:277–295.

Armitage, P., 1985, Multistage Models of Carcinogenesis. *Environ. Health Perspect.* **63**:195–201.

Crump, K. S., 1981, Investigation of the Use of Pharmacokinetic Data in Carcinogenic Risk Assessment, (Submitted to Environmental Protection Agency).

Crump, K. S., 1987, Investigation of the Incorporation of Pharmacokinetic Data for Selected Volatile Organic Chemicals into Quantitative Risk Assessment Methodology, (Submitted to State of New Jersey).

Environmental Protection Agency, (EPA), 1976, Interim procedures and guidelines for health risks and economic impact assessments of suspected carcinogens, *Fed. Reg.* **41**:21402.

Environmental Protection Agency, (EPA), Carcinogen Assessment Group, (CAG), 1978, Summary and Conclusions for Assessment of Carcinogenic Risk of Chlorobenzilate (unpublished).

Environmental Protection Agency, (EPA), 1979a, Water quality criteria: Request for comments (proposed), *Fed. Reg.* **44**:15926–15981.

Environmental Protection Agency, (EPA), 1979b, Water quality criteria: Availability (proposed), *Fed. Reg.* **44**:43660–43697.

Environmental Protection Agency, (EPA), 1979c, Water quality criteria: Availability (proposed), *Fed. Reg.* **44**:56628–56656.

Environmental Protection Agency, (EPA), 1980, Water quality criteria documents: Availability, *Fed. Reg.* **45**:79316–79379.

Environmental Protection Agency, (EPA), 1984a, Proposed guidelines for carcinogen risk assessment, *Fed. Reg.* **49**(227):46294–46301.

Environmental Protection Agency, (EPA), 1984b, Proposed guidelines for the health assessment of suspect developmental toxicants, *Fed. Reg.* **49**:46324–46331.

Environmental Protection Agency, (EPA), 1984c, Proposed guidelines for mutagenicity risk assessment, *Fed. Reg.* **49**:46312–46321.

Environmental Protection Agency, (EPA), 1984d, Proposed guidelines for exposure assessment, *Fed. Reg.* **49**:46304–46312.

Environmental Protection Agency, (EPA), 1985a, Proposed guidelines for the health risk assessment of chemical mixtures, *Fed. Reg.* **50**:1170–1176.

Environmental Protection Agency, (EPA), 1985b, Chemical Emergency Preparedness Program, Interim Guidance, Washington, D.C.

Environmental Protection Agency, (EPA), 1986a, Guidelines for carcinogen risk assessment, *Fed. Reg.* **51**:33992.

Environmental Protection Agency, (EPA), 1986b, Guidelines for health assessment of suspect developmental toxicants, *Fed. Reg.* **51**:34028.

Environmental Protection Agency, (EPA), 1986c, Guidelines for mutagenicity risk assessment, *Fed. Reg.* **51**:34006.

Environmental Protection Agency (EPA), 1986d, Guidelines for estimating exposure, *Fed. Reg.* **51**:34042.

Environmental Protection Agency, (EPA), 1986e, Guidelines for the health risk assessment of chemical mixtures, *Fed. Reg.* **51**:34014.

Interagency Regulatory Liaison Group (IRLG), 1979, Scientific bases for identification of potential carcinogens and estimation of risks, *J. Natl. Cancer Inst.* **63**:244–268.

Moolgavkar, S. H., and Venzon, D. J., 1979, Two-event models for carcinogenesis: Incidence curves for childhood and adult tumors, *Math. Biosci.* **47**:55–77.

Moolgavkar, S. H., and Knudson, A. G., 1981, Mutation and cancer: A model for human carcinogenesis, *J. Natl. Cancer Inst.* **66**:1037–1052.

Moolgavkar, S. H., 1986, Carcinogenesis modeling: From molecular biology to epidemiology, *Ann. Rev. Pub. Health* **7**:151–169.

National Academy of Sciences (NAS), 1982, *Risk and Decision Making: Perspectives and Research,* National Research Council Committee on Risk and Decision Making, National Academy of Sciences Press, Washington, D.C.

National Academy of Sciences (NAS), 1983, *Risk Assessment in the Federal Government: Managing the Process,* National Research Council Committee on Risk and Decision Making, National Academy of Sciences Press, Washington, D.C.

National Academy of Sciences (NAS), 1986, *Ecological Knowledge and Environmental Problem Solving: Concepts and Case Studies,* National Research Council Committee on Risk and Decision Making, National Academy of Sciences Press, Washington, D.C.

Office of Science and Technology Policy (OSTP), 1984, Chemical carcinogens: Notice of review of the science and its associated principles, *Fed. Reg.* **49**:21594–21661.

Thorslund, T. W., Charnley, G., and Anderson, E. L., 1986, Innovative Use of Toxicological Data to Improve

Cost-Effectiveness of Waste Cleanup. (Presented at Superfund '86: Management of Uncontrolled Hazardous Waste Sites, Washington, D.C., December 1–3, 1986.)

Thorslund, T. W., 1987, Quantitative Dose–Response Model for the Tumor Promoting Activity of TCDD, (Submitted to Environmental Protection Agency).

Thorslund, T. W., and Charnley, G., Quantitative Dose–Response Models for Tumor Promoting Agents, in: New Directions in the Qualitative and Quantitative Aspects of Carcinogen Risk Assessment, *Banbury Report* (in press).

Thorslund, T. W., Brown, C. C., and Charnley, G., 1987a, The use of biologically motivated mathematical models to predict the actual cancer risk associated with environmental exposure to a carcinogen, *J. Risk Anal.* **7**:109–119.

Thorslund, T. W., Charnley, G., Bayard, S., and Brown, R., 1987b, Quantitative Model for the Tumor Promoting Activity of 2,3,7,8-TCDD. (Presented at the Seventh International Symposium on Chlorinated Dioxins and Related Compounds, Las Vegas, Nevada, October 4–9, 1987.)

2

Current Views of the Biology of Cancer

Ronald W. Hart and Angelo Turturro

INTRODUCTION

In order to place the different methods used to estimate carcinogenic risk from chemical exposure into context, and to help decide on the best approach to improve this process, it is useful to discuss carcinogenesis with an emphasis on mechanism. Although the mechanism of action of no carcinogen is completely characterized, the efforts over the last ten years have been very fruitful, and mechanistic explanations of a number of components in the grand design that is carcinogenesis have been described in detail.

Cancer is a multistage process. That means that there are a number of steps between a carcinogenic insult and the final result, a cancer. The following themes can be thought of as "stages" in the sense that a description relating the induced cancer incidence to insult can be affected by the processes. For instance, the relationship of administered dose to effective dose can be considered a "step" since an estimation of the dynamics of the system will include the kinetics of this process. The mechanisms involved in the various processes will each contribute to the final characterization of the quantitative kinetics of the process.

There is special focus below on parameters relevant to extrapolation of risk from test systems to humans, and possible ways this can result in or influence the development of a cancer. This interaction will be followed from preabsorption of the agent, through interaction with the cells, and the biological consequence of this interaction. Finally, the progress of the tumor will be discussed.

Although the focus is on cancer induced by chemical agents, it draws freely on information derived from other types of carcinogens (e.g., viruses, radiations). Finally, this analysis is very brief. This discussion covers much the same ground as a recent consensus document on chemical carcinogenesis (Interagency Staff Group, 1986). Great-

Ronald W. Hart and Angelo Turturro • National Center for Toxicological Research, Food and Drug Administration, Jefferson, Arkansas 72079.

er detail is available in that document and in recent reviews (see Becker, 1982; Ames, 1983; Bishop, 1987).

PREABSORPTION

Humans are exposed to a chemical agent usually through dermal contact, inhalation, ingestion, or a combination of these routes of exposure. The agent is subject to modification by environmental processes, depending on its physical state and matrix, such as the bacterial content of the soil, local weather conditions, food constituents, and food preparation. Similarly, agents are subject to microenvironmental processes occurring at the interface of organism and environment. For instance, metabolic conversions by microorganisms in the gut (Goldman, 1978; Cerniglia *et al.*, 1982; Morgan and Hoffmann, 1983) have been suggested to have a potential similar to that of the liver (Goldman, 1978). Hepatic metabolism of xenobiotics is predominantly oxidative and synthetic (conjugations), while reactions by intestinal microflora are mostly of a hydrolytic and reductive nature, appearing to be most significant for agents not well absorbed from the gut and for those that are excreted, free or conjugated, in the bile (Goldman, 1978) [e.g., cycasin (Morgan and Hoffmann, 1983)]. Thus, there can be competition or cooperation between mammalian and microbial enzyme systems in sequential reactions leading to activated or deactivated chemical species, especially in the enterohepatic circulation. This interaction is further compounded by coprophagic behavior, as seen in rats (Bos *et al.*, 1986), which leads to ingestion of the products of anaerobic intestinal bacterial action subsequently exposed to oxygen.

The effects of microenvironment are especially important to consider when extrapolating the effects in test systems to humans. For instance, intra- and interspecies comparisons of microfloral metabolism of xenobiotics have been rare (for an exception, see Cerniglia *et al.*, 1982). Also, the activity is not fixed. Factors such as diet composition have also been shown to affect microbial metabolism. For example, diets with high pectin content can alter the metabolic activities of bacteria in the gut, thus directly effecting hepatic covalent binding of carcinogens (DeBethizy *et al.*, 1983). Therefore, with exposure to chemical agents, it is essential to consider the effects of environment and microenvironment in order to correctly characterize the agent of interest.

METABOLISM

Once across the interface between organism and environment, the agent undergoes metabolism. Organic chemicals, with the exception of a few direct-acting agents and agents with direct biological activity such as hormones, require activation to be toxic. The effect of activation is generally thought to result in electrophilic reactants (Miller and Miller, 1976) that bind with target intracellular nucleophilic macromolecules such as DNA. The reactive metabolites formed may also react with other nucleophiles, such as glutathione or water (Sims and Grover, 1974; Caldwell, 1982), and are usually neutralize by forming less biologically reactive metabolites that are very polar and may be more easily excreted [although sometimes reaction with glutathione enhances electrophilicity

(Williams, 1959)]. The end result of metabolism is the sum of activation, deactivation, and reactivation of the toxic metabolite of the agent at different target sites in the body.

Metabolism can be divided into two parts, organismic and cellular. Organismic metabolism can be understood as the sum of the processes leading to the toxic levels of the metabolite in the bodily fluids (e.g., blood, lymph), which in turn leads to the local (i.e., target cell) concentration of toxic metabolite. Pharmacokinetics, liver metabolism, and kidney action are examples of organismic metabolism. Cellular metabolism occurs between the local concentration and the toxic effect on the cell. The relative contribution of the two aspects of metabolism varies. When the target cell is an important part of organismic metabolism, (e.g., liver cells), or is at the contact site of chemical exposure (e.g., lung cells), the organismic aspect of metabolism becomes relatively less important. When the target is an organ exposed only by agent only systemically, the organismic aspect is more important.

In general, the enzymes involved in activation, deactivation and reactivation of an agent (as well as the production of many inactive metabolites) are part of the same mechanisms responsible for detoxification of drugs. The enzyme systems involved in biotransformation can be divided for convenience into two groups that convert a compound into either a phase 1 or phase 2 metabolite. Phase 1 metabolites are primary oxidation or reduction products, that are usually more water soluble than the parent compound and thus may generally be more easily eliminated from the body. These metabolites can then be conjugated with various soluble intracellular constituents, forming glucuronides or sulfates, and becoming even more water soluble and easily excretable. These conjugated metabolites constitute the phase 2 metabolites (Williams, 1959) that are usually excreted. The reactions that occur in the formation of either phase 1 or phase 2 metabolites require specific enzymes for their conversion, such as (phase 1) cytochrome-P450, flavin adenine dinucleotide (FAD) containing monooxygenase, epoxide hydroxylase, flavin-containing cytochrome-450 reductases, and xanthine oxidase, and (phase 2) glutathione S-transferase, uridine diphosphate (UDP) glucuronyltransferase, sulfotransferase, N-acyltransferase and N,O-acyltranferase. Interactions between a chemical carcinogen and these metabolizing systems may form a large spectrum of phase 1 and phase 2 metabolites. If the target is cellular DNA, there is an interaction between the local concentration of the appropriate metabolite and the cellular activation, deactivation, and reactivation of the chemical species that attacks the DNA.

Metabolism is an important consideration when extrapolating from test systems to man. The total enzyme level and substrate specificity of the phase 1 and phase 2 metabolizing enzymes exhibit organ, individual, and species differences (Hart *et al.*, 1982). There also exist multiple forms of different enzymes, such as the cytochrome-P450 enzymes, each of which exhibits its own specificity toward the substrate metabolized (Lu, 1979). Moreover, the activity of each metabolizing enzyme in a specific tissue of the same strain could vary widely depending on age, sex, nutritional factors, hormonal status, or other factors of the subject (Hart *et al.*, 1982). It is also useful not to forget the total potential of organismic metabolism. For example, the prolonged retention of acidic urine in dog and man, compared to the rat, can result in a very different profile of aromatic amine metabolites in dog and man than in the rat, due to the effect of a lower urine pH over a longer time on N-hydroxyarylamine conjugates (Young and Kadlubar, 1982). The important parameters in deriving local concentration in this case were not concentration of blood-borne metabolites, but the urine concentration of metabolites and the amount reactivated by the bladder conditions. Differential cellular activation, deactivation, and reactivation, may be important in understanding the differences in target organ response in different species.

Metabolism is also important in evaluating the effects of different factors that may modify metabolism and, consequently, the amount of exposure of a target to an active species. There are three general mechanisms for the modulation of metabolism by inhibitors or inducers (Wattenberg, 1980): (1) stimulation of cellular metabolism that results in an increased deactivation and/or activation (e.g., phenobarbital and flavones induce an increase in monooxygenase activity), changing the ratio of activation to deactivation (Thakker *et al.*, 1981); (2) interference with enzymatic activation of chemical carcinogens to form the ultimate carcinogenic metabolite(s) [e.g., disulfiram directly reduces the activation dimethylhydrazine (Wattenberg, 1980)]; and (3) alteration of scavenging by nucleophiles [e.g., starvation may drastically alter glutathione levels (Tateishi *et al.*, 1974; Lam *et al.*, 1981)]. As indicated above, it is the balance between the activation, detoxification and reactivation systems for a chemical carcinogen, and their interaction over time, rather than the change in one of these processes per se, that is important. If monooxygenase activity has been stimulated, resulting in increased reactive metabolite formation, a greater proportion of biologically available carcinogen will result only if the detoxification mechanisms cannot compensate or other systems are also not stimulated to compensate. Also, an alteration in metabolism may lead to a change in target organ, as the activation–deactivation–reactivation equilibrium is shifted. For instance, the coadministration of aspirin, which modulates the metabolism of *N*-[4-(5-nitro-2-furyl)-2-thiazolyl]formamide (FANFT), a potent rat urinary bladder carcinogen, will decrease the number of bladder tumors induced by FANFT; however, at the same time, it will increase the number of forestomach tumors produced (Murasaki *et al.*, 1984).

MACROMOLECULAR INTERACTIONS

The reactive species produced by metabolism attack the cells and cell components. This results in the modification of cell components, which are important to the mechanism of action of a number of carcinogens.

Modification of Cellular Components

On a molecular level, although almost any cellular component with a nucleophilic region such as RNA (Miller and Miller, 1976), protein (Ketterer, 1980), and lipid-containing membranes (Carroll, 1980), will be attacked by reactive species, it is accepted that the primary site for cancer induction is the DNA. Evidence for this includes: (1) viral carcinogens appear to need to interact with host cell DNA (Weinberg, 1982); (2) certain genetic diseases with defective DNA repair, such as xeroderma pigmentosum, are characterized by a tendency for cancer at a number of sites (Bridges, 1981; Maher *et al.*, 1982; Kraemer *et al.*, 1982); and (3) ultraviolet (254 nm) light-induced tumor formation in the gynogenetic fish, *Poecilia formosa,* is directly related to the amount of DNA damage remaining after different levels of photoreactivation repair of the DNA (Hart *et al.*, 1977).

The effect on DNA can take many forms, such as integration into DNA of viral genomes, chromosomal alterations, and damage which results in changes in the base sequence such as point mutations.

One important consequence of the integration of viral and cellular genomes is illustrated by *onc* genes. *Onc* genes were discovered in acute transforming viruses, members of the class of RNA tumor viruses known as retroviruses (for a review, see Bister and Jansen, 1986). These genes appear to have arisen by recombination of the viral genome with cellular genes, termed protooncogenes, which endow the viruses with ability to induce rapid neoplastic disease in newborn animals and to transform cells in culture (Coffin *et al.*, 1981). These protooncogenes have unknown cellular functions, although a variety of activities have been found. For example, the proto-oncogene for *erb*-A is a high-affinity thyroid hormone receptor (the viral gene lacks the thyroid hormone affinity, but maintains the nuclear binding action) (Sap *et al.*, 1986); *src* has a protein kinase activity, similar to that found when a number of growth factors bind to their receptors (Barker and Dayhoff, 1982); *ras* p21 protein seems to have a guanosine triphosphatase activity (McGrath *et al.*, 1984) similar to activity important in signal transduction (Hurley *et al.*, 1984); and *sis* has similarity to platelet derived growth factor (PDGF) (Doolittle *et al.*, 1983). Whether an *onc* gene is needed to be expressed at high levels to be correlated with the transforming activity of the virus (Trus *et al.*, 1982), or needed to be repressed (Lee *et al.*, 1987), the common thread that underlies the action important for tumorigenesis is that the *onc* gene is involved in some fashion in cellular growth control. Because of the diversity of the *onc* genes, it appears that *any* step in the growth regulation of cells, from receptor through kinase and nuclear changes, when disrupted by an *onc* gene, can have an effect significant for tumorigenesis.

Chromosomal changes can also influence tumorigenesis. For instance, in Burkitt's lymphoma, a characteristic portion of human chromosome 8 (carrying c-*myc*) is translocated to chromosome 14, the site of immunoglobulin heavy chains (Klein, 1981; Taub *et al.*, 1982). Also, c-*abl* is translocated in chronic myelocytic leukemia patients with a Philadelphia chromosome (a translocation of the gene from chromosome 9 to chromosome 22 adjacent to an immunoglobulin light-chain cluster of genes) (Taub *et al.*, 1982). Such translocations might result in the placement of an *onc* gene in an unsuitable spot, where it may be expressed or repressed inappropriately (Cory, 1986).

Direct interaction of DNA with reactive species may lead to covalently bound adducts, intercalations, strand breaks, phosphotriesters, crosslinks, apurinic sites, apyrimidinic sites, deaminations, and/or hydrations (Waring, 1981). Traditionally, however, studies of chemical carcinogenesis have focused on covalent adducts. For example, the epoxide derivatives of aflatoxin can attack the N-7 position of guanine (Lin *et al.*, 1977). The biological significance of these alterations in the DNA is not always clear, and different alterations may have very different biological effects. Some alterations may cause mutations (Magee, 1977; Radman *et al.*, 1977). For example, modification of the O-6 position of guanine will cause this base to be misread, during DNA replication, as adenine (Gerchman and Ludlum, 1973). Also, the major guanine adduct of benzo(a)pyrene, through a transversion, may be misread as a cytosine or thymine in replication (Swenson and Kadlubar, 1981; Eisenstadt *et al.*, 1982). Aromatic amines induce "base displacement" (Weinstein, 1981). Additionally, the carcinogen 2-acetylaminofluorene appears to induce a flip from a conventional right-handed DNA helix to the left-handed Z form (Grunberger and Weinstein, 1979; Weinstein, 1981), which may induce changes in gene regulation (Lipetz *et al.*, 1982).

Modulation of Cellular Component Damage

If a cell component such as DNA is damaged, cells can have three responses. They can ignore the damage, repair it, or die. Each response has consequences for carcinogenesis.

Cells Ignoring Damage. Some DNA damage is basically ignored by the cell. For instance, certain adducts, such as 3-(deoxyguanosine-N^2-yl)-acetylaminofluorene, a minor acetylated adduct of exposure to 2-acetylaminofluorene, persist in the cell (Kriek, 1972). As a result of replication over a damaged template, termed replication bypass or postreplication repair (Fujiwara and Tatsumi, 1976), damaged DNA templates can be replicated. However, because of redundancy in the genetic code, 25% of the base substitutions will have no effect on proteins derived from them. Because large portions of the genome may be inactive, redundant, or dormant, some alterations will have no consequences for tumorigenesis.

DNA Repair. Cells may attempt to repair the DNA damage (Strauss, 1985). Enzyme systems functioning before replication include nucleotide excision repair (Ahmed and Setlow, 1978), base excision repair (Ahmed and Setlow, 1978; Deutsch and Linn, 1979), direct demethylation by transfer of a methyl group to an acceptor protein (Setlow, 1980), AP site repair (direct repair of a removed base) (Linn *et al.*, 1978); strand break repair (Lindahl *et al.*, 1982); and photoreactivation (Kelner, 1949). Although there are differences, many of the processes of repair in mammalian cells are similar to those described in bacteria and it is assumed that these systems have been conserved during the course of evolution. It has been speculated that the primary role of these systems in evolution was to protect the genetic information of the species from both endogenous and naturally-occurring exogenous DNA damaging agents, long enough for the organism to replicate (Hart and Turturro, 1981; Turturro and Hart, 1984). The level of endogeneous damage should be appreciated. For instance, Lindahl and Nyberg (1972) estimated that as many as 10,000 purines may be lost from the genome of a mammalian cell per generation time. It is not surprising, therefore, that all species examined thus far possess at least one form of DNA repair (Setlow, 1980). If the DNA repair is error-free (i.e., similar in fidelity to DNA polymerase), the DNA is restored to its pristine state. However, a cell may be forced to replicate before the repair is complete, leading to mutations.

Cell Death. The cell may die, either as a result of the inability to repair a certain form of damage (especially one which blocks replication such as a double-strand crosslink), or the overwhelming of its defenses. There is some evidence that germ cells are especially susceptible to death, and this may be a self-destruct mechanism to prevent mutations from creeping into the germ line (Hart and Turturro, 1981). Much of what is considered DNA repair in culture is actually cell death, leading to removal of damaged DNA. Cell death releases contact inhibition on adjacent cells, leading to a process termed "reactive hyperplasia." This hyperplasia may play a role in "fixation" of genetic damage because, for many carcinogens, it is necessary for cellular proliferation to occur before the damage induced by a given agent is expressed. For instance, a cell replication must occur within 48 hr to express X ray induced transformation in cell culture (Terzaghi and Little, 1976). Replication must also occur *in vivo* in liver (Farber, 1984). One way to think about the process is that a cell is first "primed" for alteration by interaction with a carcinogen; cell replication then results in at least one daughter initiated cell, i.e., a cell irreversibly altered so that it can interact with the proper stimulus to form a malignant cell. Replication may play a role in stimulating postreplication repair [although this is controversial (Bowden *et al.*, 1978)], the bypass replication repair referred to above, or alterations in the genome through miscoding of DNA bases through changes in the fidelity of DNA polymerase [e.g., alterations in cellular nucleotide pool sizes and content (Peterson *et al.*, 1978), and alteration of some of the nucleotides in the pools available for replication (Topal and Baker, 1982)].

The end result of these processes is that one or more cells which are genetically altered in some fashion develops altered growth control under appropriate conditions. This "initiated" cell may or may not be expressed during the lifetime of the organism as a cancer.

CANCER FORMATION

How initiated cells express themselves as a cancer seems to be the least understood area of carcinogenesis. The process can be divided into two operational stages, promotion and progression. Promotion will be sed to describe the process(es), usually initially reversible in test systems, but later irreversible (Slaga, 1983), that results in one or more neoplastic cells,—cells with the ability to grow autonomously. Neoplastic progression will refer to the next step(s) in which cells become able to form tumors and become malignant with some potential to metastasize.

Promotion

A promoter is experimentally defined as an agent that results in an increase in cancer induction after long-term application subsequent to treatment of an animal with an initiator. Under otherwise identical conditions, neither initiator nor promoter alone induces many tumors, nor does a regimen with reversed order (treatment with promoter followed by an initiator) (Berenblum, 1982). At a particular dose level and treatment schedule, a carcinogen that does not require supplemental promoter activity is termed complete. Many or all complete carcinogens can act as both an initiator and promoter, and some act as an initiator or promoter for different tissues in the same organism at the same time (Littlefield *et al.*, 1979a,b). For the most part, the phenomenon of tumor promotion has been most carefully delineated in skin and liver carcinogenesis. Using the mouse skin system (Marks and Furstenberger, 1984), it is possible to separate promotion into two stages. Stage one is partially reversible, while stage two, which requires cell proliferation, is initially reversible and then becomes irreversible [there are other characterizations, for an example, see Farber and Cameron, (1980)]. A characteristic of promotion in skin and liver is the induction of focal masses (Marks and Furstenberger, 1984). How these nonneoplastic masses originate is not completely known, but they seem to arise through the differential stimulation of cells altered by the initiator to respond to the promoter (Marks and Furstenberger, 1984). Of the persistent masses, in all systems in which they are induced, almost all do not become neoplastic (Farber, 1984).

It is not surprising that promotion appears to operate through different alterations of growth related phenomena because, as noted above, any interference in cellular growth pattern appears to be susceptible to *onc* gene disruption. The promoter action of a complete carcinogen may not even act by the same mechanism as promoters used in initiator–promoter paradigms (Verma *et al.*, 1982). One example illustrating the complexity of the situation consists of phorbal myristate acetate (PMA) [or 12-O-tetra-decanoylphorbol-13-acetate (TPA)]. PMA binds to a receptor (Dunphy *et al.*, 1980; Farber and Cameron, 1980) that may activate protein kinase C permanently through similarity to diacylglycerol (Nishizuka, 1986). Thus, its effect may be similar to that of a constitutive growth factor. PMA produces profound biological effects *in vivo,* including edema, erythema, inflammation and cellular proliferation. It also: (1) causes dedifferentiation or inhibits terminal differentiation (Rovera *et al.*, 1977); (2) stimulates cellular differentiation (Miao *et al.*, 1978); (3) alters macrophages (Greenberger *et al.*, 1978), leading to generation of free radicals (Goldstein *et al.*, 1981); (4) induces chromosomal alterations (Emerit and Cerutti, 1982) and sister chromatid exchanges (SCE) (Nagasawa and Little, 1979); and (5) induces virus synthesis (Zur Hausen *et al.*, (1978). There are also a number of changes in metabolism (Farber and Cameron, 1980). It is not known which one(s), if any, of these effects is central to the role of promoters in carcinogenesis because a number of these same effects can be produced by agents that are not promoters (Diamond *et al.*, 1980). However, in light of the discoveries in *onc* genes, of special interest are the effects on the chromosomes and inflammation.

Phorbal myristate acetate can induce chromosomal anomalies such as SCE, although the concentrations (100 ng/ml) required for this effect are quite high (Nagasawa and Little, 1979). The activated oxygen species induced by the action of promoters, especially on inflammatory cells, can induce chromosomal damage and a soluble substance which induces chromosomal abnormalities (a clastogen) in nearby cells (Emerit and Cerutti, 1982). The inflammatory response has been shown to be critical to the development of ultraviolet-induced tumors, through an effect on T cells (Kripke, 1979). Changes in the chromosomes may rearrange genes causing inappropriate expression, and thus may simply be a nonobligatory method to achieve this inappropriate expression. Similar to the TPA effect on protein kinase C, a number of other promoter mechanisms also exhibit alteration of growth factorlike factors (or hormones). For instance, neurons control the level of thyroxine, and it has been shown that this hormone is an important factor in x-ray transformation of cells (Guernsey *et al.*, 1980). Exposure to FD&C Red No. 3 (erthyrosine) may result in elaboration of elevated amounts of thyronine stimulating hormone (TSH), leading to the induction of thyroid tumors (Ingbar *et al.*, 1984). And metallothionein gene induction by heavy metal ions (such as cadmium) and glucocorticoid receptors both work by activation of "enhancerlike" elements, leading to speculation that certain metal complexes with DNA, which appear to be act as promoters, may have effects similar to hormone or growth factor induction for gene expression (Karin *et al.*, 1984).

In this context, it is useful to look at cellular proliferation and promotion. Cellular proliferation has a role to play, as noted above, in the "fixation" of "damage." In terms of promotion, the process leading to the emergence of a neoplastic cell, the role of cellular proliferation is more complicated. Manipulation of the rate of cellular proliferation can modify tumor incidence. This has been demonstrated: (1) in partial hepatectomy for animals treated with methylnitrosourea, dimethylnistrosamine (Farber and Cameron, 1980), benzo(a)pyrene and radioactive particles that localize in the liver (Brooks *et al.*, 1982); (2) in stimulated hyperplasia resulting from a necrotizing effect (Stott *et al.*, 1981); and (3) regeneration in skin using skin abrasion (Argyris, 1982). However, many of these data are hard to evaluate because the treatments induce a chronic inflammatory response, and it is not clear whether one is studying the effects of proliferation or the inflammatory response. Inflammation results in the macrophages producing both oxygen radicals (inducing DNA damage) and growth factors such as lymphokines. Cellular proliferation by itself may stimulate the growth of initiated cells, but it should be remembered that normal cellular proliferation and differentiation in embryogenesis has the capacity to change a cancerous teratocarcinoma cell into a normal cell (Mintz and Fleischman, 1981). The differential effect on the initiated as opposed to the normal cell may be more important than a general effect on proliferation (Farber and Cameron, 1980). Some work indicates that the most important effect of replication is simply fixation (Farber and Cameron, 1980) and that "fixation" could possibly be more a part of initiation than promotion. Also, if there is a fixed probability of conversion from an initiated to a neoplastic cell, as the number of initiated cells increase the probability of the occurence of a neoplastic cell will increase. Both factors may be important in the effect of cellular proliferation on promotion.

Promotion may be significant to human carcinogenesis. Cancers in humans from causes such as exposure to cigarette smoke or exposure to benzidine in the workplace have a very long latent period. It is not clear whether this long period is the time from exposure to the production of a neoplastic cell (promotion) or the time necessary to go from a neoplastic cell to a malignant tumor (progression). Evidence that the carcinogenic risk of cigarette smoking declines with the length of time after smoking stops (Doll and Peto, 1981), suggests that most of the latent period is partially reversible and therefore probably occupied by a phenomenon similar to promotion. Standard risk assessment methodologies do not address the phenomenon of promotion, although there have been attempts to incorporate some models of this process. A special problem in incorporating this concept is that agents can be promoters *or* inhibitors, depending on when they are given in relation to other agents (Kitagawa *et al.*, 1984). This is also true with exposure to two carcinogens (Conney *et al.*, 1956). The strong tissue specificity of promoters (Diamond *et al.*, 1980), perhaps related to the specificity of numerous growth factors, also indicates that ready extrapolation, for instance of rodent liver tumors to tumors in man, will not be simple.

Neoplastic Progression

The progression of a neoplastic cell into a malignant tumor is the last major stage of cancer formation. It is probably accomplished through a number of steps, as suggested in the cascade hypothesis of metastasis (step 94).

An interesting model for the mechanism of progression of a neoplasm to malignancy (Fidler *et al.*, 1978) indicates that after a primary tumor is established, there is tumor vascularization, effected by an angiogenic factor (Folkman and Klagsburn, 1987), (by what appears to be a normal capillary growth factor), with invasion of surrounding tissue and blood vessels. This invasion seems to be accomplished through tissue damage by a number of different enzymes, such as collagenase (Liotta *et al.*, 1980) and cathepsin B (Van de Velde *et al.*, 1977). The widespread dissemination of cancer cells occurs by the lymphatic (carcinomas) and hematogenous (mesenchymal tumors) routes. During lymphatic spread, the regional lymph node is involved in the host immune responses to neoplasia. During hematogenous spread, release of tumor emboli in the bloodstream results in the destruction of most tumor cells by interaction with a number of blood elements (Warren, 1978). However,

When more emboli is released, there is a greater chance of survival to form metastases. Arrest and subsequent growth of circulating tumor cells or implantation in another site seem to be a function of tissue and metastasis, and there is some data that the site is selected by the membrane properties of the metastatic cells (Poste and Nicolson, 1980). These cells then leave the blood vessel to form micrometastases that induce blood vessel proliferation and lead to metastatic growth (Fidler *et al.*, 1978). There are a number of other models for progression that emphasize different mechanisms, such as changes in DNA methylation and tumor cell subpopulation interactions (Schirrmacher, 1985). However, there may be different mechanisms for different tumor types. This area is one of current research interest.

The route by which a neoplastic cell becomes a cancer may entail a sequence of interactions between tumor cells and both specific and nonspecific host defenses (Hart and Filder, 1980), as well as a series of events that result in the cell acquiring more characteristics of cells in a malignant neoplasm (Farber and Cameron, 1980). These selection processes are nonexclusive of each other and may involve karyotypic changes (Sandberg, 1980).

An interesting approach to this was the development of a general model for the temporal development of tumors, rooted in evolutionary theory. Based upon the observation of tumor heterogeneity, even when derived from a single clone, the "shifting balance" theory, which emphasizes that many genes with multiple pleiotropic effects mediate the expression of tumor genotype, was applied to tumor evolution (Heppner, 1984). This "microevolution" maintains a flexibility for rapid population adjustment to conditions because of a wide variety of phenotypes. "Macroevolution" occurs when a new niche is available, after the survival of a "catastrophe" for the cancer cells (resulting from clinical treatment or immunological attack), or when a new adaptive level emerges from previous microevolutionary changes. Cellular proliferation may play a role in progression perhaps even more than in promotion (or, perhaps, initiation) by increasing the number of cells and, consequently, the number of variants to be selected from.

Progression seems to be modulated by a number of factors. Important among these is the immunological system. Many tumors induced by physical and chemical agents are antigenically distinct (Kripke, 1974; Hewitt, 1978; Baldwin and Price, 1982). To overcome the defenses of an immunocompetent individual, the tumor could: (1) not be immunogenic, e.g., contain only antigens expressed normally in the body; or (2) suppress the immunological response. Lack of immunogenicity seems to be very common in spontaneous tumors in animals (Hewitt, 1978; Embleton and Middle, 1981). This also seems to be the case for humans because only cells from presumably viral induced tumors, such as Burkitt's lymphoma (McKhann, 1982), may presently be considered to be truly immunogenic. There is, however, evidence of some specific antigens associated with cells from human tumors grown in culture, such as colorectal tumor cells (Herlyn *et al.*, 1979). A tumor could also induce immunodeficiency, either general or selective. Immunosuppression could be accomplished by a variety of mechanisms, including production of circulating immune complexes to inhibit antibody response (Theofilopoulos and Dixon, 1980), or a rise in suppressor T cells to inhibit T cell response (Kripke, 1979).

CONCLUSION

Carcinogenesis is a multistage process which operates in a complex fashion. Every step in the process can be modulated, by both the effects of the agent used and the conditions important to extrapolating risk to humans, such as nutrition and changing metabolism. Compounds which have a syngeristic effect under certain circumstances can be inhibitory at others. By understanding the mechanisms which comprise the many steps in carcinogenesis we can better devise methods to limit uncertainty in our prediction of human risk, as well as discover avenues to pursue in reducing the risks to humans.

REFERENCES

Ahmed, F. E. and Setlow, R. B., 1978, Excision repair in mammalian cells, in: *DNA Repair Mechanisms* (P. C. Hanawalt, E. C. Friedberg and C. F. Fox, eds.), pp. 333–336, Academic Press, New York.

Ames, B. N., 1983, Dietary carcinogens and anticarcinogens, *Science* **221**:1256–1263.

Argyris, T. S., 1982, Epidermal tumor promotion by regeneration, in: *Carcinogenesis: A Comprehensive Survey*, Vol. 7 (E. Hecker, N. E. Fusenig, W. Kunz, F. Marks, and H. W. Thielmann, eds.), pp. 43–48, Raven Press, New York.

Baldwin, R. W., and Price, M. R., 1982, Neoantigen expression in chemical carcinogenesis, in: *Cancer: A Comprehensive Treatise Etiology, Chemical and Physical Carcinogenesis*, Vol. 1, 2nd Ed. (F. F. Becker, ed.), pp. 507–548, Plenum Press, New York.

Barker, W. C., and Dayhoff, M. O., 1982, Viral *src* gene products are related to the catalytic chain of mammalian cAMP-dependent protein kinase, *Proc. Natl. Acad. Sci. USA* **79**:2836–2839.

Becker, F. F. (ed.), 1982, *Cancer: A Comprehensive Treatise Etiology*, Vol. *1–5*, 2nd Ed., Plenum Press, New York.

Berenblum, I., 1982, Sequential aspects of chemical carcinogenesis: Skin, in: *Cancer: A Comprehensive Treatise Etiology, Chemical and Physical Carcinogenesis*, Vol. *1*: 2nd Ed. (F. F. Becker, ed.), pp. 451–484, Plenum Press, New York.

Bishop, J. M., 1987, Molecular biology of cancer, *Science* **235**:305–311.

Bister, K., and Jansen, H., 1986, Oncogenes in retroviruses and cell: Biochemical and molecular genetics, *Adv. Cancer Res.* **47**:99–188.

Bos, R. P., Koopman, J., Theuws, J., Kennis, H., and Henderson, P. Th., 1986, Appearance and reappearance of mutagens in urine from rats after oral administration of direct brown 95, due to coprophagy, *Toxicology* **39**:85–89.

Bowden, G. T., Giesselbach, B., and Fusenig, N. E., 1978, Post-replication repair of DNA in ultraviolet light-irradiated normal and malignantly transformed mouse epidermal cell cultures. *Cancer Res.* **38**:2709–2718.

Bridges, B. A., 1981, Some DNA-repair-deficient human syndromes and their implications for human health, *Proc. R. Soc. London B* **212**:263–278.

Brooks, A. L., Benjamin, S. A., James, R. K., and McClellan, R. O., 1982, Interaction of [144]Ce and partial hepatectomy in the production of liver neoplasms in the Chinese hamster, *Radiat. Res.* **91**:573–588.

Caldwell, J., 1982, Conjugation reactions in foreign-compound metabolism: Definition, consequences, and species variations, *Drug Metab. Rev.* **13**:745–777.

Carroll, K. K., 1980, Lipids and carcinogenesis, *J. Environ. Pathol. Toxicol.* **3**:253–271.

Cerniglia, C. E., Freeman, J. P., Franklin, W., and Pack, L. D., 1982, Metabolism of benzidine and benzidine-congener based dyes by human, monkey and rat intestinal bacteria, *Biochem. Biophys. Res. Comm.* **107**:1224–1229.

Coffin, J. M., Varmus, H. E., Bishop, J. M., Essex, M., Hardy, W. D., Jr., Martin, G. S., Rosenberg, N. E., Scolnick, E. M., Weinberg, R. A., and Vogt, P. K., 1981, Proposal for naming host-cell derived inserts in retrovirus genomes, *J. Virol.* **40**:953–957.

Conney, A. H., Miller, E. C., and Miller, J. A., 1956, The metabolism of methylated aminoazo dyes: V. Evidence for induction of enzyme synthesis in the rat by 3-methylcholanthrene, *Cancer Res.* **16**:450–460.

Cory, S., 1986, Activation of cellular oncogenes in hematopoietic cells by chromosome translocation, *Adv. Cancer Res.* **47**:189–234.

DeBethizy, J. D., Sherrill, J. M., Kickent, D. E., and Hamm, T. E., Jr., 1983, Effects of pectin-containing diets on the hepatic macromolecular covalent binding of 2,6-dinitro-[^{3}H]toluene in Fischer 344 rats, *Toxicol. Appl. Pharm.* **69**:369–376.

Deutsch, W. A., and Linn, S., 1979, DNA binding activity from cultured human fibroblasts that is specific for partially depurinated DNA and that inserts purines into apurinic sites, *Proc. Natl. Acad. Sci. USA* **76**:141–144.

Diamond, L., O'Brien, T. G., and Baird, W. M., 1980, Tumor promoters and the mechanism of tumor promotion, *Adv. Cancer Res.* **32**:1–74.

Doll, R., and Peto, R., 1981, The cause of cancer: Quantitative estimates of avoidable risks of cancer in the United States today, *J. Natl. Cancer Inst.* **66**:1193–1308.

Doolittle, R. F., Hunkapiller, M. W., Hood, L. E., Devare, S. G., Robbins, K. C., Aaronson, S. A., and Antoniades, H. N., 1983, Simian sarcoma virus *onc* gene, v-*sis,* is derived from the gene (or genes) encoding a platelet-derived growth factor, *Science* **221**:275–277.

Dunphy, W. G., Delclos, K. B., and Blumberg, P. M., 1980, Characterization of specific binding of [^{3}H]phorbol 12,13-dibutyrate and [^{3}H]phorbol 12-myristate-13-acetate to mouse brain, *Cancer Res.* **40**:3635–3641.

Eisenstadt, E., Warren, A. J., Porter, J., Atkins, D., and Miller, J. H., 1982, Carcinogenic epoxides of benzo(a)pyrene and cyclopenta(cd)pyrene induce base substitutions via specific transversions, *Proc. Natl. Acad. Sci. USA* **79**:1945–1949.

Embleton, M. J., and Middle, J. G., 1981, Immune responses to naturally occurring rat sarcomas, *Br. J. Cancer* **43**:44–52.

Emerit, I., and Cerutti, P., 1982, The tumor promoter phorbol-12-myristate-13-acetate induces chromosome aberrations in human lymphocytes via indirect action, in: *Mechanism of Chemical Carcinogenesis* (C. C. Harris and P. A. Cerutti, eds.), pp. 495–498, Arthur R. Liss, New York.

Farber, E., 1984, Chemical carcinogenesis: A current biological perspective, *Carcinogenesis* **5**:1–5.

Farber, E., and Cameron, R., 1980, The sequential analysis of cancer development, *Adv. Cancer Res.* **31**:125–226.

Fidler, I. J., Gersten, D. M., and Hart, I. R., 1978, The biology of cancer invasion and metastasis, *Adv. Cancer Res.* **28**:149–250.

Folkman, J., and Klagsburn, M., 1987, Angiogenic factors, *Science* **235**:442–446.

Fujiwara, Y., and Tatsumi, M., 1976, Replicative bypass repair of ultraviolet damage to DNA of mammalian cells: Caffeine sensitive and caffeine resistant mechanisms, *Mutat. Res.* **37**:91–110.

Gerchman, L. L., and Ludlum, D. B., 1973, The properties of 06-methylguanine in templates for RNA polymerase, *Biochim. Biophys. Acta* **308**:310–316.

Goldman, P., 1978, Biochemical pharmacology of the intestinal flora, *Ann. Rev. Pharmacol. Toxicol.* **18**:523–539.

Goldstein, B. D., Witz, G., Amoruso, M., Stone, D. S., and Troll, W., 1981, Stimulation of human polymorphonuclear leukocyte superoxide anion radical production by tumor promoters, *Cancer Lett.* **11**:257–262.

Greenberger, J. S., Newberger, P. E., Karpas, A., and Moloney, W. C., 1978, Constitutive and inducible granulocyte-macrophage functions in mouse, rat and human myeloid leukemia-derived continuous tissue culture lines, *Cancer Res.* **38**:3340–3348.

Grunberger, D., and Weinstein, I. B., 1979, Conformational changes in nucleic acids modified by chemical carcinogens, in: *Chemical Carcinogens and DNA* (P. L. Grover ed.), pp. 59–93, CRC Press, Boca Raton, Florida.

Guernsey, D. L., Ong, A., and Borek, C., Thyroid hormone modulation of X-ray-induced in vitro neoplastic transformation, *Nature* **288**:591–592.

Hart, I. R., and Fidler, I. J., 1980, Cancer invasion and metastasis, *Q. Rev. Biol.* **55**:121–142.

Hart, R. W., and Turturro, A., 1981, Evolution and longevity-assurance processes, *Naturwissenschaften* **68**:552–557.

Hart, R. W., Setlow, R. B., and Woodhead, A. D., 1977, Evidence that pyrimidine dimers in DNA can give rise to tumors, *Proc. Natl. Acad. Sci. USA* **74**:5574–5578.

Hart, R. W., Fu, P. P., and Chang, M. J. W., 1982, Comparative removal of polycyclic aromatic hydrocarbon-DNA adducts in vivo, in: *Sixth International Symposium on Polynuclear Aromatic Hydrocarbons: Physical and Biological Chemistry* (W. M. Cooke, A. J. Dennis, and G. L. Fisher, eds.), pp. 39–72, Battelle Press, Columbus, Ohio.

Heppner, G. H., 1984, Tumor heterogenity, *Cancer Res.* **44**:2259–2265.

Herlyn, M., Steplewski, Z., Herlyn, D., and Koprowski, H., 1979, Colo-rectal carcinoma-specific antigen: detection by means of monoclonal antibodies, *Proc. Natl. Acad. Sci. USA* **76**:1438.

Hewitt, H. B., 1978, The choice of animal tumors for experimental studies of cancer therapy, *Adv. Cancer Res.* **27**:149–200.

Hurley, J. B., Simon, M. I., Teplow, D. B., Robishaw, J. D., and Gilman, A. G., 1984, Homologies between signal transducing G proteins and *ras* gene products, *Science* **226**:860–862.

Ingbar, S. H., Bauman, A., and Braverman, L. E., 1984, *Studies of the effects of Chronic Erthyrosine Feeding on Various Aspects of Thyroid Hormone Economy in Rats.* Submitted to the Food and Drug Administration as part of "Further studies on the thyroid effects of FD&C Red No. 3," Dec. 4, 1984. FDA Color Additive Petition 96, Docket No. 76N-0366, Administrative Record Index # 299. Food and Drug Administration, Rockville, Maryland.

Interagency Staff Group, 1986, Chemical carcinogens: A review of the science and its associated principles, *Environ. Health Perspect.* **67**:201–282.

Karin, M., Haslinge, A., Holtgreve, H., Richards, R. I., Krauter, P., Westphal, H. W., and Beato, M., 1984, Characterization of DNA sequences through which cadmium and glucocorticoid hormones induce human metallothionein-IIA gene, *Nature* **308**:513–519.

Kelner, A., 1949, Effect of visible light on the recovery of *Streptomyces griseus conida* from ultraviolet irradiation injury, *Proc. Natl. Acad. Sci. USA* **35**:73–79.

Ketterer, B., 1980, Interactions between carcinogens and proteins, *Br. Med. Bull.* **36**:71–78.

Kitagawa, T., Hino, O., Nomura, K., and Sugano, H., 1984, Dose–response studies of the promoting and anticarcinogenic effects of phenobarbital and DDT in the rat hepatocarcinogenesis, *Carcinogenesis* **5**:1643–1656.

Klein, G., 1981, The role of gene dosage and genetic transpositions in carcinogenesis, *Nature* **294**:313–318.

Kraemer, K. H., Lee, M. M., and Scotto, J., 1982, Diseases of environmental–genetic interaction: Preliminary report on a retrospective study of neoplasia in 268 xeroderma pigmentosum patients, in: *Environmental Mutagens and Carcinogens* (T. Sugimura, S. Kondo, and H. Takebe, eds.), pp. 605–612, Arthur R. Liss, New York.

Kriek, E., 1972, Persistent binding of a new reaction product of the carcinogen *N*-hydroxy-*N*-2-acetylaminofluorene with guanine in rat liver DNA in vivo, *Cancer Res.* **32**:2042–2048.

Kripke, M. L., 1974, Antigenicity of murine mouse skin tumors induced by ultraviolet light, *J. Natl. Cancer Inst.* **53**:1333–1336.

Kripke, M. L., 1979, Speculations on the role of ultraviolet radiation in the development of malignant melanoma, *J. Natl. Cancer Inst.* **63**:541–548.

Lam, L. K. T., Sparnins, V. L., Hochalter, J. B., and Wattenberg, L. W., 1981, Effects of 2- and 3-tert-butyl-4-hydroxyanisole on glutathione S-transferase and epoxide hydrolase activities and sulfhydryl levels in liver and forestomach of mice, *Cancer Res.* **41**:3940–3943.

Lee, W., Bookstein, R., Hong, F., Young, L., Shew, J., and Lee, E. Y., 1987, Human Retinoblastoma susceptibility gene: Cloning, identification and sequence, *Science* **235**: 1394–1399.

Lin, J.-K., Miller, J. A., and Miller, E. C., 1977, 2,3-Dihydro-2-(guan-7-yl)-3-hydroxy-aflatoxin B1, a major acid hydrolysis product of aflatoxin B1-DNA or B1-ribosomal RNA adducts formed in hepatic microsome-mediated reactions and in rat liver in vivo, *Cancer Res.* **37**:4430–4438.

Lindahl, T., and Nyberg, B., 1972, Rate of depurination of native deoxyribonucleic acid, *Biochemistry* **11**:3610–3618.

Lindahl, T., Rydberg, B., Hjebnigren, T., Olsson, M., and Jacobson, A., 1982, Cellular defense mechanisms against alkylation of DNA, in: *Molecular and Cellular Mechanisms of Mutagenesis,* (J. Lemontt and W. M. Generoso, eds.), pp. 89–102, Plenum Press, New York.

Linn, S., Kuhnlein, U., and Deutsch, A., 1978, Enzymes from human fibroblasts for the repair of AP DNA, in: *DNA Repair Mechanisms* (P. C. Hanawalt, E. C. Friedberg, and C. F. Fox, eds.), pp. 199–203, Academic Press, New York.

Liotta, L. A., Tryggvason, K., Garbisa, S., Hart, I., Foltz, C. M., and Shafie, S., 1980, Metastatic potential correlates with enzymatic degradation of basement membrane collagen, *Nature* **284**:67–68.

Lipetz, P. D., Galsky, A. G., and Stephens, R. E., 1982, Relationship of DNA tertiary and quaternary structure to carcinogenic processes, *Adv. Cancer Res.* **36**:165–210.

Littlefield, N. A., Farmer, J. H., Gaylor, D. W., and Sheldon, W. G., 1979a, Effects of dose and time in a long-term, low-dose carcinogenic study, *J. Environ. Pathol. Toxicol.* **3**:17–34.

Littlefield, N. A., Greenman, D. L., Farmer, J. H., and Sheldon, W. G., 1979b, Effects of continuous and discontinued exposure to 2-AAF on urinary bladder hyperplasia and neoplasia, *J. Environ. Pathol. Toxicol.* **3**:35–54.

Lu, A. Y. H., 1979, Multiplicity of liver drug metabolizing enzymes, *Drug Metab. Rev.* **10**:187–208.

Magee, P. N., 1977, The relationship between mutagenesis, carcinogenesis and teratogenesis, in: *Progress in Genetic Toxicology* (D. Scott, B. A. Bridges, and F. H. Sorbels, eds.), pp. 15–27, Elsevier/North Holland Biomedical Press, Amsterdam.

Maher, V. M., Rowan, L. A., Silinskas, K. C., Kateley, S. A., and McCormick, J. J., 1982, Frequency of UV-induced neoplastic transformation of diploid human fibroblasts is higher in xeroderma pigmentosum cells than in normal cells, *Proc. Natl. Acad. Sci. USA* **79**:2613–2617.

Marks, F., and Furstenberger, G., 1984, Stages of tumor promotion in skin, *IARC Sci. Pub.* 56:13–22.

McGrath, J. P., Capon, D. J., Goeddewl, D. V., and Levinson, A. D., 1984, Comparative biochemical properties of normal and activated human *ras* p21 protein, *Nature* 310:644–649.

McKhann, C. F., 1982, Tumor immunology: Past, present and future, in: *Accomplishments in Cancer Research 1981* (J. G. Fortner and J. E. Rhoads, eds.) pp. 125–137, Lippincott, Philadelphia.

Miao, R. M., Fieldsteel, A. H., and Fodge, D. W., 1978, Opposing effects of tumour promoters on erythroid differentiation, *Nature* **274**:271–272.

Miller, E. C., and Miller, J. A., 1976, The metabolism of chemical carcinogens to reactive electrophiles and their possible mechanism of action in carcinogenesis, in: *Chemical Carcinogens* (American Chemical Society Monograph, No. 173) (C. Searle, ed.), pp. 737–762, American Chemical Society, Washington, D.C.

Mintz, B., and Fleischman, R., 1981, Teratocarcinoma and other neoplasmas as developmental defects in gene expression, *Adv. Cancer Res.* **34**:214–278.

Morgan, R. W., and Hoffmann, G. R., 1983, Cycasin and its mutagenic metabolites, *Mutat. Res.* **114**:19–58.

Murasaki, G., Zenser, T. Z., Davis, B. B., and Cohen, S. M., 1984, Inhibition by aspirin of N-[4-(5-nitro-2-furyl)-2-thiazolyl]formamide-induced bladder carcinogenesis and enhancement of forestomach carcinogenesis, *Carcinogenesis* **5**:53–55.

Nagasawa, H., and Little, J. B., 1979, Effect of tumor promoters, protease inhibitors, and repair processes on X-ray-induced sister chromatid exchanges in mouse cells, *Proc. Natl. Acad. Sci. USA* **76**:1943–1947.

Nishizuka, Y., 1986, Studies and perspectives of protein kinase C, *Science* **233**:305–312.

Peterson, A. R., Landolph, J. R., Peterson, H., and Heidelberger, C., 1978, Mutagenesis of Chinese hamster cells is facilitated by thymidine and deoxycytidine, *Nature* **276**:508–510.

Poste, G., and Nicolson, G. L., 1980, Arrest and metastasis of blood-borne tumor cells are modified by fusion of plasma membrane vesicles from highly metastatic cells, *Proc. Natl. Acad. Sci. USA* **77**:399–403.

Radman, M., Villani, G., Boiteux, S., Defais, M., Caillet-Fauquet, P., and Spadari, S., 1977, On the mechanism and genetic control of mutagenesis induced by carcinogenic mutagens, in: *Origins of Human Cancer: Mechanisms of Carcinogenesis, Vol. 4* (J. D. Watson, H. Hiatt, eds.), pp. 903–922, Cold Spring Harbor Laboratory, Cold Spring Harbor, New York.

Rovera, G., O'Brien, T. G., and Diamond, L., 1977, Tumor promoters inhibit spontaneous differentiation of Friend erythroleukemia cells in culture, *Proc. Natl. Acad. Sci. USA* **74**:2894–2898.

Sandberg, A. A., 1980, *The Chromosomes in Human Cancer and Leukemia,* Elsevier/North-Holland, Amsterdam.

Sap, J., Munoz, A., Damm, K., Goldberg, Y., Ghysdael, J., Leutz, A., Beug, H., and Vennstrom, B., 1986, The c-*erb*-A protein is a high-affinity receptor for thyroid hormone, *Nature* 324:635–640.

Schirrmacher, V., 1985, Cancer metastasis: Experimental approaches, theoretical concepts, and impacts for treatment strategies, *Adv. Cancer Res.* 43:1–74.

Setlow, R. B., 1980, DNA repair pathways, in: *DNA Repair and Mutagenesis in Eukaryotes* (W. M. Generoso, M. D. Shelby, and F. J. de Serres, eds.), pp. 45–54, Plenum Press, New York.

Sims, P., and Grover, P. L., 1974, Epoxides in polycyclic aromatic hydrocarbon metabolism and carcinogenesis, *Adv. Cancer Res.* 20:165–274.

Slaga, T. J., 1983, Overview of tumor promotion in animals, *Environ. Health Perspect.* 50:3–14.

Stott, W. T., Reitz, R. H., Schumann, A. M., and Watanabe, P. G., 1981, Genetic and nongenetic events in neoplasia, *Food Cosmet. Toxicol.* 19:567–576.

Strauss, B., 1985, Cellular aspects of DNA repair, *Adv. Cancer Res.* 45:45–106.

Swenson, D. H., and Kadlubar, F. F., 1981, Properties of chemical mutagens and chemical carcinogens in relation to their mechanisms of action, in: *Microbial Testers: Probing Carcinogenesis* (I. C. Felkner, ed.), pp. 3–33, Dekker, New York.

Tateishi, N., Higashi, T., Shinya, S., Naruse, A., and Sakamoto, Y., 1974, Studies on the regulation of glutathione level in rat liver, *J. Biochem. (Tokyo)* 75:93–103.

Taub, R., Kirsch, I., Morton, C., Lenoir, G., Swan, D., Tronick, S., Aaronson, S., and Leder, P., 1982, Translocation of the c-*myc* gene into the immunoglobulin heavy chain locus in human Burkitt's lymphoma and murine plasmacytoma cells, *Proc. Natl. Acad. Sci. USA* 79:7837–7841.

Terzaghi, M., and Little, J. B., 1976, X-radiation-induced transformation in a C3H mouse embryo-derived cell line, *Cancer Res.* 36:1367–1374.

Thakker, D. R., Levin, W., Buening, M., Yagi, H., Lehr, R. E., Wood, A. W., Conney, A. H., and Jerina, D. M., 1981, Species-specific enhancement by 7,8-benzoflavone of hepatic microsomal metabolism of benzo(e)pyrene 9,10-dihydrodiol to bay-region diol-epoxide, *Cancer Res.* 41:1389–1396.

Theofilopoulos, A. N., and Dixon, F. J., 1980, Immune complexes in human diseases: A review, *Amer. J. Pathol.* 100:531–594.

Topal, M. D., and Baker, M. S., 1982, DNA precursor pool: A significant target for N-methyl-N-nitrosourea in C3H/10T1/2 clone 8 cells, *Proc. Natl. Acad. Sci. USA* 79:2211–2215.

Trus, M. D., Sodoroski, J. G., and Haseltine, W. A., 1982, Isolation and purification of a human locus homologous to the transforming gene (v-*fes*) of feline sarcoma virus, *J. Biol. Chem.* 257:2730–2733.

Turturro, A., and Hart, R. W., 1984, DNA repair mechanisms in aging, in: *Comparative Biology of Major Age-Related Diseases: Current Status and Research Frontiers* (D. G. Sciapelli and G. Migaki, eds.), pp. 19–45, Arthur R. Liss, New York.

Van de Velde, C. J. H., Van Putten, L. M., and Zwaveling, A., 1977, A new metastasizing mammary carcinoma model in mice: Model characteristics and applications, *Eur. J. Cancer* 13:555–565.

Verma, A. K., Conrad, E. A., and Boutwell, R. K., 1982, Differential effects of retinoic acid and 7,8-benzoflavone on the induction of mouse skin tumors by the complete carcinogenesis process and by the initiation-promotion regimen, *Cancer Res.* 42:3519–3525.

Waring, M. J., 1981, DNA modification and cancer, *Ann. Rev. Biochem.* 50:159–192.

Warren, B. A., 1978, Platelet-tumor cell interactions: Morphological studies, in: *Platelets: A Multidisciplinary Approach* (G. D. Gaetano and S. Garattini, eds.), pp. 427–445, Raven Press, New York.

Wattenberg, L. W., 1980, Inhibitors of chemical carcinogens, *J. Environ. Pathol. Toxicol.* 3:35–52.

Weinberg, R. A., 1982, Oncogenes of spontaneous and chemically induced tumors, *Adv. Cancer Res.* 36:149–163.

Weinstein, I. B., 1981, Current concepts and controversies in chemical carcinogenesis, *J. Supramol. Struct. Cell Biochem.* 17:99–120.

Williams, R. T., 1959, *Detoxification Mechanisms,* 2nd Ed., Chapman and Hall, London.

Young, J. F., and Kadlubar, F. F., 1982, A pharmacokinetic model to predict exposure of the bladder epithelium to urinary N-hydroxyarylamine carcinogens as a function of urine pH, voiding interval, and resorption, *Drug. Metab. Dispos.* 10:641–648.

Zur Hausen, H., O'Neill, F. J., Freese, U. K., and Hecker, E., 1978, Persisting oncogenic herpesvirus induced by the tumor promoter TPA, *Nature* 272:373–375.

II

The Use of Scientific Data in Risk Assessment

3

Use of Short-Term Test Data in Risk Analysis of Chemical Carcinogens

W. Gary Flamm and Robert J. Scheuplein

INTRODUCTION

As the other chapters of this volume will attest, the area of risk analysis of chemical carcinogens is a new and emerging field of science that is intermingled with economic, societal, and political values. The concept that short-term tests, which will be defined and described later in this chapter, can affect the final outcome of a risk analysis is both recent and controversial. While we have not conducted a scientifically valid survey, we have done extensive sampling among highly credible and well regarded scientists whose professional activities impinge on the boundaries of the area we call risk analysis. The question asked of them was, what is the value of short-term test data in risk assessment? Approximately 10% opined that risk analysis is valueless; the remainder were evenly divided between those believing that short-term tests have no value at all to risk analysis and those who view short-term tests as holding some promise and utility for risk analysis. Among the latter group, there were those who believed that short-term tests were useful for making qualitative judgments only and they should not have an impact on quantitative risk analysis. Others felt that the main value of short-term tests in risk assessment would be for classification purposes, that is, to determine whether a substance is a genotoxic carcinogen, thus prompting the use of a conservative nonthreshold linearized extrapolation model, as opposed to a risk extrapolation approach which envisions a threshold. Finally, there were others who said they believed that short-term test data could be valuable both for qualitative and quantitative assessments, but that it is too early and scientific experience is too limited to provide general guidance on the subject. They felt,

W. Gary Flamm and Robert J. Scheuplein • Office of Toxicological Sciences, Center for Food Safety and Applied Nutrition, Food and Drug Administration, Washington, D.C. 20204.

however, that there have been and that there would be specific situations where short-term tests would prove invaluable in determining a final outcome.

In this chapter, an attempt is made to explore some of these situations, not in great depth or in detail, but only to provide some sense of the different ways in which short-term tests can be helpful. Before proceeding with the examples, the short-term tests that have been used most and are likely to prove most useful in the future are briefly described. Since there are excellent and complete descriptions of these tests and analyses elsewhere, the following descriptions will be very brief. It should be noted that the short-term tests described and included in the proffered examples are not limited to genotoxicity tests, but also include any molecular biological or biochemical test which helps to reveal the nature and degree of risk posed to human populations.

SHORT-TERM TESTS

The Ames test (Ames, 1971), which utilizes the bacterium *Salmonella typhimurium*, is certainly the most famous and most extensively used genotoxicity test. In concept, it is remarkably simple. Normal strains of the bacterium *Salmonella typhimurium* have the ability to internally synthesize histidine and thus can live in media free of histidine. Certain mutants, however, have lost this ability. These mutants of *Salmonella typhimurium* are used as the indicator organism. They are placed in a histidine-free media with a chemical mutagen, and the reverse mutations induced in the histidine operon (a series of linked genes) are readily demonstrable because of the ability of the mutants to synthesize histidine and grow in histidine-free media. The indicator organism is combined with a liver homogenate of rats that have been treated with the chemical, arochlor. This preparation is rich in induced microsomal enzymes able to metabolize substances that are not themselves carcinogenic or mutagenic, but are rendered active by microsomal metabolism. Several different mutant strains are used as indicator organisms in order to measure the full range of mutagenic events that can occur. The test has the advantage of being simple to use, and it is rapid and inexpensive. However, it has the disadvantage of being able to measure only certain genetic events and not others, of utilizing a procaryotic genome, and of not possessing mammalian DNA repair.

Mammalian cell test systems that measure forward mutations in mammalian cells grown in tissue culture are also available. These include Chinese hamster cells (Chu and Malling, 1968), mouse lymphoma cells (Clive *et al.*, 1973) and a variety of human cells (DeMars, 1974), to mention a few. These forward mutation systems tend to make use of purine and pyrimidine salvage pathways as a convenient way of detecting forward mutations. For example, 6-thioguanine is used to poison normal wild-type cells capable of metabolizing 6-thioguanine to the ribosyl phosphate through the enzyme, hypoxanthine guanine phosphoribosyl transferase (HGPRT). This conversion allows the 6-thioguanine ribosyl phosphate to be incorporated into DNA and results in the eventual death of the cell. Those cells which lack HGPRT (mutants of the wild-type) are unable to metabolize and incorporate 6-thioguanine into their DNA and therefore continue to survive. Other similar forward mutational assays have been developed using thymidine kinase and bromodeoxyuridine (BUDR) resistance. BUDR, if phosphorylated by thymidine kinase, will be incorporated into DNA, thus killing the affected cell. Mutants lacking thymidine kinase cannot incorporate BUDR into their DNA and, hence, are able to survive. In theory, these forward mutational assays should be able to measure any kind of genetic event which can destroy the gene specified function. Consequently, in theory at least, these forward mutational assays should be able to measure a broader spectrum of events and chemicals that cause these events than would be possible of those tests that measure only reversions.

A third category of short-term tests are those that measure damage to DNA (Bradley *et al.*, 1985). Methods are available to measure DNA damage either indirectly or directly. The indirect methods tend to focus on DNA repair replication as a measure of DNA damage (McQueen and Williams, 1985). DNA repair replication is an enzyme mediated process whereby chemical damage to DNA is repaired by cutting out a small piece of DNA and replacing it with new nucleotides. There are various ways of measuring DNA repair replication, but they can be subdivided into two categories. One such method involves cytologic techniques and is usually referred to as unscheduled DNA synthesis (UDS). This is carried out in several different ways, but fundamentally it involves the measurement of the incorporation of tritiated thymidine into DNA as a response to DNA damage. It is necessary, however, that normal DNA replication be distinguished from DNA repair replication. This can be carried out in several ways. Normal DNA replication can be inhibited without inhibiting unscheduled DNA synthesis so that all radiolabeling is attributable to repair replication. Another way involves taking into account the fact that the distribution and intensity of radiolabeling differs between unscheduled and normal replication.

The other methods for measuring DNA repair involve biochemical techniques that can include any aspect of the DNA repair process. It is possible to imagine hundreds, if not thousands, of different assays able to measure different aspects of repair at the biochemical level. Indeed, the number and variety of tests that could be developed for measuring DNA repair biochemically is limited only by one's imagination.

A fourth category of short-term tests involves measuring normal DNA synthesis that is the result of cell death accompanied by cell proliferation, often leading to hyperplasia. This is normally and simply accomplished by measuring the rate of incorporation of tritiated thymidine into cellular DNA. Both autoradiographic and direct biochemical isolation techniques can be used, as in the measurement of DNA repair. These tests can be conducted in a matter of days, though the period of time in which the animal and its tissue is exposed to the chemical is variable, ranging from just several days to one year.

The above short-term tests all measure the biological or chemical effects on the target cell or molecule. There are also short-term tests which measure effective dose (Stern, 1986). It is obvious that dose is as important a parameter of risk as the biological effect or the strength of the biological effect. Dose is often a problem for the risk assessor because, while the administered dose may be known, the actual dose to the target tissues or target molecules that are at issue in the risk assessment is ordinarily not known. This is illustrated later by an example of the physiologically-based pharmacokinetic models for determining effective dose, a newly emerging technique that is gaining popularity. These models are heavily dependent upon computers and computer time for solving a myriad of simultaneous equations. The physiologically-based model recognizes that there are many physiological compartments into which the chemical and its metabolites may enter and pass. To assess their presence and levels in these compartments, it is necessary to solve these simultaneous equations or to gather a host of data on a large number of compartments at many different time points. Clearly, the former alternative is the least labor intensive and the route most investigators are likely to elect.

PREDICTION OF CARCINOGENICITY

Massive studies with hundreds of chemicals have been conducted in order to determine how well mutagenicity tests correlate with the ability of a substance to induce cancer in rats and mice. The effort began in the early 1970s and focused initially on the Ames test using *Salmonella typhimurium*. It was later joined with other studies using mutagenicity tests in fungi, mammalian cells grown in culture, DNA repair, and other systems. There was much federal support and fanfare—surely, the prophets of mutagenicity tests said, toxicology and safety evaluation stood at the threshold of a new area when it would be possible to test thousands of compounds for their intrinsic potential to produce cancer (Flamm and Lorentzen, 1986). Indeed, there is little question that for many classes of chemicals, mutagenicity tests do a commendable job; tests on aromatic amines, polynuclear aromatic hydrocarbons, and nitrosamine are a few examples. However, a large federally sponsored testing program, the National Toxicology Program, has revealed that a growing number of nonmutagenic compounds are capable of inducing cancer in the test animals, rats and mice. Debate rages on whether these nonmutagenic compounds accomplish their cancer induction by some secondary process, such as, cellular injury, hormonal imbalance, or metabolic overload. If so, the supporters of short-term predictive tests argue that these secondary carcinogens are not actual carcinogens and affect cancer response only at doses that cause other toxic effects. On the other hand, the vast majority of substances shown to be mutagenic are capable of inducing cancer in rats and mice.

After hearing for more than a decade that the correlation or predictiveness of mutagenicity tests for predicting carcinogenicity in rodents is 90% or some other percentage, the middle 1980s are flooded with arguments and counterarguments as to the usefulness or lack of usefulness of mutagenicity for predicting carcinogenicity. Many of these arguments are likely to never be resolved, but this should not cloud the importance and real power of *in vitro* methodology. Its importance comes from several sources: Cells, tissues, and organs can be isolated from the rest of the organism and studied in isolation without interference; molecular studies can be more easily and readily performed *in vitro;* and it is often possible to achieve far greater sensitivity in the measurements that are made on *in vitro* systems than on *in vivo*. These advantages can also be disadvantages, and are often cited as reasons why certain *in vitro* results should be ignored or not accorded much weight in safety evaluation. This merely proves that *in vitro* systems, like those *in vivo*, can easily be misused and the inferred data misinterpreted. The fact remains, however, that *in vitro* tests provide important information. For this information to contribute to knowledge about a compound, it requires the application of scientific judgment.

More recently, scientists have argued that the potency of chemicals in short-term acute toxicity tests in animals is a good measure of carcinogenic potency. For instance, saccharin is a chemical of low acute toxicity and is similarly a weak carcinogen. On the other hand, dioxin (TCDD) is acutely toxic, as well as a very potent carcinogen in rodents. In fact, the empirical correlation in potency is claimed to be excellent (Zeise *et al.*, 1986). Parodi *et al.* (1982) compared carcinogenicity with acute toxicity and three different measures of mutagenicity, and found acute toxicity the most strongly correlated with carcinogenic potency. The reasons for this are unclear, but the high degree of correlation seems to support the idea that the relationship is more than spurious. One possible explanation is that many of the compounds which help to establish the relationship are in fact secondary carcinogens and their carcinogenic activity depends upon toxicity. Three facts need to be borne in mind when considering the relationship: (1) many highly toxic compounds have never been demonstrated to be carcinogenic; (2) some compounds like ethylene dibromide are highly carcinogenic at doses which produce no acute toxicity; and (3) there is no reason to believe that acute toxicity shares commonality with carcinogenicity in biological or mechanistic terms.

CASE EXAMPLES

The following are the five major objectives for using short-term tests in the risk assessment of chemical carcinogens: (1) it is cheaper and faster to use these tests than to rely exclusively upon carcinogen bioassay, which takes a minimum of three years; (2) short-term methods may help to elucidate the mechanism by which a compound is carcinogenic and thereby be more applicable to defining human risk than traditional studies; (3) short-term studies can assist in better defining the mathematical relationship between administered dose and biological response; (4) short-term tests can help to determine the existence of thresholds and the levels at which they exist; and (5) short-term tests can be used to determine the effective dose to target tissue.

At least one example is given below for each objective. The examples are intended for illustrative purposes only, and no attempt is made here to judge whether the responsible investigator(s) was correct either in judgment or the application of short-term test data to risk analysis.

Objective 1: Cheaper and Faster

Several years ago, in the wake of the energy and fuel crisis, the American automotive industry, in conjunction with the Environmental Protection Agency (EPA), attempted to determine whether it should move toward dieselization of automotive engines, that is, the equipping of American cars with diesel rather than gasoline engines. The advantage of the diesel engine is its fuel efficiency, while the disadvantage is its emissions. Gasoline engines with catalytic converters have become incredibly clean, with virtually no particulates or hydrocarbons. The automotive industry needed to decide whether to make a major commitment toward building small diesel engines, and was compelled to weigh the fuel economy advantages against the potential environmental and health problems posed by diesel emissions. What was needed was a rapid assay which could estimate the lifetime risks of cancer from lifetime exposure to diesel fuel emissions. What was available was the traditional carcinogen bioassay which takes years to complete. To solve this problem, EPA scientists were challenged to become highly creative (Lewtas *et al.*, 1981). In reviewing the carcinogenicity and mutagenicity data for roofing tar, coke oven emissions, and cigarette smoke, they found that the relative toxicities of the mixtures were reasonably constant regardless of the bioassay utilized. For example, the ratio of the activity of

*Table 1. Comparison of Relative Potencies
of Emission Extracts*

	Coke oven	
Bioassay	Roofing tar	Cigarette
Human lung capacity	0.39	0.0024
Tumor initiation	0.20	0.0011
Ames test	0.78	0.52
Mouse lymphoma	1.4	0.066

roofing tar to the activity of coke oven emissions was approximately the same for tumor initiation in animals, for the mouse lymphoma assay, for the Ames test, and for *human lung cancer* (Table 1). When such relationships occur, it is possible to calculate a proportionality constant to use in estimating the human cancer risk from, say, diesel and gasoline automotive emissions for which no human data are available.

There are many scientists who would object to this approach and would argue that comparing very simple biological systems to highly complex ones ignores important pharmacokinetic considerations such as absorption and absorption barriers, metabolic activation and deactivation mechanisms, tissue distribution, repair mechanisms, conjugation, and elimination. In any case, the investigators involved deserve credit for attempting to provide a creative solution to a formidable toxicological problem.

Objective 2: Mechanism of Action

Nowhere in toxicology is the importance of understanding mechanisms of action better illustrated than it is for saccharin. The artificial sweetener saccharin is known to produce bladder cancer in rats under certain conditions of dose, time, and age of exposure (Arnold *et al.*, 1977). It also has been shown to act as an effective promoter or enhancer of bladder carcinogenicity when administered after other known bladder carcinogens (Cohen *et al.*, 1979). But, again, this occurs only in the rat and not in the mouse. The reason for the species difference is unknown. Obviously, if we were to know the mechanism by which saccharin induces bladder cancer in rats, we would be able to determine whether that mechanism is operable in mice, and perhaps come to fully understand the reasons for the species difference. Without such information, it is not possible to determine whether saccharin poses a risk of bladder cancer in humans. Are humans like rats or like mice in regard to saccharin-induced bladder carcinogenicity? Thus far, all the short-term tests have shown is that saccharin appears not to be genotoxic and not to be metabolized. Why saccharin should act so differently in the rat than in the mouse is even more difficult to explain, given the knowledge that it is not metabolized.

A number of epidemiology studies have been conducted that have succeeded in showing that past consumption of saccharin in the United States does not constitute a significant risk factor for bladder cancer in the United States. The studies, however, are not powerful enough to demonstrate that humans are less sensitive to the carcinogenic effects of saccharin than rats. The question therefore remains open as to whether humans are more like mice or more like rats. Only mechanistic studies can answer that question.

An example of where the mechanistic question has been answered is the case of melamine. Melamine (Lorentzen, 1983), like saccharin, is not metabolized, is not genotoxic, and yet produces bladder cancer. However, unlike saccharin, melamine at doses high enough to produce bladder cancer, also produces crystals of melamine in the urinary bladder of the animals administered melamine in their diet. Bladder crystals or stones have been shown to be capable of inducing bladder hyperplasia, tumors, and cancer. In the case of melamine, both the time as well as the dose relationships for the development of melamine crystals in the urinary bladder were such as to strongly support the concept that it was the crystals of melamine acting as bladder stones that were ultimately responsible for the development of bladder cancer. This assumption then leads to the conclusion that as long as exposures to melamine do not exceed the solubility of melamine in urine, there would be no crystals or stones of melamine to contend with and, consequently, no risk of cancer.

Objective 3: Defining Better the Mathematical Relationship between Administered Dose and Biological Response

Formaldehyde vapors have been shown to cause nasal cancer in rats at a concentration in air of 14.3 part per million (ppm) (Swenberg, *et al.*, 1983). The affected cells giving rise to nasal cancer are at the interface between the environment and the body. No other cancers of any other tissues have been found, despite the fact the concentrations used were high enough to cause a high incidence of extremely rare squamous cell carcinoma of the nasal turbinates. It is also apparent that the dose–response curve for the induction of these cancers is extremely steep. At 14 ppm for six hr, five days a week, formaldehyde induced a 50% incidence in nasal cancer, but at approximately one-half that dose, only a 1% incidence of cancer was seen. Formaldehyde is mutagenic at high concentrations in certain test systems and is known to react with DNA, preferentially with single-stranded DNA, and to form crosslinks between DNA and nuclear protein. Given these facts, the questions which arise are, why is formaldehyde's carcinogenicity limited to just those cells that come into direct contact with formaldehyde and why is the dose–response so steep? In order to answer these questions, the Chemical Institute of Industrial Toxicology (CIIT) has undertaken extensive studies which include careful analysis of the rate of formation of formaldehyde-induced DNA adducts from the mucosal cells of rats exposed to formaldehyde.

As with the incidence of nasal cancer, the dose-response relationship between formaldehyde and formaldehyde-induced DNA adducts is steep and nonlinear (Fig. 1). In contrast, it is of importance to know that the relationship between formaldehyde concentration and the induction of protein adducts is linear. One explanation as to why fewer DNA adducts are induced at lower concentrations (e.g., 1 ppm) of formaldehyde than would be predicted based on linear extrapolation of data from higher concentrations (e.g., 15 ppm) is that higher concentrations of formaldehyde are highly toxic to the nasal cells, causing them to synthesize DNA and undergo cell proliferation. During DNA synthesis, more of the DNA becomes single-stranded than in resting cells, thus making more DNA available to react with formaldehyde. It is known that these adducts are reparable, though the possibility exists that repair becomes less efficient as more of the DNA reacts with formaldehyde. Furthermore, in rapidly replicating cells, there is a greater chance that the

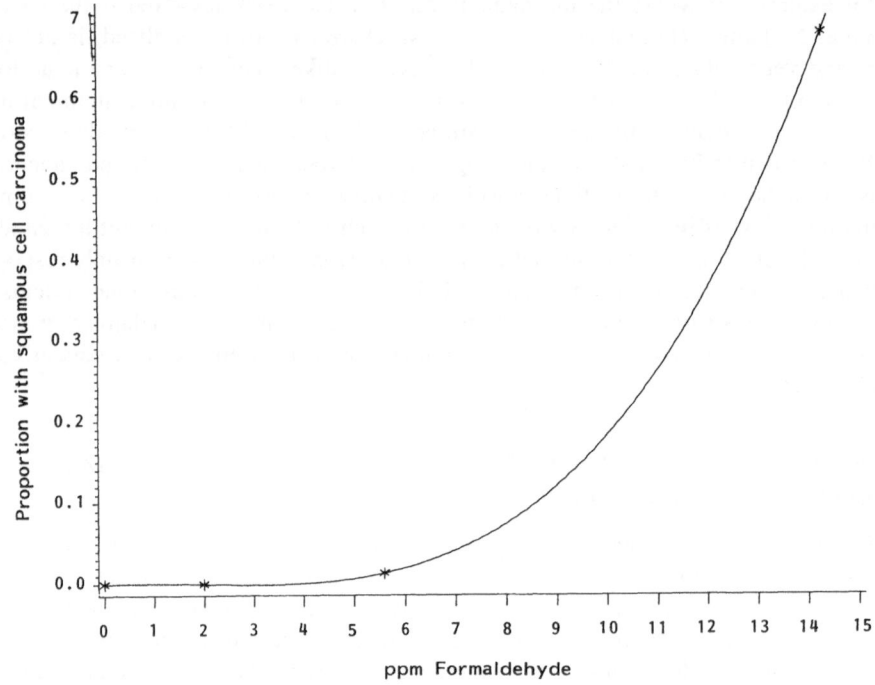

Figure 1. Dose–response relationship for formaldehyde.

formaldehyde adducts will lead to a mutagenic/carcinogenic change prior to the ability of the cell to repair the damage.

The picture then is one where at low concentrations of formaldehyde, little of the gas reacts with DNA, in part because most of the DNA in the nasal cells is double-stranded and unavailable to react with formaldehyde, and possibly because of formaldehyde's greater affinity to react with mucous secretions and cellular proteins. These reactions may be saturable so that at higher concentrations of formaldehyde, little or no protection of DNA is provided. Even though some DNA adducts have been formed at the lower concentrations of formaldehyde, these adducts are reparable and at the low concentrations they are presumably efficiently repaired. As the concentration of formaldehyde is increased, several things begin to happen. Any protection to the DNA that mucous secretions or protein provides is gradually lost as these processes saturate. Nasal cells are induced to divide and synthesize DNA, making more single-stranded DNA available, and leading to the induction of more DNA adducts per unit concentration of formaldehyde. As more and more adducts are induced, the efficiency of repair decreases and the effectiveness of each adduct for causing mutation or neoplastic transformation is significantly increased. This theory is consistent with the finding that the toxicity of formaldehyde is much more dependent upon the concentration of formaldehyde than the cumulative dose. For example, if the cumulative dose to rats exposed to 15 ppm formaldehyde six hr/day, five days/week (450 ppm-hr/wk) is compared with that of rats exposed to 3 ppm for 22 hr/day, seven days/wk (462 ppm-hr/wk), it is apparent that similar cumulative doses of

*Table 2. The Effects of Concentration Versus Dose in Rats Exposed
to Formaldehyde*

Dose (ppm-hr/wk)	Concentration (ppm)	Time (hr/day)	Time (days/wk)	Cytotoxicity	Cell proliferation
450	15	6	5	+ + + +	+ + + +
462	3	22	7	—	—

formaldehyde resulted, yet the incidence of the lesions which resulted were vastly different (Table 2).

Based on a consideration of all the scientific evidence available, it seems likely that the DNA adducts (which are actually methylene bridges crosslinking DNA to nuclear protein) and toxicity (cell turnover) are critically and causally involved in the induction of nasal cancer. These adducts can therefore be used to help in determining (or predicting) the carcinogenic effects of formaldehyde at concentrations that are below those that can be practically measured by animal/cancer experiments. It should be remembered, however, that the efficiency with which these adducts can induce nasal cancer probably diminishes at lower doses where DNA repair is likely to be more effective in preventing premutational DNA lesions from expressing their biological effect.

Objective 4: Help to Determine the Existence of Thresholds and the Level at Which They Exist

The widely used antioxidant food additive, butylated hydroxyanisole (BHA) was demonstrated to induce a 100% incidence of rare squamous cell carcinomas and papillomas of the forestomach of Fischer 344 rats when fed BHA at 2% in their diets for 24 months (Ito *et al.*, 1983). At one-quarter of that level in feed, 0.5%, no tumors or carcinomas were observed after 24 months, indicating an extremely steep dose–response curve for the carcinogenic effect of BHA. The results, while quite reproducible, appear somewhat surprising in light of the fact that BHA has been shown to inhibit or prevent chemical carcinogenesis in a variety of biomodels, including those in which tumors of the forestomach are induced by known carcinogens. Further, BHA does not appear to be a mutagen in any of several gene mutational assays in both bacteria and mammalian cells.

Why should a nongenotoxic antioxidant compound which inhibits chemically induced carcinogenesis under a variety of situations induce cancer in the forestomach of rodents without inducing any systemic cancers and only when fed at extremely high levels? And, why should it exhibit such a steep dose–response curve? The answers to these questions are not known with absolute certitude, but one fact stands out clearly. At doses which induce cancer, BHA administration in the diet results in a greatly (appropriately eight-fold) increased rate of cell turnover among the squamous cells of the forestomach as measured by the incorporation of tritiated thymidine into DNA of these cells (Iverson *et al.*, 1985). Accompanying the enhanced incorporation of tritiated thymidine into DNA, were marked signs of hyperplasia occurring at the junction of the forestomach with the glandular stomach, the site of origin of the papillomas and carcinomas. Both the enhanced incorporation of tritiated thymidine and hyperplasia occurred within days after feeding levels of BHA that produced either cancer or hyperplasia in chronic studies. At slightly lower levels (of 0.25% BHA or below in the diet) no enhancement of thymidine incorporation was observed at any time during the feeding of BHA, evidencing an apparent no-observed-effect level (NOEL). Whether substantially increased cell turnover alone is both necessary and sufficient for the development of cancer of the forestomach is not known with certainty, though the question is testable. Nevertheless, cell turnover and hyperplasia appear to be tightly linked to the process which leads ultimately to cancer of the forestomach. Without such increased cell turnover or hyperplasia, it is doubtful that BHA would induce cancer of the forestomach. Consequently, doses or dietary levels of BHA which are below those required to stimulate cell turnover at any time during the course of the animal's life may represent a threshold dose for the induction of forestomach cancer. How can an increased rate of cell turnover by itself contribute to an increased incidence of cancer? There are two plausible explanations. One, the greatly increased number of cell divisions increases the likelihood of genetic mistakes which may lead to neoplastic transformation and, secondly, the cells may be reaching the end of their normal ability to divide and must either die or undergo changes that result in neoplastic transformation. This latter explanation has an *in vitro* parallel with so-called "late-passage" cultures (those that have already undergone many cell divisions) which are known to undergo neoplastic transformation far more readily than "early-passage" cells.

Objective 5: Effective Dose

The quantitative results of animal bioassays, even when free of the problems associated with sensitivity and tumor identification, are still difficult to project reliably to humans. One major issue is the appropriate dose-scaling factor to be used between animals and humans. Do animals and humans respond comparably on the basis of mg/kg per day, mg/cm^2 per day, mg/kg per lifetime or to some other scaling metric? A related issue is that of administered versus effective dose. It is generally believed that it is the concentration of the chemical that is seen by the target tissue and not the administered dose that is relevant to toxicity. If this tissue concentration, of perhaps a short-lived electrophilic metabolite of the parent substance, happens to be proportional to the administered dose, then a straightforward projection of risk between species seems possible. Under these conditions, we may expect the administered dose to be a reasonable surrogate for the effective dose, and to be proportional to the observed risk. If a comparable proportionality exists in humans, a simple interspecies extrapolation is possible—assuming the appropriate dose scaling is used. But in the typical case, the relationship between administered and effective dose is probably nonlinear in both species, and depends upon species-specific biochemical, metabolic, and physiological processes.

Over the last few years, much effort has been directed into incorporating this mechanistic information into cancer risk extrapolation models (Gerlowski and Jain, 1983; Lutz and Dedrick, 1985). One of the more promising approaches is physiologically-based pharmacokinetic (PBPK) modeling. A PBPK mathematical model is a series of conceptualized lumped compartments (body regions) representing organs or tissues of uniform concentration, connected by a hypothetical blood supply analogous in flow rate and anatomy to the species under study. A series of ordinary differential equations, amenable to solution by computer, describe the system, which is detailed enough to incorporate such data as organ blood flows and volumes, organ metabolism, partition coefficients, protein binding and other biological information. Such models can provide, ideally, an excellent approximation of the time course of the concentration of the chemical and its metabolites in the blood and organs of interest (i.e., the effective dose). In addition, animal scale-up is included automatically because once an accurate description of the distribution of the substance is developed in one species, the same model should be capable of predicting the correct tissue concentrations for a different species as long as the anatomy, physiology, and metabolism are *qualitatively* the same, and *quantitative* differences are adequately reflected by the different model parameters (such as, organ sizes, metabolic constants, and plasma binding) (Dedrick, 1973).

Andersen *et al.* constructed a PBPK model of the disposition of methylene chloride (MC) in four mammalian species (rats, mice, hamsters and humans) (Andersen *et al.*, 1986). Since MC caused malignang lung and liver tumors in mice, the PBPK model included both lung and liver as distinct, metabolically active compartments. Evidence indicates that MC is metabolized by the same two pathways in each species, but the extent of metabolism and the relative contribution of each pathway varies from species to species. The model was constructed to calculate the contributions from the two pathways of metabolism in lung and liver tissue in an effort to explain the lack of liver or lung carcinogenicity in rats and hamsters and to predict any risk for humans.

The tumor incidence in mice correlated with the tissue AVC (area under the concentration/time curve) for both parent MC and the amount of MC metabolized by the glutathione *S*-transferase (GST) dependent pathway, but not with the amount of MC metabolized by the mixed function oxidase (MFO) dependent pathway. Because MC was considered unlikely on chemical grounds to be directly involved in carcinogenesis, the metabolism of MC by GST was indicted as the important pathway for carcinogenesis. In vitro metabolism of MC in rat, mouse, hamster and human liver fractions indicated a lower level of GST dependent metabolism in both hamsters and humans, thus tending to confirm the negative findings in hamsters and indicating a low carcinogenic risk to humans from MC exposure despite the positive findings in mice. Target tissue doses in humans were calculated to be 140- to 170-fold lower (inhalation) or 50- to 210-fold lower (drinking water) than would be expected from direct linear extrapolation using surface area scaling.

CONCLUSIONS

A variety of short-term tests both *in vivo* and *in vitro* can contribute vitally important information to the risk assessment process. At present, there are only a few good examples of how these tests are impacting on risk assessment and the final numerical outcome. It is to be expected that industry and government will take the lead in developing an understanding of how to use short-term tests for improving the scientific assumptions on which risk assessments are based. Eventually this process can only improve the quality of science on which risk assessments depend.

REFERENCES

Ames, B. N., 1971, The detection of chemical mutagens with enteric bacteria, in: *Chemical Mutagens* (A. Hollaender, ed.), pp. 267–281, Plenum Press, New York.

Andersen, M. E., *et al.*, 1986, Physiologically-based pharmacokinetics and the risk assessment process for methylene chloride (submitted to TAP on January 19, 1986, draft subject to revision).

Arnold, D. L., Moodie, C. A., Stavric, B., Stoltz, D., Grice, H. C., and Munro, I. C., 1977, Canadian saccharin study, *Science* **197**:320.

Bradley, M. O., Sina, J. F., and Erickson, L. C., 1985, Measurements of chemical interaction with DNA, in: *Mechanisms and Toxicity of Chemical Carcinogens and Mutagens* (W. G. Flamm and R. J. Lorentzen, eds.), pp. 99–127, Princeton Scientific Publishing, Princeton.

Chu, E. H. Y., and Malling, H. V., 1968, Mammalian cell genetics II: Chemical induction of specific locus mutations in Chinese hamster cells *in vitro*, *Proc. Natl. Acad. Sci. USA* **61**:1306–1312.

Clive, D., Flamm, W. G., and Patterson, J. B., 1973, Specific-locus mutational assay system for mouse lymphoma cells, in: *Chemical Mutagens* (A. Hollaender, ed.), pp. 79–103, Plenum Press, New York.

Cohen, S. M., Arai, M., Jacobs, J. B., and Friedell, G. H., 1979, Promoting effects of saccharin and DL-tryptophan in urinary bladder carcinogenesis, *Cancer Res.* **39**:1207–1217.

Dedrick, R. L., 1973, Animal scale-up, *J. Pharmacokinet. Biopharm.* **1**:435–461.

DeMars, R., 1974, Resistance of cultured human fibroblasts and other cells to purine and pyrimidine analogs in relation to mutagenesis detection, *Mutat. Res.* **24**:335–364.

Flamm, W. G., and Lorentzen, R. J., 1986, The use of *in vitro* methods in safety evaluation, *In Vitro Toxicol.* **1**:1–4.

Gerlowski, L. E., and Jain, R. K., 1983, Physiologically-based pharmacokinetic modeling: Principles and applications, *J. Pharm. Sci.* **72**:1103–1126.

Ito, N., Fukushima, S., Hagiwara, A., Shibata, M., and Ogiso, T., 1983, Carcinogenicity of butylated hydroxyanisole in F344 rats, *J. Natl. Cancer Inst.* **70**:343–352.

Iverson, F., Lok, E., Nera, E., Karpinski, K., and Clayson, D. B., 1985, A 13 week feeding study of butylated hydroxyanisole: The subsequent regression of the induced lesions in male Fischer 344 rat forestomach epithelium, *Toxicology* **35**:1–11.

Lewtas, J., Bradow, R. L., Jungers, R. H., Harris, B. D., Zweidinger, R. B., Cushing, K. M., Gill, B. E., and Albert, R. E., 1981, Mutagenic and carcinogenic potency of extracts of diesel and related environmental emissions, *Environ. Int.* **5**:383–387.

Lorentzen, R. J., 1983, Melamine. (Memorandum of Conference of the Cancer Assessment Committee, March 17, 1983.)

Lutz, R. J., and Dedrick, R. L., 1985, Physiological pharmacokinetics: Relevance to human risk assessment, in: *Toxicity Testing: New Approaches and Application in Human Risk Assessment* (T. L. Black, D. K. Flaherty, W. E. Ribelin, and A. G. E. Wilson, eds.), pp. 129–149, Raven Press, New York.

McQueen, C. A., and Williams, G. M., 1985, Mammalian cell DNA repair assays for carcinogens, in: *Mechanisms and Toxicity of Chemical Carcinogens and Mutagens* (W. G. Flamm and R. J. Lorentzen, eds.), pp. 129–151, Princeton Scientific Publishing, Princeton.

Parodi, S., Taningher, M., Boero, P., and Santi, L., 1982, Quantitative correlations amongst alkaline DNA fragments, DNA binding, mutagenicity in the Ames tests, and carcinogenicity for 21 cpds, *Mutat. Res.* **93**:1–24.

Stern, R. M., 1986, The management of risk for industrial metallic aerosols: *In vitro* assessment of delivered dose per unit exposure, in: *Risk and Reason* (P. Ottedal and A. Brogger, eds.), pp. 121–124, Alan R. Liss, New York.

Swenberg, J. A., Gross, E. A., Martin, J., Popp, J. A., 1983, Mechanisms of formaldehyde toxicity, in: *Formaldehyde Toxicity* (James E. Gibson, ed.), Hemisphere Publishing, New York.

Zeise, L., Crouch, E. A. C., and Wilson, R., 1986, A possible relationship between toxicity and carcinogenicity, *J. Am. Coll. Tox.* **5**:137–150.

4

Use of Animal Bioassay Data in Carcinogen Risk Assessment

Elizabeth K. Weisburger

INTRODUCTION

Risk assessment generally comprises some or all of the following factors: hazard identification, dose–response assessment, exposure assessment, and risk characterization (National Research Council, 1983). Animal bioassays are fundamental in furnishing information directly relevant to the first two of these factors, identification of the hazard and dose–response assessment.

The bioassay program which has been most used (or misused) for purposes of risk assessment was originally that of the National Cancer Institute (NCI), now under the auspices of the National Toxicology Program (NTP). The concept for the program originated about 1960 with Michael Shimkin, then Director of the Field Studies Area of NCI. He considered that there was a need for more systematic investigation of chemical carcinogenesis in animals, for at that time only a few compounds had been tested for possible carcinogenicity in a sufficient number of animals and at more than one dose level (Weisburger, 1983). The purpose of the NCI effort was to gather facts and acquire knowledge, allowing a clarification of the process of carcinogenesis in both humans and experimental animals. A consequence would be an increased comprehension of the etiology and pathogenesis of cancer. The original bioassay program was not intended to be a medium for large-scale bioassay of industrial or environmental materials. Instead, priority was given to study of chemicals where the results would most likely contribute to knowledge of the etiology of cancer or to understanding the mechanism of action of carcinogens. A second aim was to test representative compounds from classes of chemicals which had not yet been tested for carcinogenic activity. It was considered that the results of such studies

Elizabeth K. Weisburger • Division of Cancer Etiology, National Cancer Institute, Bethesda, Maryland 20892.

should permit more intelligent choices as to which chemical structures require further scrutiny. Obviously, the original bioassay program was highly research-oriented, with a great deal of emphasis on chemical structures and structural classes. Furthermore, when the bioassay program began, use of the data for risk analysis was not even considered because this area did not come into prominence until the late 1970s or early 1980s (Scientific Committee, Food Safety Council, 1978; Richmond, 1981).

Bioassay projects were accomplished through a contract program due to a lack of resources and personnel at NCI. Initially, contracts were reviewed by the Branch Advisory Panel, but later proposed contracts were discussed by a committee of NCI personnel before review by an advisory panel.

HISTORY OF BIOASSAY PROGRAM

The first projects in the bioassay program were largely devoted to model studies, attempting to find which animal systems should be used, what protocols were feasible, and the spontaneous tumor incidence in the available strains of mice and rats. Publications from these projects included several on the use of the strain A mouse in testing alkylating agents and various environmental materials (Shimkin *et al.*, 1966; Stoner *et al.*, 1973; Shimkin and Stoner, 1975; Theiss *et al.*, 1977), use of Fischer (F344) rats for testing numerous compounds at five dose levels (Hadidian *et al.*, 1968), tests of many compounds with induction of mammary tumors in virgin female Sprague–Dawley rats as an endpoint (Griswold *et al.*, 1966, 1968), the use of Charles River rats and HaM/ICR mice (Russfield *et al.*, 1975; Weisburger *et al.*, 1978, 1981), tests of over 100 pesticides and related materials in two hybrid strains of mice (Innes *et al.*, 1969), studies on cancer chemotherapeutic agents (Weisburger, 1977), and several papers on the spontaneous tumor incidence in the control animals (Prejean *et al.*, 1973; Homburger *et al.*, 1975). In all these projects, publication in a scientific journal was usually the final product, indicating the research-oriented aspect of the bioassay program. There was relatively little interaction with regulatory agencies. However, appointment of a new leader for the program led to several changes: (1) Further developmental efforts were to cease and future tests were to be done according to the relatively standardized FDA–UICC protocols (Association of Food & Drug Officials, 1959; Berenblum, 1969); (2) There was to be greater cooperation with the regulatory agencies and data were to be shared with them as expeditiously as possible.

The formation of a commission (MRAK Commission) in April of 1969 to investigate the benefits and risks of pesticides and to report their recommendations and findings, led to the realization that an appreciable number of pesticides used then had not been adequately tested (U.S. Department of Health, Education, and Welfare, 1969). The Environmental Protection Agency (EPA) requested NCI to take the lead in initiating studies of pesticides and other environmental materials because NCI was the one agency with a viable operating bioassay system.

Consequently, the NCI bioassay program initiated long-term studies on approximately 40 pesticides, the results of which appeared later as technical reports. The Osborne–Mendel rat was used for a few tests, because of its reported sensitivity to chlorinated compounds (Fitzhugh and Nelson, 1947; Reuber and Glover, 1970). Nevertheless, the decision was made that the Fischer (F344) rat and the C57BL/6XC3H/Anf (B6C3F$_1$) mouse would be the standard animals for bioassays. This was based both on the experience with these strains and that the studies using other strains had shown certain deficiencies, such as very large size in some rats and early deaths in mice. There was, however, an appreciable difference between the protocol actually adopted for the bioassay program and that recommended by the FDA and UICC. Three dose levels were recommended, but the NCI guidelines called for only two dose levels, the maximum tolerated dose (MTD) and half the MTD (Sontag *et al.*, 1976). One reason was that there were many compounds to test, and the purpose was to demonstrate that compounds either did or did not have the capability of acting as carcinogens. Dose–response relationships were not considered within the province of the program. Another reason was in the exploratory contract where five dose levels were tested in rats (Hadidian *et al.*, 1968); only the most potent carcinogens showed an effect at the lower doses. Thus, an impetus to test compounds at multiple dose levels was diminished because testing in this manner greatly increased the cost without providing much in the way of return. The NCI studies therefore provided two points, defining a straight-line relationship, whereas three points or more are needed to define a curve, the usual shape resulting from a dose–response plot.

The passage of the National Cancer Act in 1971 led to allocation of greater funds for research so that new contracts to test compounds could be negotiated. As a consequence, over 60 full-scale long-term studies were initiated in 1971 and over 200 in 1972, the peak year for such efforts.

RESULTS OF BIOASSAY PROGRAM

Among the chemicals entered on test in 1971 there was an appreciable number of the simpler halogenated compounds. Many of these were used extensively as degreasing agents and solvents for varied types of applications; most had had no long-term toxicity tests or else only fragmentary studies had been done. When the bioassays showed that mice receiving trichloroethylene or chloroform developed liver tumors and that rats had kidney tumors from chloroform (NCI, 1976a,b), a good deal of regulatory action began. A paradox was that such efforts concentrated on the weaker carcinogens trichloroethylene and chloroform (Seltzer, 1975; NIOSH, 1975). The more potent carcinogens 1,2-dibromo-3-chloropropane and 1,2-dibromoethane (Olsen *et al.*, 1973) received relatively little attention until several years later. Trichloroethylene, besides being a major degreasing agent, was also employed to decaffeinate coffee. Because traces of the compound remained in the coffee, FDA took regulatory action to prevent this use of trichloroethylene. The coffee industry then converted to dichloromethane (methylene chloride), which had not been tested at that time. Presently, extensive tests in different species and by various routes of administration have been reported on dichloromethane, both by industry and by government through the NTP (Burek *et al.*, 1984; NTP, 1986). These tests have shown that dichloromethane is clearly carcinogenic in mice and to some extent in rats also. The FDA has decided to allow continued use of dichloromethane as a decaffeinating agent because a risk analysis based on the trace amounts remaining in the coffee showed a

Table 1. Chemicals Shown to be Carcinogenic in Mice and Rats in NCI Bioassay Program

Compound	Site affected	
	Mice	Rats
Aromatic amines		
2-Aminoanthraquinone	Liver (M + F)	Liver (M)
	Lymphoma (F)	
1-Amino-2-methylanthraquinone	Liver (F)	Liver (M + F)
		Kidney (M)
o-Anisidine HCl	Bladder (M + F)	Bladder (M + F)
		Kidney (M)
		Thyroid (M)
p-Cresidine	Bladder (M + F)	Bladder (M + F)
	Liver (F)	Liver (M)
		Nasal cavity (M + F)
Cupferron	Blood vessels (M + F)	Blood vessels (M + F)
	Liver (F)	Liver (M + F)
	Zymbal's gland (F)	Forestomach (M + F)
		Zymbal's gland (F)
4-Chloro-o-phenylenediamine	Liver (M + F)	Bladder (M + F)
		Forestomach (M + F)
2,4-Diaminoanisole · H_2SO_4	Thyroid (M + F)	Skin and associated glands (M + F)
		Thyroid (M + F)
2,4-Diaminotoluene	Liver (F)	Liver (M + F)
	Lymphoma (F)	Mammary gland (F)
Hydrazobenzene	Liver (F)	Liver (M + F)
		Mammary gland (F)
		Zymbal's gland (M)
4,4'-Methylenebis(N,N-dimethyl)-benzenamine	Liver (F)	Thyroid (M + F)
Michler's ketone	Blood vessels (M)	Liver (M + F)
	Liver (F)	
5-Nitro-o-anisidine	Liver (F)	Skin and associated structures (M + F)
4,4'-Oxydianiline	Liver (M + F)	Liver (M + F)
	Thyroid (F)	Thyroid (M + F)
	Harderian gland (M + F)	
4,4'-Thiodianiline	Liver (M + F)	Liver (M)
	Thyroid (M + F)	Thyroid (M + F)
		Zymbal's gland (M + F)
		Colon (M)
		Uterus (F)
o-Toluidine HCl	Liver (F)	Spleen (M + F)
	Blood vessels (M)	Bladder (F)
		Subcutaneous tissue (M)
		Mammary gland (F)
Halogenated compounds		
Chloroform	Liver (M + F)	Kidney (M)
1,2-Dibromo-3-chloropropane	Stomach (M + F)	Stomach (M + F)
		Blood vessels (M + F)
		Mammary gland (F)

Table 1. (Continued)

Compound	Site affected	
	Mice	Rats
1,2-Dibromoethane	Stomach (M + F)	Stomach (M + F)
	Lung (M + F)	Liver (F)
		Blood vessels (M)
Tris(2,3-dibromopropyl)phosphate	Stomach (M + F)	Kidney (M + F)
	Lung (M + F)	Liver (M)
	Kidney (M)	
	Liver (F)	
2,4,6-Trichlorophenol	Liver (M + F)	Lymphoma (M)

minimal risk to the users (Department of Health and Human Services, 1986). Other intermediates that were carcinogenic in both mice and rats, with the sites affected, are listed in Table 1.

CHLOROFORM

The results of the bioassay on chloroform led FDA to prohibit its use in toothpaste, cough syrup, liniments, and similar products (Davidson *et al.*, 1982). The EPA also became involved, for traces of chloroform and many other halogenated compounds are formed during chlorination of water supplies (Rook, 1980; Glaze *et al.*, 1980; Briley *et al.*, 1980). Haloforms, including chloroform, are also produced by edible red seaweeds (*Asparagopsis taxiformis* and related algae) (Burreson *et al.*, 1975; Siuda, 1980), demonstrating a natural occurrence. The EPA used the NCI data, after extrapolation from the high levels given the animals, to calculate a risk assessment for humans from ingestion of chloroform in drinking water. However, there are outstanding differences between mice and humans with respect to chloroform (Table 2). One is that in mice, more of a dose of chloroform is metabolized to reactive entities (Brown *et al.*, 1974), including phosgene, which may attack cellular proteins (Pohl *et al.*, 1981) or lipids (Cowlen *et al.*, 1984). However, attachment of chloroform or its metabolites to the cellular nucleic acids is minimal. Another difference between the bioassay animals and the human situation is that

Table 2. Comparative Metabolism of Chloroform

Species	Oral dose (mg/kg)	Excretion (%)		
		Expired as $CHCl_3$	Expired as CO_2	Urine and feces
Human	7	40.3 (18–66)	49.5	—
Mouse	60	6.1	85.1	2.6
Rat	60	19.7	65.9	7.6
Squirrel monkey	60	78.7	17.6	2.0

Table 3. Comparative Intake of Chloroform

Species		Daily intake (mg/kg)	
Human (50 kg)		Air	0.011
		Food	0.00087
		Water	0.0188[a]
		Total	0.0307
Mouse[b]	Male		138;277
	Female		238;477
Rat[b]	Male		90;180

[a]Highest level
[b]Bioassay.

even assuming the highest level of chloroform found in drinking water (Kraybill, 1985), the exposure of most humans to this compound is thousands of times lower than that received by the mice and rats in the NCI study (Table 3).

DOSE–RESPONSE RESULTS

Inspection of the data on kidney tumors in male rats from the NCI study on chloroform shows that there was a relatively low response. In mice, it appears that liver tumor response may show a very steep drop from that seen at the levels tested in the bioassay (Fig. 1). As mentioned, the NCI bioassay studies were done at only two dose levels, sufficient only to determine a straight line. However, toxicological responses generally follow a curved-line relationship; three points or more are required to determine such an element. Inspection of various dose–response curves (Scientific Committee, Food Safety Council, 1978) shows that except for hexachlorobenzene, where the dose–response plot is a straight line to the origin, for all other compounds a variety of curves was evident. Some curves, as for nitrilotriacetic acid and saccharin, show a lack of response until fairly high doses were attained. Others indicate a small region of no response, followed by a steep rise with an increase in dose, specifically for aflatoxin and dimethylnitrosamine. Overall, there is considerable variation in dose–response relationships and no set pattern or a single equation is followed (Scientific Committee, Food Safety Council, 1978).

Furthermore, the responses to carcinogens, as with any xenobiotic, are influenced by many factors. In animals the species, strain, sex, age, diet, rate of metabolism, hormonal status, presence of enzyme inducers, immune status, and the spontaneous tumor incidence in a given animal model are some of the most prominent factors (Scientific Committee, Food Safety Council, 1978; Weisburger, 1981). For the human situation there are many uncertainties regarding the influences specific factors bear on cancer (Phillips, 1975; Lyon *et al.*, 1976; National Research Council, 1982; Marchetto *et al.*, 1983; Morin *et al.*, 1984). However, the models used by EPA for estimating the risk to man at low doses of chloroform did not consider any of these parameters. More realistic methods for quantitative cancer risk assessment, which allow the application of pharmacokinetic data in the process, have now been proposed (Sielken, 1986).

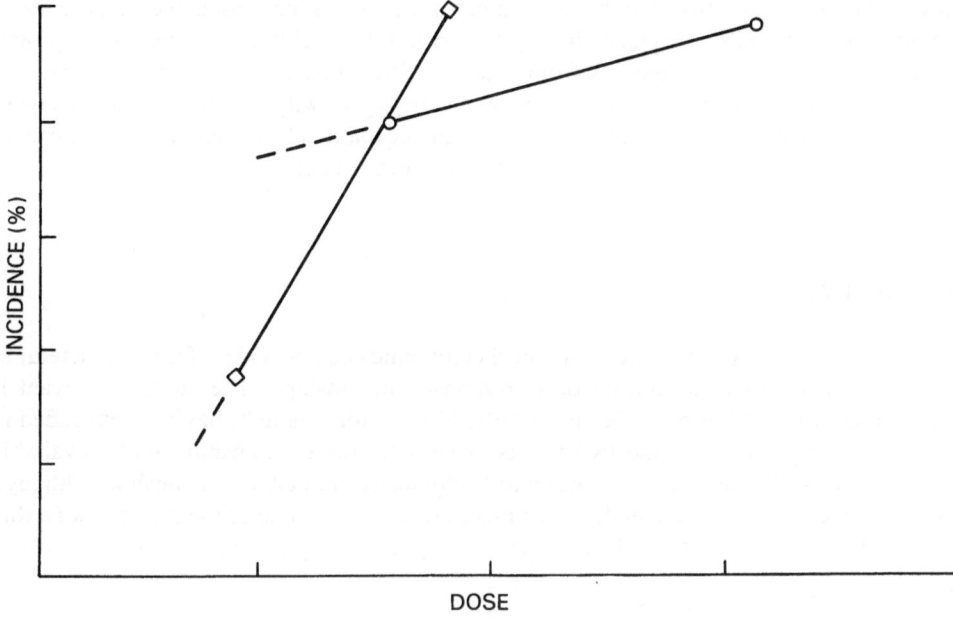

Figure 1. Dose–response plot for liver cancer in mice given chloroform. Male mice, □–□; female mice, O–O.

IMPROVEMENTS IN THE BIOASSAY PROGRAM

Therefore, the former bioassays and the process which used the data for risk assessment are lacking for several reasons, including, too few points on the dose response curve and rigid, unrealistic models. To remedy these deficiencies, different methods for risk assessment are needed and are now available. To obtain a better dose–response curve, EPA is requesting in the Toxic Substance Control Act Test Guidelines that toxicity tests of various types be done at three dose levels, spaced in order to afford a dose–response curve (EPA, 1985). The NTP, the agency which has the main responsibility (and funds) to conduct bioassays in new forthcoming tests, will convert from bioassays at two levels to those at three levels. The levels will be chosen based on pharmacokinetic considerations, probable levels of human exposure, minimally toxic doses as derived from prechronic studies, and any other relevant factors.

In the design of new bioassays, because most effects are seen at the MTD or half the MTD, inclusion of smaller groups of animals, such as 25 males and 25 females, at levels which are suitable fractions of the MTD, should allow better definition of the dose–response curve without greatly increasing the cost of the bioassay. Certainly the somewhat increased expense would be less than the total cost incurred for the travel and support expenses of the many meetings focusing on which extrapolation model to use and the discussions on the models. With more data points, more reasonable risk estimates could be done, based on data from animal experiments rather than on conjecture. Combined with more realistic models for risk assessment, the overall evaluation should represent a reasonable case rather than worst case estimates for risk. Such reasonable risk estimates are important in order to place the relative risk for developing cancer in its proper perspective—compared to the risk from other activities such as driving an automobile, or taking an airplane trip. Some risk is associated with any activity (Environ, 1986). However, some lifestyle factors are more important than occupational exposure in causing cancer in humans (Higginson and Muir, 1979; Doll and Peto, 1981).

SUMMARY

Animal bioassays of discrete chemical compounds can provide information useful in identification of a hazard and on dose–response relationships. The latter is relevant if compounds are tested at multiple dose levels. Much effort, though, has been expended in trying to extrapolate from the two points or straight-line relationship usually available from the NCI/NTP bioassays to a more toxicologically creditable relationship. Although some risk factors have come under government regulation, some of the major risk factors for human cancer are not regulated, because they are lifestyle factors.

REFERENCES

Association of Food & Drug Officials of the United States, 1959, *Appraisal of the Safety of Chemicals in Foods, Drugs, and Cosmetics,* Editorial Committee, Baltimore.

Berenblum, I. (ed.), 1969, *Carcinogenicity testing.* A report of the panel on carcinogenicity of the Cancer Research Commission of UICC, Vol. 2, Geneva, UICC.

Briley, K. F., Williams, R. F., Longley, K. E., and Sorber, C. A., 1980, Trihalomethane production from algal precursors, in: *Water Chlorination: Environmental Impact and Health Effects,* Vol. 3 (R. L. Jolley, W. A. Brungs, and R. B. Cumming, eds.), pp. 117–129, Ann Arbor Science, Ann Arbor, Michigan.

Brown, D. M., Langley, P. F., Smith, D., and Taylor, D. C., 1974, Metabolism of [^{14}C]chloroform by different species, *Xenobiotica* **4**:151–163.

Burek, J., Nitschke, K., Bell, T., Wackerle, D., Childs, R., Beyer, J., Dittenber, D., Rampy, L., and McKenna, M., 1984, Methylene chloride: A two-year inhalation toxicity and oncogenicity study in rats and hamsters, *Fundam. Appl. Toxicol.* **4**:30–47.

Burreson, B. J., Moore, R. E., and Roller, P., 1975, Volatile halogen compounds in the algae *Asparagopsis taxiformis* (Rhodophyta), *J. Agric. Food Chem.* **24**:856–861.

Cowlen, M. S., Hewitt, W. R., and Schroeder, F., 1984, 2-Hexanone potentiation of [^{14}C]chloroform hepatotoxicity: Covalent interaction of a reactive intermediate with rat liver phospholipid, *Toxicol. Appl. Pharmacol.* **73**:478–491.

Davidson, I. W. F., Sumner, D. D., and Parker, J. C., 1982, Chloroform: A review of its metabolism, teratogenic, mutagenic, and carcinogenic potential, *Drug Chem. Toxicol.* **5**:1–87.

Department of Health and Human Services, Food and Drug Administration, 1986, Cosmetics: proposed ban on the use of methylene chloride as an ingredient of aerosol cosmetic products; extension of comment period, *Fed. Regist.* **51**:6494.

Doll, R., and Peto, R., 1981, The causes of cancer: Quantitative estimates of avoidable risks of cancer in the United States today. *J. Natl. Cancer Inst.* **66**:1191–1308.

Environ, 1986, *Elements of Toxicology and Chemical Risk Assessment,* Washington, D.C.

Environmental Protection Agency (EPA), 1985, Toxic Substance Control Act Test Guidelines: Final Rules, *Fed. Regis.* **50**:39252–39516.

Fitzhugh, O. G., and Nelson, A. A., 1947, The chronic oral toxicity of DDT (2,2-bis(p-chlorophenyl)-1,1,1-trichloroethane), *J. Pharmacol. Exp. Ther.* **89**:18–30.

Glaze, W. H., Saleh, F. Y., and Kinstley, W., 1980, Characterization of nonvolatile halgenated compounds formed during water chlorination, in: *Water Chlorination: Environmental Impact and Health Effects,* Vol. 3 (R. L. Jolley, W. A. Brungs, and R. B. Cumming, eds.), pp. 99–108, Ann Arbor Science, Ann Arbor, Michigan.

Griswold, D. P., Casey, A. E., Weisburger, E. K., and Weisburger, J. H., 1968, The carcinogenicity of multiple intragastric doses of aromatic and heterocyclic nitro or amino derivatives in young female Sprague–Dawley rats, *Cancer Res.* **28:**924–933.

Griswold, D. P., Casey, A. E., Weisburger, E. K., Weisburger, J. H., and Schabel, F. M., Jr., 1966, On the carcinogenicity of a single intragastric dose of hydrocarbons, nitrosamines, aromatic amines, dyes, coumarins, and miscellaneous chemicals in female Sprague–Dawley rats, *Cancer Res.* **26:**619–625.

Hadidian, Z., Fredrickson, T. N., Weisburger, E. K., Weisburger, J. H., Glass, R. M., and Mantel, N., 1968, Tests for chemical carcinogens: Report on the activity of derivatives of aromatic amines, nitrosamines, quinolines, nitroalkanes, amides, epoxides, aziridines, and purine antimetabolites, *J. Natl. Cancer Inst.* **41:**985–1036.

Higginson, J., and Muir, C. S., 1979, Environmental carcinogenesis: Misconceptions and limitations to cancer control, *J. Natl. Cancer Inst.* **63:**1291–1298.

Homburger, F., Russfield, A. B., Weisburger, J. H., Lim, S., Chak, S., and Weisburger, E. K., 1975, Aging changes in CDR-1 HaM/ICR mice reared under standard laboratory conditions, *J. Natl. Cancer Inst.* **55:**37–46.

Innes, J. R. M., Ulland, B. M., Valerio, M. G., Petrucelli, L., Fishbein, L., Hart, E. R., Pallotta, A. J., Bates, R. R., Falk, H. L., Gart, J. J., Klein, M., Mitchell, I., and Peters, J., 1969, Bioassay of pesticides and industrial chemicals for tumorigenicity in mice: A preliminary note. *J. Natl. Cancer Inst.* **42:**1101–1114.

Kraybill, H. F., 1985, Assessment of human exposure to environmental contaminants with special reference to cancer, in: *Toxicological Risk Assessment,* Vol. II (D. B. Clayson, D. Krewski, and I. Munro, eds.), pp. 17–42, CRC Press, Boca Raton, Florida.

Lyon, J. L., Klauber, M. R., Gardner, J. W., and Smart, C. R., 1976, Cancer incidence in Mormons and non-Mormons in Utah, 1966–1970, *N. Engl. J. Med.* **294:**129–133.

Marchetto, D., Li, F. P., and Henson, D. E., 1983, Familial carcinoma of ureters and other genitourinary organs, *J. Urol.* **130:**772–773.

Morin, M. M., Pickle, L. W., and Mason, T. J., 1984, Geographic patterns of ethnic groups in the United States, *Am. J. Public Health* **74:**133–139.

National Cancer Institute (NCI), 1976a, *Report on Carcinogenesis Bioassay of Chloroform,* March 1, 1976.

National Cancer Institute (NCI), 1976b, *Carcinogenesis Bioassay of Trichloroethylene,* Carcinogenesis Technical Report Series No. 2, Bethesda, Maryland, DHEW Publication No. (NIH) 76–802.

National Institute of Occupational Safety and Health (NIOSH), 1975, *Current Intelligence Bulletin 2: Trichoroethylene,* June 6, 1975.

National Research Council, 1982, *Diet, Nutrition and Cancer.* National Academy Press, Washington, D.C.

National Research Council, 1983, *Risk Assessment in the Federal Government: Managing the Process.* National Academy Press, Washington D. C.

National Toxicology Program (NTP), 1986, *Toxicology and carcinogenesis studies of dichloromethane (methylene chloride) (CAS No. 75-09-2) in F344/N rats and B6C3F$_1$ mice (inhalation studies).* Technical Report Series No. 306.

Olson, W. A., Habermann, R. T., Weisburger, E. K., Ward, J. M., and Weisburger, J. H., 1973, Brief communication: Induction of stomach cancer in rats and mice by halogenated aliphatic fumigants, *J. Natl. Cancer Inst.* **51:**1993–1995.

Phillips, R. L., 1975, Role of life-style and dietary habits in risk of cancer among Seventh-Day Adventists, *Cancer Res.* **35:**3513–3522.

Pohl, L. R., Branchflower, R. V., Highet, R. J., Martin, J. L., Nunn, D. S., Monks, T. J., George, J. W., and Hinson, J. A., 1981, The formation of diglutathionyl dithiocarbonate as a metabolite of chloroform, bromotrichloromethane, and carbon tetrachloride, *Drug Metab. Dispos.* **9:**334–339.

Prejean, J. D., Peckham, J. C., Casey, A. E., Griswold, D. P., Weisburger, E. K., and Weisburger, J. H., 1973, Spontaneous tumors in Sprague–Dawley rats and Swiss mice, *Cancer Res.* **33:**2768–2773.

Reuber, M. D., and Glover, E. L., 1970, Cirrhosis and carcinoma of the liver in rats given subcutaneous carbon tetrachloride, *J. Natl. Cancer Inst.* **44:**419–423.

Richmond, C. R., 1981, Health Risk Analysis: A challenge for the 1980's, in: *Health Risk Analysis: Proceed-*

ings of The Third Life Sciences Symposium, Health Risk Analysis, Gatlinburg, Tennessee, Oct. 27–30, 1980. Franklin Institute Press, Philadelphia.

Rook, J. J., 1980, Possible pathways for the formation of chlorinated degradation products during chlorination of humic acids and resorcinol, in: *Water Chlorination: Environmental Impact and Health Effects,* Vol. 3 (R. L. Jolley, W. A. Brungs, R. B. Cumming, eds.), pp. 85–98, Ann Arbor Science, Ann Arbor, Michigan.

Russfield, A. B., Homburger, F., Boger, E., Van Dongen, C. G., Weisburger, E. K., and Weisburger, J. H., 1975, The carcinogenic effect of 4,4′-methylene-bis-(2-chloroaniline) in mice and rats, *Toxicol. Appl. Pharmacol.* **31**:47–54.

Scientific Committee, Food Safety Council, 1978, Proposed system for food safety assessment, *Food Cosmet. Toxicol.* **16**(Suppl. 2):1–136.

Seltzer, R. J., 1975, Reactions grow to trichloroethylene alert, *C&E News* (May 19), pp. 41–43.

Shimkin, M. B., and Stoner, G. D., 1975, Lung tumors in mice: Application to carcinogenesis bioassay, *Adv. Cancer Res.* **21**:1–58.

Shimkin, M. B., Weisburger, J. H., Weisburger, E. K., Gubareff, N., and Suntzeff, V., 1966, Bioassay of 29 alkylating chemicals by the pulmonary tumor response in strain A mice, *J. Natl. Cancer Inst.* **36**:915–936.

Sielken, R. L., Jr., 1986, An individualized response model for quantitative cancer risk assessment. (Presentation at meeting of AIHC and CMA, Washington, D.C., June 27.)

Siuda, J. F., 1980, Natural production of organohalogens, in: *Water Chlorination: Environmental Impact and Health Effects,* Vol. 3 (R. L. Jolley, W. A. Brungs, and R. B. Cumming, eds.), pp. 63–72, Ann Arbor Sciences, Ann Arbor, Michigan.

Sontag, J. M., Page, N. P., and Saffiotti, U., 1976, *Guidelines for Carcinogen Bioassay in Small Rodents,* Carcinogenesis Program, National Cancer Institute, Bethesda, Maryland, DHEW Publication No. (NIH) 76–801.

Stoner, G. D., Shimkin, M. B., Kniazeff, A. J., Weisburger, J. H., Weisburger, E. K., and Gori, G. B., 1973, Test for carcinogenicity of food additives and chemotherapeutic agents by the pulmonary tumor response in strain A mice, *Cancer Res.* **33**:3069–3085.

Theiss, J. C., Stoner, G. D., Shimkin, M. B., and Weisburger, E. K., 1977, Test for carcinogenicity of organic contaminants of United States drinking waters by pulmonary tumor response in strain A mice, *Cancer Res.* **37**:2717–2720.

U.S. Department of Health, Education, and Welfare, 1969, *Report of the Secretary's Commission on Pesticides and Their Relationship to Environmental Health.* Washington, D.C.

Weisburger, E. K., 1977, Bioassay program for carcinogenic hazards of cancer chemotherapeutic agents, *Cancer* **40**:1935–1949.

Weisburger, E. K., 1981, Techniques for carcinogenicity studies, *Cancer Res.* **41**:3690–3694.

Weisburger, E. K., 1983, History of the Bioassay Program of the National Cancer Institute, *Prog. Exp. Tumor Res.* **26**:187–201.

Weisburger, E. K., Russfield, A. B., Homburger, F., Weisburger, J. H., Boger, E., Van Dongen, C. G., and Chu, K. C., 1978, Testing of twenty-one environmental aromatic amines or derivatives for long-term toxicity or carcinogenicity, *J. Environ. Pathol. Toxicol.* **2**:325–356.

Weisburger, E. K., Ulland, B. M., Nam, J., Gart, J., and Weisburger, J. H., 1981, Carcinogenicity tests of certain environmental and industrial chemicals, *J. Natl. Cancer Inst.* **67**:75–88.

III

Exposure Assessment

5

Assessing the Extent of Human Exposure to Organics

Curtis C. Travis and Holly A. Hattemer-Frey

INTRODUCTION

Risk analysis consists of two basic components, exposure assessment and health effects assessment. Exposure assessment involves determining the pathways and extent of human exposure to toxic chemicals. Because of the complex processes involved, exposure assessment is often the most resource demanding part of evaluating the risks of human exposure to environmental pollutants (Office of Science and Technology Policy, 1985). This chapter provides an overview of some of the important aspects of exposure assessment.

EXPOSURE ASSESSMENT METHODOLOGY

Evaluating the risks of chemical exposure involves identifying: (1) the sources and magnitude of environmental input; (2) the pathways of human exposure; and (3) the extent of exposure to populations at risk (EPA, 1986).

Sources of Environmental Input

To monitor the environmental fate of a chemical, it is necessary to identify the sources and rates at which it enters the environment (EPA, 1986). To adequately assess human exposure from all media, care must be taken not to overlook important sources of

Curtis C. Travis and Holly A. Hattemer-Frey • Office of Risk Analysis, Health and Safety Research Division, Oak Ridge National Laboratory, Oak Ridge, Tennessee 37831-6109.

environmental contamination. Consider, for example, hazardous waste landfills. The potential threat of groundwater contamination from landfills is well documented (Travis and Etnier, 1984). Moreover, volatile organics in landfills can be transported through the soil and substantially contribute to atmospheric pollution (CARB, 1982). It has been estimated that the quantity of chemicals volatilized from waste disposal sites in Southern California is equal to the atmospheric releases from all local industrial atmospheric sources (CARB, 1982). This source of environmental contamination has received little attention in the literature.

Pathways of Human Exposure

Principal pathways of human exposure include inhalation, ingestion, and dermal absorption. Again, care must be taken in identifying pathways of human exposure. Consider, for example, human exposure from contaminated drinking water. Recent studies indicate that ingestion may not be the sole or even primary route of human exposure to organics distributed in drinking water supplies (Brown *et al.*, 1984; Wallace, 1986). Both dermal absorption and inhalation could also be major pathways of exposure. For example, showerhead and tub-faucet aeration of water can increase the indoor air concentration of certain organics (EPA, 1984; Wallace *et al.*, 1985). Preliminary investigations show that for some chemicals, inhalation exposure from showering could equal exposure from ingestion of contaminated drinking water (EPA, 1984). In addition, Brown *et al.* (1984) estimated that dermal exposure to some organics during showering could account for 91% of total daily exposure.

Extent of Human Exposure

There are two basic methods of determining the extent of human exposure to chemicals: measurement and prediction. A direct approach is to measure the concentration of a substance in various environmental media and then calculate the average daily intake. This procedure is often done in occupational and urban settings where chemicals are concentrated enough to allow direct measurement. In other situations, however, direct measurement is not feasible because background concentrations are too low (below detection limits) or direct measurement would be prohibitively costly or impractical. Under these circumstances, indirect methods must be used to estimate human exposures. For example, past human exposure to some chemicals can be extrapolated from measured concentrations of organics in human tissue, hair, blood, and urine samples (Murphy *et al.*, 1983; Patterson *et al.*, 1986; van den Berg *et al.*, 1986). In addition, biological markers can be used to identify and quantify past human exposure (Perera, 1986; Perera *et al.*, 1982; Perera and Weinstein, 1982; Shugart, 1986; Shugart *et al.*, 1983; Vainio *et al.*, 1983). These two techniques for indirectly estimating past human exposure to chemical carcinogens, however, are currently only applicable to a small number of chemicals. Hence, other predictive methods, such as the use of computer transport models and predictive equations must also be used to evaluate the risks of human exposure to chemical carcinogens.

PATHWAY PROCESSES

The basic processes that control the environmental fate of a compound are transport, transformation, and cross-media transfer.

Transport

Transport is the movement of chemicals *within* a particular environmental medium due to natural forces. For example, atmospheric transport is frequently controlled by ambient winds. The direction and speed of the winds determine where a chemical will be found. Similarly, chemicals found in surface and groundwater can be carried by water movements, currents, or by sediment suspended in the water.

Transformation

Transformation is any process that changes the physical or chemical structure of a compound. A chemical may be physically transformed (e.g., volatilize from a solid to a gaseous form) or may undergo chemical transformation (e.g., hydrolysis, oxidation, or reduction) or biotransformation (e.g., biodegradation or bioaccumulation). Transformation may involve interaction with other pollutants, such as the reaction of nitrogen oxides, hydrocarbons, and sunlight to form ozone. Transformation processes can also increase or decrease the biotoxicity of a chemical. For example, certain atmospheric photochemical reactions can increase the mutagenicity of some fractions of smoke released from residential wood stove fires, while the mutagenicity of other smoke fractions can be decreased due to chemical transformation (Kamens *et al.*, 1985). Of the three processes that influence the environmental fate of and human exposure to pollutants, transformation processes are the least understood.

Cross-Media Transfer

Cross-media transfer is the movement of pollutants *between* the environmental media of air, water, soil, and biota. For example, an airborne pollutant can be transferred from the atmosphere to the earth's surface through gravitational settling or be washed out by rain. A chemical in a river system may transfer to the atmosphere through volatilization, or it may sorb onto suspended sediment and be deposited on the river bottom. A pollutant in soil can volatilize to the atmosphere or leach into groundwater supplies.

Cross-media transfer can result in the wide distribution of pollutants throughout the environment and, consequently, enhance the potential for human exposure from multiple sources. For example, although organics entering water supplies via industrial discharge are treated at treatment plants, up to 99% of the organics present in the water can be lost to the atmosphere. A Philadelphia study found that volatilization of organics at water treatment plants accounted for almost half of the total human exposure to chemical carcinogens (Haemisegger *et al.*, 1985).

BIOCHEMICAL AND PHYSICOCHEMICAL PROPERTIES

Many chemical, physical, and environmental parameters, such as water solubility, vapor pressure, octanol–water partitioning, and bioaccumulation, influence the behavior and fate of organics released into the environment. The importance of these factors and how they influence each other is often inadequately understood. However, the examination of a few basic physicochemical properties can provide insight into the behavior and fate of chemicals released into the environment.

Water Solubility

Water solubility is the maximum amount of a chemical that will dissolve in pure water at a specific temperature and pH. A chemical's solubility in water affects its fate and transport in all environmental media and significantly influences human exposure to organics through aquatic pathways. Highly soluble compounds tend to leach rapidly from soil into groundwater and surface water supplies. In addition, they tend to be less volatile (Menzer and Nelson, 1980), more biodegradable (Lyman *et al.*, 1982), and more mobile (Briggs, 1981) than nonsoluble chemicals.

Vapor Pressure

Vapor pressure measures the relative volatility of a chemical in its pure state and is useful for determining the extent to which a chemical will be transported into air from soil and water surfaces. Volatilization is a major route for the distribution of many chemicals in the environment (Dobbs and Cull, 1982). A chemical's volatility is affected by its solubility, vapor pressure, and molecular weight, as well as the nature of the air-to-water or soil-to-water interface through which the chemical must pass (Lyman *et al.*, 1982). For example, chemicals that have a low vapor pressure and a high affinity for soil or water are less likely to vaporize than chemicals that have a high vapor pressure and a weak affinity for soil or water.

Bioconcentration and Biotransfer Factors

Assessing the environmental fate of chemicals depends largely on being able to predict the extent to which they will bioaccumulate in living organisms, including fish, cattle, and humans. Organisms can concentrate chemicals in their tissues at levels substantially higher than a chemical's concentration in water (in the case of aquatic organisms) or in food (in the case of terrestrial organisms). A traditional measure of a chemical's potential to accumulate in biota is the bioconcentration factor (BCF), which is defined as the equilibrium concentration of organic in an organism or tissue (mg/kg) divided by the concentration of organic (mg/kg) in water (for aquatic organisms), soil (for vegetation), or food (for terrestrial organisms). This concept, however, is not readily applied to humans, because the amount of chemical in various food items of the human diet can vary markedly. Hence, for risk assessment purposes, it is more efficacious to examine the biotransfer factor (BTF), which is defined as the equilibrium concentration of organic in an organism or tissue (mg/kg) divided by the average daily intake of organic (mg/day) (Travis *et al.*, 1987b).

Octanol–Water Partition Coefficient

Organisms tend to accumulate chemicals in the lipid portions of their tissues. Thus, one way to determine the bioaccumulation potential of a chemical is to measure how lipophilic it is. Since it is difficult to directly measure a chemical's lipophilicity, researchers typically use the octanol–water partition coefficient (K_{ow}) to predict a chemical's tendency to partition between an octanol component (a good surrogate for fat) and water. The octanol–water partition coefficient is defined as the ratio of a chemical's concentration in the octanol phase to its concentration in the aqueous phase (Lyman *et al.*, 1982). It is directly related to a chemical's tendency to bioconcentrate in biota (Chiou *et al.*, 1982; Chou and Griffin, 1986; Geyer *et al.*, 1982, 1987; Kenaga, 1980; Kenaga and Goring, 1980; Travis and Arms, 1987b) and inversely correlated with water solubility (Chiou *et al.*, 1982; Kenaga and Goring, 1980). Hence, the octanol–water partition coefficient is used extensively to estimate the bioconcentration potential of organics in biological systems. Chemicals with large K_{ow} values tend to accumulate in soil, sediment, and biota, but not in water. For example, lipophilic compounds such as dioxin, dichlorodiphenyltrichloroethane (DDT), and polychlorinated biphenyls (PCBs) are most soluble in organic matter. This class of chemicals tends to bioaccumulate in biota and vegetation, sorb strongly onto soil, sediment, and vegetation, and transfer to humans through the food chain. Conversely, chemicals with small K_{ow} values tend to partition mostly into air or water. For example, volatile organics such as trichloroethylene and tetrachloroethylene, tend to be widely distributed in air and inhalation is the primary pathway of human exposure.

EVALUATING THE PATHWAYS OF HUMAN EXPOSURE

For risk assessment purposes, an important objective in evaluating the environmental behavior and fate of various pollutants is predicting the major pathways and extent of human exposure. Many chemicals cycle in the environment with cross-media transfers occurring between air, water, soil, and biota. As a result of this cycling behavior and a chemical's presence in various environmental media, human exposure often results from multiple sources. Travis *et al.* (1987a) found that 50–80% of all chemicals released into the environment result in human exposure through multiple media.

Chemicals released into the environment may pose health risks to humans via inhalation, ingestion, or dermal absorption. The relative importance of an exposure pathway depends upon the concentration of a chemical in the relevant medium and the rate of intake by exposed individuals. Thus, total exposure is the sum of exposures from all media into which a chemical partitions.

Uptake of Organics from Air

Humans are exposed to organics present in air via inhalation and absorption through the lung. The amount of chemical taken in during inhalation depends upon: (1) the background concentration of a chemical in inspired air; (2) the amount of air inspired per unit time; and (3) the percent of chemical in inspired air that is absorbed through the lung. Thus, daily intake of a chemical in air can be estimated using the equation:

$$
\begin{aligned}
\text{Intake (mg/day)} =\ & \text{Concentration of chemical in air (mg/m}^3) \\
& \times \text{ amount of air inhaled (20 m}^3\text{/day)} \\
& \times \text{ percent absorption through lungs}
\end{aligned}
$$

The atmosphere also plays an important role in dispersing organics throughout the environment (Atlas and Giam, 1981). Stable compounds, such as PCBs, can be transported thousands of miles from their original source of release (Atlas *et al.*, 1986; Travis *et al.*, 1987a). Because PCBs have low vapor pressures and high octanol–water partition coefficients, they are expected to be found mostly in soil. However, volatilization of PCBs from spills, landfills, road oils, and other sources results in small but measurable releases into the atmosphere (Lewis and Martin, 1985; Weaver, 1984). Despite the fact that these emissions account for less than 1% of the total amount of PCBs released into the environment (Holton *et al.*, 1987), atmospheric transport is considered the primary mode of global transport of PCBs and atmospheric deposition the major source of PCB contamination of unpolluted areas (Atlas *et al.*, 1986). Eisenreich *et al.* (1981) reported that atmospheric deposition accounts for 60% of PCB input to the Great Lakes. Atlas *et al.* (1986) estimated that 98% of the PCBs entering ocean waters are deposited from the atmosphere. Furthermore, PCBs have a large bioconcentration potential. The BCF of PCBs in fish and shellfish ranges from 27,000 to 60,000 (Bruggeman *et al.*, 1984; Geyer *et al.*, 1982). Thus, once deposited, they tend to accumulate in biota and have a large potential of transferring to humans through the food chain.

Indoor air pollution has recently been recognized as another potentially important source of inhalation exposure (Wallace *et al.*, 1982, 1985). More than 250 volatile organics have been detected at part per billion (ppb) levels in urban residences and office buildings (Meyer, 1983). Many of these organics are components of consumer products and building materials commonly found in the home and office. For example, paradichlorobenzene is used in moth crystals and deodorants, benzene and tetrachloroethylene are used in dry cleaning processes, and vinylidene chloride, styrene, and xylenes are found in paint. Because they have high vapor pressures, these compounds readily volatilize and contaminate indoor air. Wallace *et al.* (1985) continuously monitored individuals for exposure to 20 organic compounds and concluded that, in both industrial and rural areas, the major sources of inhalation exposure are found indoors. Wallace (1986) reported that mean personal air exposures to 11 prevalent chemicals were greater than mean outdoor air concentrations.

Uptake of Organics from Water

The principal exposure route from contaminated drinking water is ingestion. The amount of chemical ingested can be estimated from the concentration of chemical in the water supply, the amount of water consumed daily, and the percent of chemical absorbed through the gastrointestinal (GI) tract. Thus, the daily intake of a chemical present in drinking water can be estimated using the equation:

Intake (mg/day) = Concentration of pollutant in water (mg/liter)
× amount of water ingested (2 liter/day)
× percent absorbed through GI tract

The case of aldicarb use on Long Island illustrates the importance of water as an exposure pathway for many environmental pollutants. Aldicarb is a relatively new pesticide marketed under the trade name, Temik, and is widely used in the United States for application to potatoes, cotton, sugar beets, and other farm crops. Temik was used by many potato farmers on Long Island since the early 1970s. Although it is highly soluble, researchers expected that, under normal conditions, aldicarb and its highly toxic residues would be degraded to innocuous forms before reaching groundwater supplies. Hence, no assessment of its impact on groundwater supplies was done for several years. In August 1979, however, 8000 private wells located in the potato farming region of Long Island were sampled (Harris and Davids, 1982). Of the 1832 wells sampled in Southhampton, 29% were contaminated with aldicarb and 15% exceeded the New York State Department of Health (NYSDOH) standard of 7 ppb for safe drinking water (Harris and Davids, 1982). Although agricultural use of Temik was banned in 1980, a study conducted by the Cornell University Center for Environmental Research estimated that aldicarb concentrations in Long Island's drinking water supplies could exceed the NYSDOH limit of 7 ppb for another 100 to 140 years (McIntyre, 1983).

In addition to direct exposure through ingestion of contaminated drinking water, the presence of pollutants in ocean and coastal waters can result in their bioaccumulation in aquatic and terrestrial organisms. Many organochlorines have been detected in deep-sea fish, sediment, and subsurface ocean waters (Tanabe and Tatsukawa, 1986). Sauer (1981) reported that concentrations of 35 volatile organics in coastal and ocean surface waters ranged from nondectable, at parts per trillion (ppt) detection limits, to 210 ppt.

Uptake of Organics Through the Food Chain

The food chain is a primary source of human exposure for a large class of organics, including DDT, dioxin, and most pesticides (Travis and Arms, 1987a). Assessing the magnitude of exposure to this group of chemicals depends largely on being able to predict their bioaccumulation in the food chain. Direct evidence of human exposure to organics through the food chain is limited (Office of Technology Assessment, 1979). The extent of human exposure to chemicals present in food can be estimated in three ways: (1) determining body burdens through examination of human tissue, hair, blood, breast milk, and urine samples (Murphy *et al.*, 1983; Patterson *et al.*, 1986; van den Berg *et al.*, 1986); (2) estimating dietary intake from measured concentrations of organics in food (Gartrell *et al.*, 1985, 1986; McConnell *et al.*, 1975); and (3) estimating human intake by evaluating the bioaccumulation of organics in the food chain (Geyer *et al.*, 1987; Travis *et al.*, 1987b). Although studies have been conducted to determine the levels of organics in human tissues and food items, these analyses are usually limited to a few chemicals. Thus, for most organics, estimating human exposure to chemicals present in food is accomplished by using predictive equations that estimate exposure from ingestion of contaminated agricultural produce (fruits, vegetables, and grains), meat, milk, and fish.

Vegetation

Accumulation of organics in vegetation is a complex process that involves root uptake, foliar uptake, and adherence of organics deposited from the atmosphere. Root uptake of organics has been correlated with K_{ow} (Baes, 1982; Briggs *et al.*, 1982) and can be estimated using B_v, the soil-to-plant BCF for vegetation. B_v is defined as the equilibrium concentration of organic in plant tissue (mg/kg dry weight) divided by the concentration of organic in soil (mg/kg dry weight). Travis and Arms (1987b) developed the following regression equation to estimate B_v:

$$B_v = 38.9 \, K_{ow}^{-0.58}$$

Since B_v is inversely related to K_{ow}, lipophilic compounds are not likely to be taken up through the roots. Helling *et al.* (1973) and Isensee and Jones (1971) reported that only 0.15% of the dioxin available in the soil was taken up by oats and soybeans.

While some organics are taken up by plants directly from contaminated soil and translocated to upper plant parts, other compounds volatilize from the soil, and their vapors are absorbed by aerial plant parts (Bacci and Gaggi, 1985, 1986, 1987; Beall and Nash, 1971). Volatilization of organics from polluted soil may be as or more important than root uptake as a source of plant contamination. Buckley (1982) and Nash and Beall (1970) reported that PCB and DDT residues present in plant foliage were mainly due to vapor transport from the soil. The absorption of volatilized organics by upper plant parts can be estimated from B_{va}, the air-to-plant BCF for vegetation, which is defined as the equilibrium concentration of organic in upper plant parts (mg/g dry weight) divided by the concentration of organic in air as a vapor (mg/g). B_{va} can be estimated from the following regression equation developed by Travis and Hattemer-Frey (1987b):

$$B_{va} = 9.1 \, K_{ow}^{0.71}$$

Thus, foliar uptake of volatilized organics is positively correlated with K_{ow}.

Deposition or direct application of organics onto outer plant surfaces can also contribute substantially to vegetative contamination. Isensee and Jones (1971) demonstrated that 94% of the dioxin applied to soybeans and 63% of the dioxin applied to oats remained on the leaves for 21 days, indicating that most of the dioxin deposited from the atmosphere onto outer plant surfaces is likely to persist until the plant is harvested or consumed by animals. In the absence of specific data, it is generally assumed that organics deposited onto plant surfaces have a 14-day weathering half-life (Baes *et al.*, 1984).

Beef and Milk

Kenaga (1980) and Travis and Arms (1987b) showed that a positive correlation exists between K_{ow} and the bioconcentration of organics in cow tissue and milk. Biotransfer factors for organics in cow tissue (B_b) and milk (B_m) are defined as the equilibrium concentration of organic in cow whole tissue or milk (mg/kg) divided by the average daily intake of organic (mg/day). Travis and Arms (1987b) developed the following regression equations to estimate the biotransfer of organics in cow tissue and milk:

$$B_b = 2.5 \times 10^{-8} K_{ow}$$

and

$$B_m = 8.1 \times 10^{-9} K_{ow}$$

Ingestion of contaminated plants and soil can be a major exposure pathway for terrestrial organisms. Lipophilic compounds, such as DDT and dioxin, tend to accumulate in soil and on outer plant surfaces. Travis and Hattemer-Frey (1987a) showed that the ingestion of contaminated soil and vegetation accounted for 99% of the total daily intake of dioxin by cattle.

Fish

Fish can take up organics directly from contaminated water or from ingesting contaminated food items and concentrating them in their tissues at levels thousands of times greater than their concentration in the water in which they live (Isensee and Jones, 1975). The BCF for a chemical in fish (B_f) is defined as the equilibrium concentration of organic in fish tissue (mg/kg) divided by the concentration of organic in water (mg/l). If measured BCFs for fish are not available, they can be estimated from the following equation derived by Mackay (1982):

$$B_f = 0.048 \, K_{ow}$$

Table 1 lists the BCFs for some ubiquitous environmental pollutants in fish. A high BCF indicates that a compound is likely to accumulate in fish and that the aquatic food chain will be an important exposure pathway for humans.

Table 1. Bioconcentration Factors for Organics in Fish

Chemical	BCF	Reference
Aldicarb	42	Garten and Trabalka (1983)
Benzo(a)pyrene (BaP)	11,100	EPA (1980a)
DDT	51,286	Garten and Trabalka (1983)
Dieldrin	14,125	Garten and Trabalka (1983)
Hexachlorobenzene (HCB)	12,300	Garten and Trabalka (1983)
PCBs	60,000	Bruggeman et al. (1984)
TCDD	49,000	Mehrle et al. (1987)
Trichloroethylene	17	EPA (1980c)
Tetrachloroethylene	17	EPA (1980b)

MULTIMEDIA TRANSPORT MODELS

Multimedia transport models estimate the concentration of a pollutant in various environmental media and then use those concentrations to predict the amount of pollutant to which humans are exposed. The models divide the environment into six compartments: air, water, soil, sediment, suspended sediment, and biota. The air, water, and soil compartments are interactively connected, while the sediment, suspended sediment, and biota compartments are connected with the water compartment only (Mackay et al., 1985a,b; Travis et al., 1987a). Some multimedia models can also account for uptake through the food chain by estimating the bioaccumulation of materials in aquatic and terrestrial organisms, including humans. While multimedia transport models should not be viewed as exact replicas of the environment, they are considered acceptable for predicting the equilibrium partitioning of nonparticulate chemicals (Cohen and Ryan, 1985; Eberhardt et al., 1976; Hushon et al., 1983; Mackay et al., 1985a,b; Mackay and Paterson, 1982). The validity of transport model predictions can be evaluated by determining if predicted concentrations are of the same order of magnitude as measured background concentrations. Thus, multimedia transport models represent a useful tool for estimating human exposure to organics from multiple media.

Application of a Multimedia Transport Model: TCDD

Although there are actually more than 75 different molecular forms of dioxin, 2,3,7,8-tetrachlorodibenzo-*p*-dioxin (TCDD) is often referred to as dioxin. Dioxins are highly lipophilic, extremely persistent compounds. Because of their extreme toxicity, much debate has arisen about the environmental fate and extent of human exposure to dioxins. TCDD has been measured in air, soil, sediment, suspended sediment, fish, and human adipose tissue samples (Crummett, 1987; Czuczwa et al., 1984; Eitzer and Hites, 1986; O'Keefe et al., 1983; Patterson et al., 1986). Although the magnitude of the source term remains unknown, principal environmental releases of TCDD are suggested to be: (1) incineration of municipal and chemical wastes (Czuczwa and Hites, 1985; Lao et al., 1985); (2) automobile exhaust (Marklund et al., 1987); and (3) discharge from routine chlorination processes at waste water treatment facilities (Bumb et al., 1980; Esposito et al., 1980). In addition, Agent Orange, used widely as a defoliant in Vietnam, contained about 2 parts per million TCDD (Czuczwa and Hites, 1986). The application of pesticides containing small quantities of TCDD, however, is not considered a major source of environmental input (Mill, 1985; Podoll et al., 1986).

The low water solubility, low vapor pressure, and high K_{ow} of TCDD result in its partitioning mainly between soil (85.3%) and sediment (14.3%) with less than 1% distributing into air, water, suspenced sediment, and biota (Travis and Hattemer-Frey, 1987a). Most of the TCDD released into the atmosphere is eventually deposited onto plant, water, and soil surfaces. Because of its high lipophilicity, TCDD sequesters almost completely in soil and biota and, hence, the food chain is the major pathway of human exposure. Table 2 gives the predicted average daily intake of TCDD by humans.

These data show that the food chain, especially meat and dairy products, accounts for 98% of human exposure to TCDD. Consumption of contaminated fish and shellfish does not comprise a major source of human exposure to TCDD. The model estimated the

Table 2. Predicted Average Daily Intake of TCDD
by Humans

Source	Daily intake (ng/day)	Percentage of total daily intake
Air	0.001	2%
Water	6.5×10^{-6}	<0.01%
Food (total)	0.046	98%
Vegetables	0.005	11%
Milk	0.013	27%
Meat	0.023	50%
Fish	0.005	10%

avarage daily intake of TCDD for the general population of the United States to be 0.05 ng per day.

CONCLUSIONS

Exposure assessment involves determining the pathways and extent of human exposure to toxic chemicals. Various measurement and predictive techniques can be used to evaluate the movement and transfer of chemicals within and between environmental media, as well as the concentration of organics to which humans are exposed. Evaluating the risks associated with exposure to environmental pollutants involves identifying the sources and magnitude of environmental input, the transport and transformation of chemicals released into the environment, the pathways of human exposure, and the extent of exposure for populations at risk.

Since organic chemicals tend to end up in the media in which they are most soluble, a few basic physicochemical properties can be used to predict the behavior and fate of chemicals released into the environment. Highly lipophilic compounds tend to sequester in soil, sediment, and biota, and the food chain is the primary pathway of human exposure. Highly soluble compounds are found in water, and ingestion of contaminated water is usually the primary pathway of human exposure. Volatile compounds tend to partition almost exclusively into air, and inhalation is the major source of human exposure.

REFERENCES

Atlas, E., and Giam, C. S., 1981, Global transport of organic pollutants: Ambient concentrations in the remote marine atmosphere, *Science.* **211**:163–165.

Atlas, E., Bidleman, T., and Giam, C. S., 1986, Atmospheric transport of PCBs to the oceans, in: *PCBs and the Environment*, Vol. I (J. S. Waid, ed.), pp. 79–100, CRC Press, Boca Raton, Florida.

Bacci, E., and Gaggi, C., 1985, Polychlorinated biphenyls in plant foliage: Translocation or volatilization from contaminated soils? *Bull. Environ. Contam. Toxicol.* **35**(5):673–681.

Bacci, E., and Gaggi, C., 1986, Chlorinated pesticides and plant foliage: Translocation experiments, *Bull. Environ. Contam. Toxicol.* **37**(6):850–857.

Bacci, E., and Gaggi, C., 1987, Chlorinated hydrocarbon vapors and plant foliage: Kinetics and applications, *Bull. Environ. Contam. Toxicol.* (manuscript submitted).

Baes, C. F., III, 1982, Prediction of radionuclide K_d values from soil–plant concentration ratios. *Trans. Amer. Nuclear Soc.* **41**:53–54.

Baes, C. F., III, Sharp, R. D., Sjoreen, A., and Shor, R., 1984, *A Review and Analysis of Parameters for Assessing Transport of Environmentally Released Radionuclides Through Agriculture.* U.S. Department of Energy, Oak Ridge National Laboratory Report ORNL–5786, Oak Ridge, Tennessee.

Beall, M. L., Jr., and Nash, R. G., 1971, Organochlorine insecticide residues in soybean plant tops: Root vs. vapor sorption, *Agron. J.* **63**:460–464.

Briggs, G. C., 1981, Theoretical and experimental relationships between soil adsorption, octanol–water partition coefficients, water solubilities, bioconcentration factors, and the parachor, *J. Agric. Food Chem.* **29**:1050–1059.

Briggs, G. G., Bromilow, R. H., and Evans, A. A., 1982, Relationships between lipophilicity and root uptake and translocation of non-ionized chemicals by barley, *Pest. Sci.* **13**:495–504.

Brown, H. S., Bishop, D. R., and Rowan, C. A., 1984, The role of skin absorption as a route of exposure for volatile organic compounds (VOCs) in drinking water, *Amer. J. Public Health.* **74**(5):477–484.

Bruggeman, W. A., Opperhuizen, A., Wybenga, A., and Hutzinger, O., 1984, Bioaccumulation of super-lipophilic chemicals in fish, *Toxicol. Environ. Chem.* **7**:173–189.

Buckley, E. H., 1982, Accumulation of airborne polychlorinated biphenyls in foliage, *Science* **216**:520–522.

Bumb, R. R., Crummett, W. B., Cutie, S. S., Gledhill, J. R., Hummel, R. H., Kagel, R. O., Lamparski, L. L., Luoma, E. V., Miller, D. L., Nestrick, T. J., Shadoff, L. A., Stehl, R. H., and Woods, J. S., 1980, Trace chemistries of fire: A source of chlorinated dioxins, *Science* **210**:385–390.

California Air Resources Board (CARB), 1982, *Assessment of the Volatile and Toxic Organic Emissions from Hazardous Waste Disposal in California.*

Chiou, C. T., Schmedding, D. W., and Manes, M., 1982, Partitioning of organic compounds in octanol–water systems, *Environ. Sci. Technol.* **16**(1):4–10.

Chou, S. F. J., and Griffin, R. A., 1986, Solubility and soil mobility of polychlorinated biphenyls, in: *PCBs and the Environment,* Vol. I (J. S. Waid, ed.), pp. 101–120, CRC Press, Boca Raton, Florida.

Cohen, Y., and Ryan, P. A., 1985, Multimedia modeling of environmental transport: Trichloroethylene test case, *Environ. Sci. Technol.* **19**:412–417.

Crummett, W. B., 1987, Dow Chemical Co., personal correspondence.

Czuczwa, J. M., and Hites, R. A., 1985, Dioxins and dibenzofurans in air, soil, and water, in: *Dioxins in the Environment* (M. A. Kamrin and P. W. Rodgers, eds.), pp. 85–99, Hemisphere Press, Washington, D.C.

Czuczwa, J. M., and Hites, R. A., 1986, Airborne dioxins and dibenzofurans: Sources and fates, *Environ. Sci. Technol.* **20**(2):195–200.

Czuczwa, J. M., McVeety, B. D., and Hites, R. A., 1984, Polychlorinated dibenzo-p-dioxins in sediments from Siskiwit Lake, Isle Royale, *Science* **226**:568–569.

Dobbs, A. J., and Cull, M. R., 1982, Volatilization of chemicals—Relative loss rates and the estimation of vapor pressures, *Environ. Poll.* (Series B) **3**:289–298.

Eberhardt, L. L., Gilbert, R. O., Hollister, H. L., and Thomas, J. M., 1976, Sampling for contaminants in ecological systems, *Environ. Sci. Technol.* **10**:917–925.

Eisenreich, S. J., Looney, B. B., and Thornton, J. D., 1981, Airborne organic contaminants in the Great Lakes ecosystem, *Environ. Sci. Technol.* **19**:413–417.

Eitzer, B. D., and Hites, R. A., 1986, Concentrations of dioxins and dibenzofurans in the atmosphere, *Inter. J. Environ. Anal. Chem.* **27**:215–230.

Environmental Protection Agency (EPA), 1980a, *Ambient Water Quality Criteria for Polynuclear Aromatic Hydrocarbons,* EPA-440/5-80-069, Washington, D.C.

Environmental Protection Agency (EPA), 1980b, *Ambient Water Quality Criteria for Tetrachloroethylene,* EPA-440/5-80-073, Washington, D.C.

Environmental Protection Agency (EPA), 1980c, *Ambient Water Quality Criteria for Trichloroethylene,* EPA-440/5-80-077, Washington, D.C.

Environmental Protection Agency (EPA), 1984, *Techniques for the Assessment of the Carcinogenic Risk to the U.S. Population Due to Exposure from Selected Volatile Organic Compounds from Drinking Water via the Ingestion, Inhalation, and Dermal Routes,* Office of Drinking Water, Washington, D.C.

Environmental Protection Agency (EPA), 1986, Guidelines for exposure assessment, *Fed. Regist.* **51**(185):34042–34054.

Esposito, M. P., Tiernan, T. O., and Dryden, F. E., 1980, *Dioxins*. U.S. Environmental Protection Agency Report No. EPA 600/2-80-197. Office of Research and Development, Cincinnati, Ohio.

Garten, C. T., and Trabalka, J. R., 1983, Evaluation of models for predicting terrestrial food chain behavior of Xenobiotics, *Environ. Sci. Technol.* **17**:590–595.

Gartrell, M. J., Craun, J. C., Podrebarac, D. S., and Gunderson, E. L., 1985, Pesticides, selected elements, and other chemicals in adult total diet samples, October 1978–September 1979, *J. Assoc. Off. Anal. Chem.* **65**(5):862–875.

Gartrell, M. J., Craun, J. C., Podrebarac, D. S., and Gunderson, E. L., 1986, Pesticides, selected elements, and other chemicals in adult total diet samples, October 1980–March 1982, *J. Assoc. Off. Anal. Chem.* **69**(1):146–161.

Geyer, H., Sheehan, P., Kotzias, D., Freitag, D., and Korte, F., 1982, Prediction of ecotoxicological behavior of chemicals: Relationship between physico-chemical properties and bioaccumulation of organic chemicals in the mussel *Mytilus edulis, Chemosphere* **11**(11):1121–1134.

Geyer, H. J., Scheunert, I., and Korte, F., 1987, Correlation between the bioconcentration potential of organic environmental chemicals in humans and their n-octanol/water partition coefficients. *Chemosphere* **16**(1):239–252.

Haemisegger, E. R., Jones, A. D., and Reinhardt, F. L., 1985, EPA's experience with assessment of site-specific environmental problems: A review of IEMD's geographic study of Philadelphia, *J. Air Poll. Control Assoc.* **35**(8):809–815.

Harris, D., and Davids, H. W., 1982, *Report on the Occurrence and Movement of Agricultural Chemicals in Groundwater: South Fork of Suffolk County,* Bureau of Water Resources, Suffolk County Department of Health Services, Long Island, New York.

Helling, C. S., Isensee, A. R., Woolson, E. A., Ensor, P. D. J., Jones, G. E., Plummer, J. R., and Kearney, P. C., 1973, Chlorodioxins in pesticides, soils, and plants, *J. Environ. Qual.* **2**(2):171–178.

Holton, G. A., Travis, C. C., and Eitner, E. L., 1985, A comparison of human exposures to PCB emissions from oceanic and terrestrial incineration, *Hazardous Waste Hazardous Mater.* **2**:453–471.

Hushon, J. M., Klein, A. W., Strachan, W. J. M., and Schmidt-Bleeh, F., 1983, Use of OECD premarket data in environmental exposure analysis for new chemicals, *Chemosphere* **12**(6):887–910.

Isensee, A. R., and Jones, G. E., 1971, Absorption and translocation of root and foliage applied 2,4 di-chlorophenol, 2,7-dichlorodibenzo-p-dioxin, and 2,3,7,8-dichlorodibenzo-p-dioxin, *J. Agric. Food Chem.* **19**(6):1210–1214.

Isensee, A. R., and Jones, G. E., 1975, Distribution of 2,3,7,8-Tetrachlorodibenzo-p-dioxin (TCDD) in aquatic model ecosystem, *Environ. Sci. Technol.* **9**(7):668–672.

Kamens, R., Bell, D., Dietrich, A., Goodman, R., Claxton, L., and Tejada, S., 1985, Mutagenic transformations of dilute wood smoke systems in the presence of ozone and nitrogen dioxide: Analysis of selected high-pressure liquid chromatography fractions from wood smoke particulate extracts, *Environ. Sci. Technol.* **19**(1):63–69.

Kenaga, E. E., 1980, Correlations of bioconcentration factors in aquatic and terrestrial organisms with their physical and chemical properties, *Environ. Sci. Technol.* **14**:553–556.

Kenaga, E. E., and Goring, C. A. I., 1980, Relationship between water solubility, sorption, octanol–water partitioning, and concentration of chemicals in biota, in: *Aquatic Toxicology* (J. E. Eaton, P. R. Parrish, and A. C. Hendricks, eds.), American Society for Testing Materials STP 707, Philadelphia.

Lao, R. C., Thomas, R. S., Chiu, C., Li, K., and Lockwood, J., 1985, Analysis of PCDD-PCDF in environmental samples, in: *Chlorinated Dioxins and Dibenzofurans in the Total Environment II,* (L. H. Keith, C. Rappe, and G. Choudhary, eds.), pp. 65–78, Butterworth Publishers, Boston.

Lewis, R. L., and Martin, B. E., 1985, Measurement of fugitive atmospheric emissions of polychlorinated biphenyls from hazardous waste landfills, *Environ. Sci. Technol.* **19**(10):986–991.

Lyman, W. J., Reehl, W. F., and Rosenblatt, D. H., 1982, *Handbook of Chemical Property Estimation Methods,* McGraw-Hill, New York.

Mackay, D., 1982, Correlation of bioconcentration factors, *Environ. Sci. Technol.* **16**:274–278.

Mackay, D., and Paterson, S., 1982, Calculating fugacity, *Environ. Sci. Technol.* **15**:1006–1014.

Mackay, D., Paterson, S., Cheung, B., and Neely, W. B., 1985a, Evaluating the environmental fate of chemicals with a level III model, *Chemosphere.* **14**(3/4):335–374.

Mackay, D., Paterson, S., and Cheung, B., 1985b, Evaluating the environmental fate of chemicals: The fugacity level III approach as applied to 2,3,7,8-TCDD, *Chemosphere* **14**(6/7):859–863.

Marklund, S., Rappe, C., and Tysklind, M., 1987, Identification of polychlorinated dibenzofurans and dioxins in exhausts from cars run on leaded gasoline, *Chemosphere* **16**(1):29–36.

McConnell, G., Ferguson, D. M., and Pearson, C. R., 1975, Chlorinated hydrocarbons and the environment, *Endeavour* **34**:13–18.

McIntyre, M., 1983, Report sees 140-year temik peril, *Newsday*, April 28.

Mehrle, P., Buckler, D. R., Little, E. E., Smith, L. M., Petty, J. D., Peterman, P. H., Stalling, D. L., DeGraeve, G. M., Kyle, J. J., and Adams, W. J., 1987, Toxicity and bioconcentration of 2,3,7,8-Tetrachlorodibenzodioxin and 2,3,7,8-Tetrachlorodibenzofuran in rainbow trout, *Environ. Toxicol. Chem.* (manuscript submitted).

Menzer, R. E., and Nelson, J. O., 1980, Water and soil pollutants, in: *Toxicology* (J. Doull, C. D. Klaassen, and M. D. Amdur, eds.), Macmillan, New York.

Meyer, B., 1983, *Indoor Air Quality*, Addison Wesley, Massachusetts.

Mill, T., 1985, Prediction of the environmental fate of tetrachlorodibenzodioxin, in: *Dioxins in the Environment* (M. A. Kamrin and P. W. Rodgers, eds.), pp. 173–193, Hemisphere Press, Washington, D.C.

Murphy, R. S., Kutz, F. W., and Strassman, S. C., 1983, Selected pesticide residues or metabolites in blood and urine specimens from a general population survey, *Environ. Health Perspect.* **48**:81–86.

Nash, R. G., and Beall, L. M., Jr., 1970, Chlorinated hydrocarbon insecticides: Root uptake versus vapor contamination of soybean foliage, *Science* **210**:1109–1111.

Office of Science and Technology Policy, 1985, Chemical carcinogens: A review of the science and its associated principles, *Fed. Regist.* **50**:10372–10422.

Office of Technology Assessment (OTA), 1979, *Environmental Contaminants in Food*, U.S. Government Printing Office, Washington, D.C.

O'Keefe, P., Meyer, C., Hilker, D., Aldous, K., Jelus-Tyror, B., Dillon, K., Donnelly, R., Horn, E., and Sloan, R., 1983, Analysis of 2,3,7,8-tetrachlorodibenzo-p-dioxin in Great Lakes fishes, *Chemosphere* **12**(3):325–332.

Patterson, D. G., Jr., Hoffman, R. E., Needham, L. L., Roberts, D. W., Bagby, J. R., Pirkle, J. L., Falk, H., Sampson, E. J., and Houk, V. N., 1986, 2,3,7,8-Tetrachlorodibenzo-p-dioxin levels in adipose tissue of exposed and control persons in Missouri, *JAMA* **256**(19):2683–2686.

Perera, F., 1986, New approaches in risk assessment for carcinogens, *Risk Anal.* **6**(2):195–201.

Perera, F., and Weinstein, I. B., 1982, Molecular epidemiology and carcinogen–DNA adduct detection: New approaches to studies of human cancer causation, *J. Chronic Dis.* **35**:581–600.

Perera, F., Poirier, M. C., Yuspa, S. H., Nanayama, J., Jaretzki, A., Curnen, M. M., Knowles, D. M., and Weinstein, I. B., 1982, A pilot project in molecular epidemiology: Determination of benzo(a)pyrene–DNA adducts in animal and human tissues by immunoassay, *Carcinogenesis* **3**:1405–1410.

Podoll, R. T., Jaber, H. M., and Mill, T., 1986, Tetrachlorodibenzodioxin: Rates of volatilization and photolysis in the environment, *Environ. Sci. Technol.* **20**(5):490–492.

Sauer, T. C., Jr., 1981, Volatile organic compounds in open ocean and coastal surface waters, *Org. Geochem.* **3**:91–101.

Shugart, L., 1986, Covalent binding of benzo(a)pyrene diol epoxide to DNA of mouse skin—in vivo persistence of adduct formation, *J. Toxicol. Environ. Health.* **15**(2):225–263.

Shugart, L., Holland, J. M., and Rahn, R. O., 1983, Dosimetry of PAH skin carcinogenesis—covalent binding of benzo(a)pyrene to mouse epidermal DNA, *Carcinogenesis* **4**(2):195–198.

Tanabe, S., and Tatsukawa, R., 1986, Distribution, behavior, and load of PCBs in the oceans, in: *PCBs and the Environment*, Vol. I (J. S. Waid, ed.), pp. 143–162, CRC Press, Boca Raton, Florida.

Travis, C. C., and Arms, A. D., 1987a, The food chain as a source of toxics exposure, in: *Toxic Chemicals, Health and the Environment* (L. B. Lave and A. C. Upton, eds.), pp. 95–113, Praeger, New York.

Travis, C. C. and Arms, A. D., 1987b, Bioconcentration of organics in beef, milk, and vegetation, *Environ. Sci. Technol.* (in press).

Travis, C. C., and Etnier, E. L. (eds.), 1984, *Groundwater Pollution: Environmental and Legal Problems*, Westview Press, Boulder, Colorado.

Travis, C. C., and Hattemer-Frey, H. A., 1987a, Human exposure to 2,3,7,8-TCDD, *Chemosphere* (in press).

Travis, C. C., and Hattemer-Frey, H. A., 1987b, Uptake of organics by aerial plant parts: A call for research, *Chemosphere* (in press).

Travis, C. C., Dennison, J. W., and Arms, A. D., 1987a, The extent of multimedia partitioning of organic chemicals, *Chemosphere* **16**(1):117–125.

Travis, C. C., Hattemer-Frey, H. A., and Arms, A. D., 1987b, Relationship between dietary intake of organics and their concentrations in human adipose tissue and breast milk, *Arch. Environ. Contam. Toxicol.* (in press).

Vainio, H., Sorsa, M., and Hemminki, K., 1983, Biological monitoring in surveillance of exposure to genotoxicants, *Am. J. Indus. Med.* **4**:87–103.

van den Berg, M., van der Wielen, F. W. M., Olie, K., and van Boxtel, C. J., 1986, The presence of PCDDs and PCDFs in human breast milk from the Netherlands, *Chemosphere* **15**(6):693–706.

Wallace, L. A., 1986, Personal exposures, indoor and outdoor air concentrations, and exhaled breath concentrations of selected volatile organic compounds measured for 600 residents of New Jersey, North Dakota, North Carolina and California, *Toxicol. Environ. Chem.* **12**:215–236.

Wallace, L., Zweidinger, R., Erickson, M., Cooper, S., Whitaker, D., and Pellizzari, E., 1982, Monitoring individual exposure measurements of volatile organic compounds in breathing-zone air, drinking water, and exhaled breath, *Environ. Inter.* **8**:269–282.

Wallace, L. A., Pellizzari, E. D., Hartwell, T. D., Sparacino, C. M., Sheldon, L. S., and Zelon, H., 1985, Personal exposures, indoor–outdoor relationships, and breath levels of toxic pollutants measured for 355 persons in New Jersey, *Atmos. Environ.* **19**(10):1651–1661.

Weaver, G., 1984, PCB contamination in and around New Bedford, Massachusetts, *Environ. Sci. Technol.* **18**(11):22A–27A.

6

Partitioning Models

Donald Mackay and Sally Paterson

INTRODUCTION

An essential component of any chemical risk assessment is quantifying the nature and extent of exposure expressed in terms of concentration, dosage, or duration. In this chapter, we outline the structure of such exposure assessments using relatively simple partitioning models and provide an illustration of the underlying concepts. A full-scale exposure analysis may involve an extensive program of data collection, determination, and interpretation involving chemical analyses of various biotic and abiotic media, calculation of the rates of emission into, and migration between, environmental media, and estimation of the toxic effects on organisms, populations, communities, and ecosystems. Examples are the series of reports published in the United States by the National Academy of Sciences/National Research Council and in Canada by the Environmental Secretariat of the National Research Council.

The exposure analysis process is essentially an exercise in mathematical modeling, usually formulated and implemented as a computer program. These programs may range from simple "back-of-the-envelope" calculations that can be done on a hand calculator to very complex, lengthy programs involving predictions of chemical migration in the atmosphere, lakes, rivers, soils, and groundwater, through food chains and even to the target organs or tissues within the victim organisms. Such processes are best understood by conducting and illustrating a relatively simple but comprehensive calculation which includes all the essential components. More complex and detailed assessments could be viewed as substitution of one component or module for another.

The approach taken here is to present a specimen calculation in its entirety, then discuss its application and how the descriptive equations for various components could be modified to improve the model's fidelity and reliability.

Donald Mackay and Sally Paterson • Institute for Environmental Studies, University of Toronto, Toronto, Ontario M5S 1A4, Canada.

Environmental partitioning calculations have been reviewed by several authors. Pa-terson (1985) has described several of these models and in particular has highlighted the fugacity approach. Various chapters in the two volume text by Neely and Blau (1985) treat aspects of this issue. Cohen (1986) has recently given an account of the structure and purpose of these models and refers to many recent papers. Other useful accounts are to be found in the compilations edited by Dickson *et al.* (1982), Swann and Eschenroeder (1983), Sheenan *et al.* (1985), and Proceedings of the GSF Workshop held in Munich (1985).

THE MODEL

We consider a hypothetical region illustrated in Figure 1 consisting of defined volumes of air, water, soil, and sediment. In the interests of simplicity all these media are assumed to be homogeneous or well mixed. Chemical is emitted into the region at a steady rate of *E* mole/day. Concentrations have built up to steady state in all media to values such that the total rate of removal equals the emission rate. Two removal mechanisms exist, reaction or degradation and advective outflow in air and water. These advection rates correspond to residence times of 20 days for air and 100 days for water, the assumption

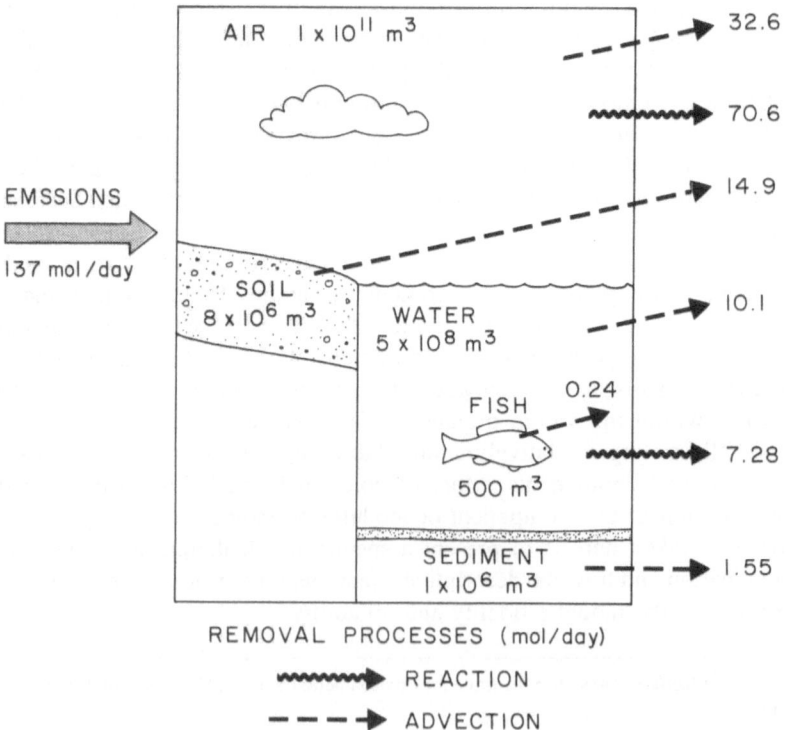

Figure 1. Hypothetical environment with mass balance (mole/day) for illustrative chemical.

being, for example, that 5×10^9 m³/day of clean air (G_1) blow into the air medium of volume 10^{11} m³ (yielding a residence time of $10^{11}/(5 \times 10^9)$ or 20 days) and that there is an equal outflow of air containing the prevailing concentration C_1 mole/m³, thus the removal rate is G_1C_1 or $5 \times 10^9 C_1$ mole/day. The water is treated similarly. The reaction rates are chemical-specific and are estimated from the persistence half-lives for each medium. For example, if the half-life in water is 10 days the corresponding rate constant k is 0.693/10 or 0.069 days^{-1} and the rate of reaction is VCk mole/day where V is the volume (m³) of water and C the concentration (mole/m³) in water.

The overall mass balance is thus

$$E = \Sigma G_i C_i + \Sigma V_i C_i k_i$$

where the summations are over the relevant media. If the air blowing into the system contains a concentration of the chemical, a GC term to incorporate this inflow must be added to the left side of the above equation.

The remaining undetermined variables are the concentrations C_i. These can be determined if it is assumed that all concentrations are in equilibrium such that partition coefficients K_{ij} apply, i.e.,

$$C_i/C_j = K_{ij}$$

Because there are five media, there are four independent partition coefficients, each of which generates an equation, thus when combined with the overall mass balance

Table 1. Description of Hypothetical Chemical Properties

Properties		Partition coefficients		Fugacity capacities (mole/m³ per Pa)	
Molecular weight (g/mole):	200	K_{AW}:	0.00969	Z_A:	4.04×10^{-4}
Solubility (mole/m³):	0.125	K_{SW}:	184.5	Z_W:	0.0417
Vapor pressure (Pa):	3.0	K_{BW}:	307.5	Z_S:	7.69
Log octanol/water partition		K_{FW}:	480.0	Z_B:	12.8
coefficient:	4.0			Z_F:	20.0

Advective processes

	Flow rate (m³/day)	D (mole/Pa per day)
Air:	$G_A = 5.0 \times 10^9$	$D_{AA} = G_A Z_A = 2.02 \times 10^6$
Water:	$G_W = 5.0 \times 10^6$	$D_{AW} = G_W Z_W = 2.08 \times 10^5$

	Rate constants (days^{-1})	D (mole/Pa per day)	Total
k_A:	0.0531 (reaction) + 0.020 (advection)	$k_A V_A Z_A$	9.324×10^5
k_W:	0.0139 (reaction) + 0.010 (advection)	$k_W V_W Z_W$	2.89×10^5
k_S:	0.00693 (reaction)	$k_S V_S Z_S$	4.26×10^5
k_B:	0.00347 (reaction)	$k_B V_B Z_B$	4.44×10^4
k_F:	0.139 (reaction)	$k_F V_F Z_F$	1.39×10^3
		Total	3.92×10^6

equation the number of concentrations equals the number of equations and solution is possible. It is most convenient if all partition coefficients are defined with respect to water in the denominator, i.e., K_{AW} (air–water), K_{SW} (soil–water), etc. This enables all concentrations except that of water to be eliminated. Rearranging the equations gives

$$E = C_W \left(\Sigma G_i K_{iw} + \Sigma V_i K_{iw} k_i \right)$$

where K_{iw} are the partition coefficients (K_{ww} being unity). This can be solved directly for C_W. The other concentrations can then be deduced and the entire mass balance assembled.

The partition coefficients can be calculated from the chemical's properties of solubility, vapor pressure, and octanol–water partition coefficient, and the environmental properties of temperature, organic carbon contents in soil and sediment, and fish lipid content, as discussed by Mackay and Paterson (1982).

Table 1 gives properties, partition coefficients and reaction rate constants for a hypothetical chemical; Tables 2 and 3 and Fig. 1 give the calculation and mass balance. The significance of this calculation is that the dominant phases into which the chemical partitions become apparent. A "behavior profile" emerges. As shown in Table 3 most of the chemical partitions into soil (45%), air (30%), and water (15%), with only 9% in sediment and a negligible amount in fish. The total amount of chemical present is 947 kg, which is equivalent to emissions over 35 days. Thus, the average residence time or persistence is 35 days. It is also possible to calculate where the dominant reactions occur and how significant advection is as a removal mechanism. In this case the primary removal process is reaction in air as indicated in Figure 1.

Table 2. Calculation of Exposure

Conventional format

$$E = \Sigma G_i C_i + \Sigma V_i C_i k_i$$

but

$$C_i = K_{iw} C_W$$

$$E = C_W (\Sigma G_i K_{iw} + \Sigma V_i K_{iw} k_i)$$

$$C_W = E / (\Sigma G_i K_{iw} + \Sigma V_i K_{iw} k_i)$$

and $\quad C_A = K_{AW} C_W, \; C_S = K_{SW} C_W, \; C_B = K_{BW} C_W, \; C_F = K_{FW} C_W$

Process rates

   Advection: $G_i C_i$ mole/day

   Reaction: $V_i K_{iw} C_w k_i$ mole/day

Fugacity format

$$C_i = f Z_i$$

$$E = f \Sigma G_i Z_i + f \Sigma V_i Z_i k_i$$

$$f = E / (\Sigma D_{Ai} + \Sigma D_{Ri})$$

where

$$D_{Ai} = G_i Z i$$

and

$$D_{Ri} = V_i Z_i k_i$$

Process rates

   Advection: $f D_{Ai} = f G_i Z_i$ mole/day

   Reaction: $f D_{Ri} = f V_i Z_i k_i$ mole/day

Table 3. Concentrations, Amounts, and Percentages of Chemical in Each Phase[a]

	Volume (m³)	Concentration (g/m³)	Amount (g)	Percent
Air	1×10^{11}	2.82×10^{-6}	2.82×10^5	29.8
Water	5×10^8	2.91×10^{-4}	1.46×10^5	15.4
Soil	8×10^6	5.37×10^{-2}	4.30×10^5	45.4
Sediment	1×10^6	8.96×10^{-2}	8.96×10^4	9.45
Fish	500	0.140	70	0.01
Total			9.47×10^5	100

[a]Production = 1×10^5 kg/year = 1370 mole/day, Fraction entering environment = 0 1; Total emissions = $1 \times 10^5 \times 0$ 1 $\times$ 1000/365 = 2.74×10^4 g/day; Residence time = (total amount)/(emissions) = $(9\ 47 \times 10^5)/(2.74 \times 10^4)$ = 34.6 days; Prevailing fugacity = $3\ 5 \times 10^{-5}$ Pa

THE FUGACITY APPROACH

Another, algebraically identical but more elegant method of solving this problem is to use the fugacity approach as described in a series of papers by Mackay and co-workers (1979, 1981, 1982, 1985, 1986).

Fugacity, like chemical potential, is a criterion of equilibrium, thus when a chemical is at equilibrium between two phases its fugacities in each are equal. In the region considered, this implies that a single chemical fugacity prevails over all media. Fugacity (*f*) is substituted for concentration using the relationship

$$C = fZ$$

where Z is a "fugacity capacity" which is unique for each chemical in each medium. When two phases are in equilibrium they share a common fugacity thus

$$C_i/C_j = fZ_i/fZ_j = Z_i/Z_j = K_{ij}$$

The Z term is thus essentially half the partition coefficient K_{12}.

Rates of reaction, advection, or transfer are expressed as products of fugacity f and a D value with dimension of mole/Pa per day, i.e.,

$$\text{Rate} = f_i D_i$$

Rates of various processes can thus be expressed as D values and added and compared directly. The overall mass balance equation thus becomes

$$E = \Sigma f D_i = f \Sigma D_i$$

where ΣD_i is the sum of all the D values representing processes causing the chemical to be removed from the system. Definitions of D are given and discussed elsewhere (Mackay *et al.*, 1985), but in this situation are defined summarily as *VZk* for reaction and as *GZ* for advection. The estimated fugacity can thus be converted into various concentrations. As before, the amounts and persistence can be estimated.

The analogous fugacity version of the conventional partition coefficient calculation is given in Tables 1 and 2 with, of course, identical results. The advantage of the fugacity approach is that it becomes much simpler for multimedia systems, especially when intermedia transfer resistances are present. The fugacity approach is particularly useful because the rates of the various removal processes by reaction and advection from all phases can be compared and determined directly. Each process rate is proportional to the corresponding *D* value. It is clear from Table 1 that the largest *D* value is in the air and that it consists primarily of a reaction term. This reaction rate constant of 0.053 corresponds to a half-life of 13 days. The overall chemical persistence of 35 days is longer by a factor of approximately 3 because only approximately one-third of the chemical is in the air and thus susceptible to this removal process at any time.

The essential point is that from input data consisting of emission rate, properties of the chemical, and properties of the environment, it is possible to calculate where the chemical partitions, its concentrations in various phases, its persistence or lifetime, and where most of it reacts or advects from the system.

FROM CONCENTRATIONS TO EXPOSURE AND EFFECTS

Subsequent calculations can take one or both of two directions. First, target concentrations may be defined for each medium. For example, from considerations of toxicity or aesthetics it may be possible to suggest that water concentrations should be maintained below 1 μg/liter, air below 1 μg/m^3, and fish below 1 mg/kg. These target concentrations can then be compared as a ratio or quotient to the estimated environmental concentrations. A hypothetical example is given in Table 4 showing the application of the quotient method. In this case it is apparent that the primary concern is with air and fish ingestion. The proximities of the estimated prevailing concentrations to the targets are expressed as these quotients, a large value implying a large safety factor. The high-risk situations correspond to low quotients. The concentration level in fish is not directly toxic to the fish but poses a possible threat to humans if consumed on a regular basis.

There are often problems associated with suggesting target concentrations in soil and sediment because these media are not normally consumed directly by organisms. Whereas simple lethality experiments can be designed using air, water, or food as vehicles of toxicant administration, it is not always clear how concentrations in the solid matrices of soils and sediments relate to exposure or intake of a chemical by organisms. It is even difficult to design meaningful bioassays involving interaction between organisms, soils, and sediments. A second approach is to use these media concentrations to calculate dosages to human and other organisms, as illustrated in Table 4 and Fig. 2.

An average human inhales some 20 m^3 of air per day, thus the associated amount of chemical can be easily calculated. Not all this chemical may be absorbed, but at least a maximum dosage can be evaluated. The same human may consume 2 liters/day of water with its chemical, enabling this dosage to be estimated. Food, the other vehicle, is more

Table 4. Comparison of Environmental Concentrations and Human Intake Rates with Effect Levels

Comparison of environmental effect concentrations with predicted concentrations

	Effect level	Actual level	Quotient or ratio
Air pollution (μg/m^3)	15	2.82	5.3
Fish toxicity (g/m^3)	5	2.91×10^{-4}	17,160
Soil contamination (μg/g)	5	3.58×10^{-2}	140

Comparison of allowable human intake with predicted intakes[a]

	Concentration (g/m^3)	Volume of intake (m^3)	Actual intake (μg/day)	Percent of permissible intake	Percent of actual intake
Ingestion of food and water					
Fish	0.140	0.00025	35	0.7	34
Meat products	0.140	0.00005	7	0.14	6.8
Dairy products	2.9×10^{-4}	0.00025	0.073	0.001	0.07
Vegetable products	2.9×10^{-4}	0.00045	0.13	0.003	0.13
Water	2.9×10^{-4}	0.002	0.58	0.012	0.56
Air inhalation	2.82×10^{-6}	20	56	1.1	54.4
Domestic exposure			1	0.02	1
Occupational exposure			3	0.06	3
Total			103[b]	2.04	100

[a]Average daily intake (ADI) = 5000 μg/day
[b]Ratio of ADI/intake = 5000/103 = 48.5

difficult to treat. An average diet may consist of 1 kg/day broken down as shown in Table 4. Fish concentrations can be estimated directly from the model, but meat, vegetable, and dairy product concentrations are still poorly understood functions of the concentrations of chemical in air, water, soil, animal feeds, and of agrochemical usage. It is likely that techniques will emerge for calculating food–environment concentration ratios, but at present the best approach is to analyze a typical "food basket." The food concentrations used here are illustrative and were obtained by assuming that meat consumed had partitioning properties similar to fish, and that dairy and vegetable products consisted largely of water. This issue is complicated by the fact that much food is grown at distant locations and imported. Beverages, food, and water may also be treated for chemical removal commercially or domestically.

Much chemical exposure may also occur in occupational (e.g., factory) and institutional or commercial (e.g., schools, stores, cinemas) settings, and at home, but these exposures vary greatly from individual to individual and depend on lifestyle. For illustrative purposes and to give a complete picture, exposures from these sources are included in Table 4.

The picture that emerges is a profile of relative exposures by various routes from which the dominant route(s) can be elucidated. If desired, appropriate measures can be taken to reduce certain critical exposures. For example, fish consumption could be re-

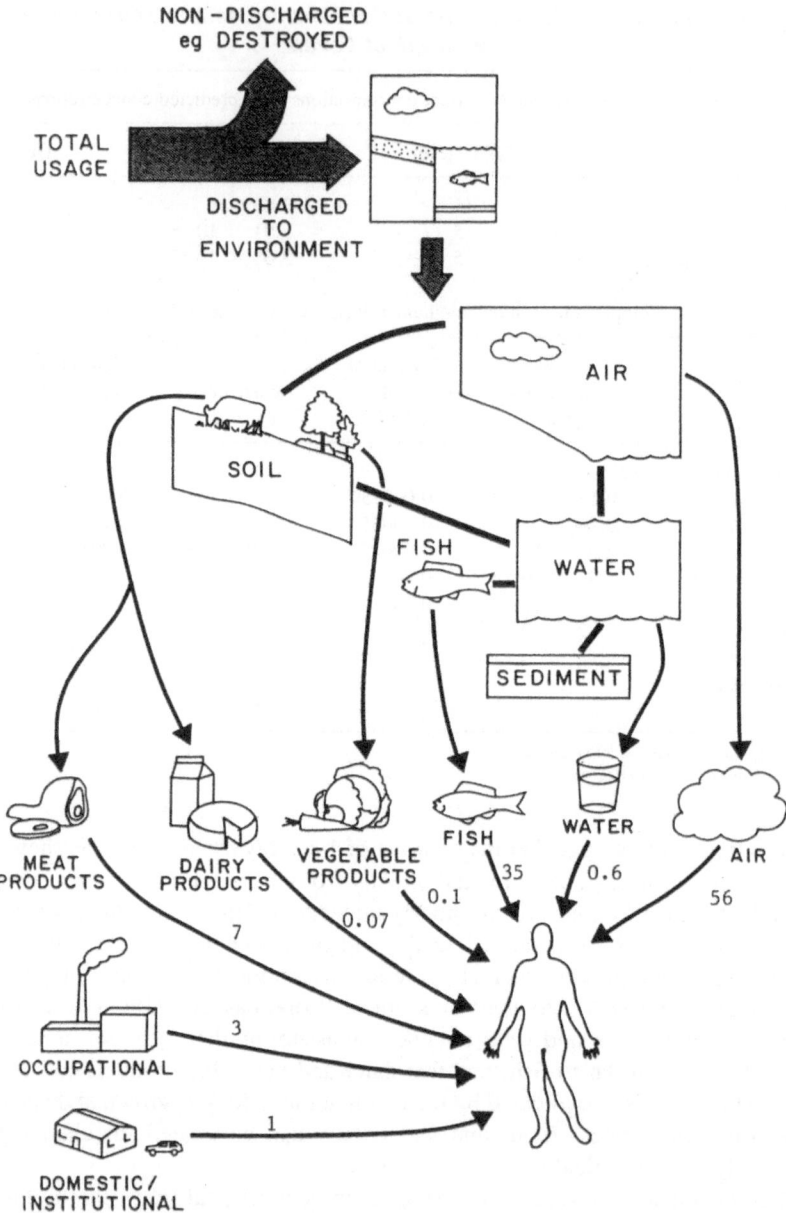

Figure 2. Predicted routes of human exposure to a hypothetical compound (µg/day).

duced. An advantage of this approach is that it places the entire spectrum of exposure routes in perspective. There is little merit in reducing an already small exposure.

As illustrated in Table 4 and Fig. 2, the dominant routes in the case of this chemical are consumption of fish and air inhalation. These routes vary greatly in magnitude and relative contribution from chemical to chemical.

DISCUSSION

This simple model has a number of obvious weaknesses. In all cases appropriate "corrections" can be introduced, albeit at the cost of increased mathematical complexity and the need for additional input data. Perhaps there are three major deficiencies.

1. *Variation of concentration in time*. In most cases the prevailing environmental condition is dynamic; improving or deteriorating, it is a reflection of past history of emissions as well as current emission rates. In the case of agrochemicals, application may be during a short intense period. Spills result in similarly intense but irregular and unpredictable pulse inputs. Degradation rates are usually temperature dependent and thus vary seasonally.
2. *Variation of concentration in space*. In reality, concentrations in these media are variable from place to place with "hot spot" regions of relatively high contamination as well as more pristine regions. Variations can be quantified by using various statistical distribution functions (Mackay and Paterson, 1984), but the parameters defining the distribution of skewness or standard deviation require experimental determination.
3. *Transport resistances*. Environmental media are rarely in equilibrium with the rate of transport controlled by various processes such as diffusion, rainfall, sedimentation, and volatilization. The model can be expanded to include a mathematical description of these rates and resistances but this involves a significant increase in complexity and data needs.

In many cases other environmental media such as groundwater, atmospheric particles, suspended aquatic matter, and terrestrial and aquatic vegetation play an important role in determining chemical fate. Again, these media can be included with the associated cost in complexity.

Perhaps most difficult is the issue of estimating the nature and magnitude of the toxic effect at the low concentrations which generally prevail in the environment, an issue which is beyond the scope of this chapter. It is sufficient to note that the errors or uncertainty in estimating toxic effects (especially for carcinogens) are probably as large or larger than those associated with exposure estimation. Clearly, there is a need to "match" the accuracy of the exposure and effects components. There is little merit in estimating exposures to an accuracy of a factor of 2 if there is a factor of 100 accuracy in effects, and vice versa. Fortunately, it often transpires that accurate exposure estimates are not needed because the concentrations are many orders of magnitude lower than "effect levels." Partitioning exposure models can therefore be viewed as a method of identifying with order of magnitude accuracy, the critical media and exposure routes, as a preamble to more accurate quantitative, site specific estimations.

Finally, presenting the data from the partitioning model, assessing the quotients, and highlighting the dominant exposure routes provides a sound basis for estimating risk. The chemical's behavior profile emerges clearly. If such profiles can be presented to the public the individual is then able to choose or modify a lifestyle which minimizes exposure and presumably risk. Individuals then have, in principle, the freedom and information to judge and respond to the acceptability of risk from this chemical compared to the other voluntary and involuntary risks to which they are subject.

REFERENCES

Cohen, Y., 1986, Organic pollutant transport, *Environ. Sci. Technol.* **20**:538–544.

Dickson, K. L., Maki, A. W., and Cairns, J., Jr. (eds.), 1982, *Modeling the Fate of Chemicals in the Environment,* Ann Arbor Science, Ann Arbor, Michigan.

GSF, *Gessellschaft für Stahlen und Umweltforschung mbH München,* Projektgruppe, Umweltgefährdung-spotentiale von Chemikalien (Ed.), Environmental Modelling for Priority Setting Among Existing Chemicals. (Proceedings of a Workshop held in München, Neuherberg, Nov. 11–13, 1985.)

Mackay, D., 1979, Finding fugacity feasible, *Environ. Sci. Technol.* **13**:1218.

Mackay, D., and Paterson, S., 1981, Calculating fugacity, *Environ. Sci. Technol.* **15**(9):1006–1014.

Mackay, D., and Paterson, S., 1982, Fugacity revisited, *Environ. Sci. Technol.* **16**:654–660.

Mackay, D., and Paterson, S., 1984, Spatial concentration distributions in evaluative chemical fate models, *Environ. Sci. Technol.* **18**:207A–214A.

Mackay, D., Paterson, S., Cheung, B., and Neely, W. B., 1985, Evaluating the environmental behavior of chemicals with a level III fugacity model, *Chemosphere* **14**:335–374.

Mackay, D., Paterson, S., and Schroeder, W. H., 1986, Model describing the rates of transfer processes of organic chemicals between atmosphere and water, *Environ. Sci. Technol.* **20**:810–816.

Neely, W. B., and Blau, G. E. (eds.), 1985, *Environmental Exposure from Chemicals,* Vol. I, CRC Press, Boca Raton, Florida.

Paterson, S., 1985, Equilibrium models for the initial integration of physical chemical properties, in: *Environmental Exposure from Chemicals,* Vol. I (W. B. Neely and G. E. Blau, eds.), pp. 217–233, CRC Press, Boca Raton, Florida.

Sheehan, P., Korte, F., Klein, W., Bourdeau, P. (eds.), 1985, *Appraisal of tests to predict the environmental behaviour of chemicals,* SCOPE 25, J. Wiley and Sons, New York.

Swann, R. L., and Eschenroeder, A. (eds.), 1983, *Fate of Chemicals in the Environment,* ACS Symposium Series 225, American Chemical Society, Washington, D. C.

7

Pharmacokinetics

Curtis C. Travis

INTRODUCTION

Growing public awareness of the potential risk to humans from hazardous chemicals in the environment has led to increased concern about the effects of these chemicals on animals and man. This awareness has generated a demand for a rational means of estimating risk and of limiting exposure where risk is judged excessive. An outcome of this awareness has been the emergence of the field of risk assessment. Risk assessment synthesizes all available data on exposure to chemicals and combines it with the best scientific judgment to estimate the associated risk.

While prediction of human risk due to chemical exposure should be based on human data, adequate human data are rarely available. Consequently, experimental animal data are the common alternatives upon which analyses of risk are based. Estimations of risk from this type of data involve a series of judgmental decisions concerning unresolved issues in risk assessment. The major assumptions arise from the necessity to extrapolate experimental results (1) across species from rats or mice to humans; (2) from the high-dose regions to which animals are exposed in the laboratory to the low-dose regions to which humans are exposed in the environment; and (3) across routes of administration. Development of tools and methodologies which can help evaluate the scientific bases of these assumptions will reduce the uncertainties in the risk assessment process. Pharmacokinetic models are one such tool.

Pharmacokinetics is the study of the absorption, distribution, metabolism, and elimination of chemicals in animal systems. As such, it provides a means of resolving some of the ambiguities in risk assessment and of evaluating the scientific assumptions upon which risk assessment is based. A recent development in the area of pharmacokinetics is the advent of physiologically-based pharmacokinetic (PBPK) models. Relying on actual

---

Curtis C. Travis • Office of Risk Analysis, Health and Safety Research Division, Oak Ridge National Laboratory, Oak Ridge, Tennessee 37831-6109.

physiological parameters such as body weight, cardiac output, breathing rates, blood flow rates, and tissue volumes to describe the metabolic process, the PBPK models relate exposure concentrations to organ concentration over a range of exposure intervals (Ramsey and Andersen, 1984; Andersen *et al.*, 1987; Ward *et al.*, 1987; Travis *et al.*, 1987a). The physiological parameters are coupled with chemical-specific parameters and metabolic constants to predict the dynamics of a compound's movement through an animal system. By simply changing the parameters, the model can predict substance transport and metabolism via several routes of administration, across species, and through temporal variations in exposure (Travis, 1987). Continual development and sophistication of these models will correspondingly reduce the uncertainties involved in risk assessment.

This chapter examines PBPK models and their role in the risk assessment process. Beginning with a general description of PBPK models, the chapter discusses their use in determining transport of parent compound, in describing metabolite formation, and in extrapolating associated risks to untested doses and routes of exposure.

PHARMACOKINETIC MODELS

A pharmacokinetic model is a set of equations that can be used to describe the time course of a parent chemical or metabolite in an animal system. There are two types of pharmacokinetic models: data-based and physiologically-based (NRC, 1986).

Data-Based Models

A data-based model divides the animal system into a series of compartments which, in general, do not represent real, identifiable anatomic regions of the body. Figure 1 shows a simple data-based model that has been used to describe the pharmacokinetics of styrene (a volatile organic) in rats (Young *et al.*, 1979) and humans (Ramsey *et al.*, 1980). The body has been divided into two compartments: a central compartment and a peripheral compartment. Reitz *et al.* (1982) used a similar model to describe ethylene dichloride kinetics. In applying these models, time–course concentration curves are first determined from *in vivo* animal experiments. Then, model compartment volumes and rate

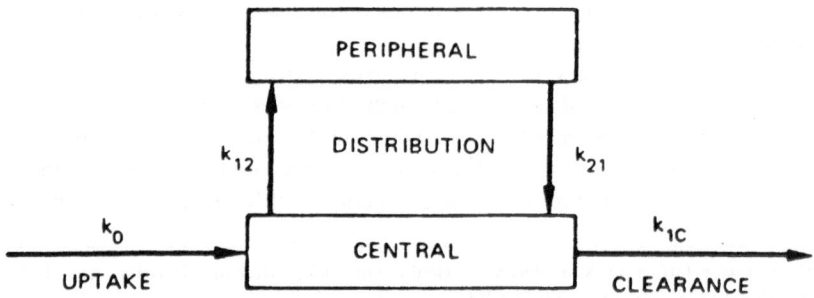

Figure 1. A data-based compartmental model that has been used to describe the pharmacokinetics of organics. The model has a central blood compartment and a peripheral tissue compartment. The compartment volumes and rate constants are adjusted to give model-generated curves that fit the experimental data.

constants are determined by trial and error so that the model predictions fit the empirical data. These models are useful for interpolation and limited extrapolation in the *same* animal species. However, since the parameters in these data-based models generally do not correspond to physiologically-identifiable entities, they do not allow for extrapolation *across* animal species.

Physiologically-Based Models

A PBPK model is comprised of series of compartments representing organs or tissue groups with realistic weights and blood flows determined from the literature (Arms and Travis, 1987). These models require a variety of physiological information: tissue volumes, blood flow rates to tissues, cardiac output, alveolar ventilation rates (for volatile compounds) and, possibly, membrane permeabilities. The models also utilize biochemical information such as air–blood partition coefficients, and metabolic parameters. The uniqueness of the physiologically-based approach is this reliance on measured physiological and biochemical parameters. An appealing aspect of these physiological models is that they allow ready extrapolation from a test species to an untested species simply by placing the appropriate physiological and biochemical parameters in the model (Dedrick, 1973; Ward *et al.*, 1987; Travis, 1987). Similarly, the effect of route of administration can be investigated by allowing for several different input functions.

It should be pointed out that no one PBPK model can be used to determine the distribution of all chemicals. Like any other tool, the primary rule in model selection is that the model should provide the simplest description consistent with its intended purpose. The number of compartments and the way they are connected will vary from chemical to chemical depending upon the chemical's metabolic behavior and the nature of the carcinogenic bioassay data available for the chemical.

EXAMPLE OF A PHYSIOLOGICALLY-BASED MODEL

A physiologically-based model which has found frequent application in the description of the inhalation of volatile organics is shown in Fig. 2 (Ramsey and Andersen, 1984; Andersen *et al.*, 1987; Ward *et al.*, 1987; Travis *et al.*, 1987a). Tissue groups utilized in the model include (1) organs such as brain, kidney, and viscera, (2) muscle, (3) fat, and (4) metabolic organs (principally liver). The model is described mathematically by a set of differential equations which calculate the rate of change of the amount of chemical in each compartment. Metabolism in this model occurs only in the liver. If metabolism depends on an enzyme whose supply is limited with respect to the time of the reaction, the rate of the metabolism will saturate as a function of time. This is referred to as Michaelis–Menten metabolism and is described by the following equation:

$$\frac{dA_m}{dt} = \frac{V_{max}C_{ven}}{(K_m + C_{ven})} \tag{1}$$

where A_m is the amount of metabolite, C_{ven} is the concentration of the parent compound in the venous blood, V_{max} is the maximum metabolic (mg/hr) rate and K_m, the Michaelis constant, is the venous blood concentration (mg/liter blood) at which the metabolic rate is half of V_{max}.

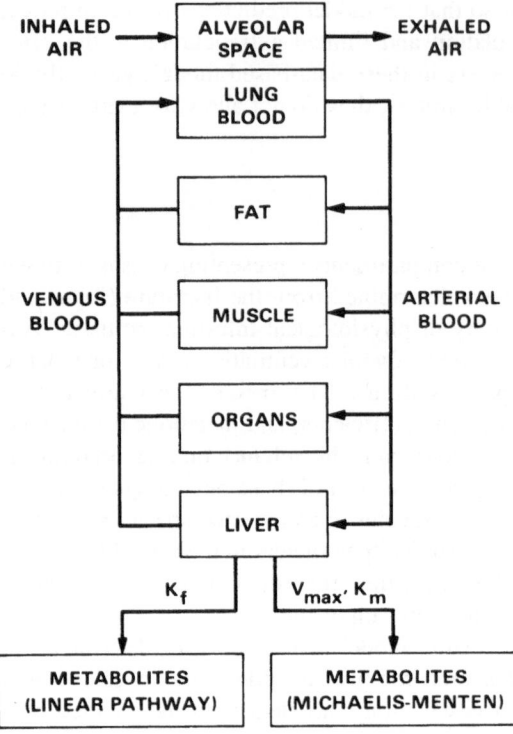

Figure 2. Diagram of a physiologically based pharmacokinetic model. The tissue groups are fat, muscle, organs, and liver. These groups are connected by blood flow to each tissue group.

When the rate of metabolite formation is nonsaturable and depends linearly on the venous blood concentration, C_{ven}, then a second mathematical description of metabolism is used:

$$\frac{dA_m}{dt} = K_f V C_{ven} \tag{2}$$

where V is the volume of the tissue compartment in which the metabolism occurs (the liver in the present model) and K_f is the linear metabolic rate constant. Linear (nonsaturable) metabolism will occur whenever there is an endless supply of compounds required by the metabolic reaction. There are, therefore, three kinetic constants describing metabolism: the linear metabolic constant K_f (hr^{-1}) and the two Michaelis–Menten metabolic constants V_{max} (mg/hr) and K_m (mg/liter blood).

The parameters used in a physiologically-based model can be divided into three classes: physiological, biochemical, and metabolic. The physiological parameters (such as breathing rates, blood flow rates, and tissue volumes) have been well-characterized for mice, rats, and humans (Arms and Travis, 1987) and are fixed *a priori* before using the model (see Table 1). The biochemical parameters describe the partitioning of a given chemical between air and blood, and blood and tissues. These can be determined in the laboratory using a vial equilibration technique (Sato and Nakajima, 1979). The metabolic parameters to be used in the model for a particular chemical can either be determined through closed chamber studies (Andersen *et al.*, 1980; Filser and Bolt, 1979; Gargas *et*

Table 1. Physiological Parameters for Use in Pharmacokinetics

	Mouse	Rat	Human
Body weight (kg)	0.024	0.25	70.0
Alveolar ventilation (liter/hr)	1.33	7.96	353.5
Total blood flow rate (liter/hr)	1.33	5.16	371.6
Blood flow fractions			
Blood flow fraction in liver	0.25	0.25	0.25
Blood flow fraction in fat	0.09	0.09	0.05
Blood flow fraction in organs	0.51	0.51	0.51
Blood flow fraction in muscle tissues	0.15	0.15	0.19
Tissue group volume fractions			
Volume fraction in liver	0.06	0.04	0.04
Volume fraction in fat	0.10	0.07	0.20
Volume fraction in organs	0.05	0.05	0.05
Volume fraction in muscle tissues	0.70	0.75	0.62

al., 1986) or through optimization techniques to find the best metabolic parameters consistent with empirical data.

APPLICATION OF A PHYSIOLOGICALLY-BASED MODEL

Ward *et al.* (1987) have developed a physiologically-based pharmacokinetic model to describe the metabolism of tetrachloroethylene in mice, rats, and humans. Tetrachloroethylene (also known as perchloroethylene, perc, and PCE) is a nonflammable, colorless liquid, relatively insoluble in water, with a chloroformlike odor. PCE is extensively used in the textile industry as a dry cleaning aid, constituting more than 65% of the total dry cleaning solvent usage in the United States. PCE is also used as an industrial metal cleaner, heat exchange fluid, and therapeutic drug in the treatment of hookworms and some nematodes (IARC, 1979). PCE has been shown to be a hepatocellular carcinogen in mice following both inhalation and gavage exposures (NCI, 1977; NTP, 1985). Ward *et al.* (1987) determined the metabolic parameters of PCE by fitting model predictions to species-specific empirical data. These parameters are given in Table 2. Comparison of model results with independent empirical data on inhalation and gavage exposures in mice, rats, and humans, demonstrates that the pharmacokinetic model can be used to determine the time course of PCE in these species.

Table 2. Metabolic Parameters Used in
Describing the Behavior of Tetrachloroethylene

Parameter	Mouse	Rat	Human
Body weight (kg)	0.024	0.25	70.0
V_{max} (mg/hr)	0.11	0.068	3.5
K_m (mg/liter blood)	0.4	0.3	0.3
K_f (hr^{-1})	1.84	2.73	0.0

Mice

The extent of PCE metabolism in mice (B6C3F$_1$) was investigated by Schumann *et al.* (1980). Mice were exposed for 6 hr by inhalation to 10 part per million (ppm) (67.8 mg/m^3) ^{14}C-labeled PCE and to a single oral dose of 500 mg ^{14}C-labeled PCE/kg body weight. Following inhalation of 10 ppm ^{14}C-labeled PCE, total metabolites were observed to account for 88% of total radioactivity recovered, while unchanged PCE in expired air accounted for 12%. The reverse situation was observed after a single oral dose of 500 mg/kg. Approximately 83% was detected unchanged in expired air, while 17% appeared as metabolites. This shift in the major route of elimination is a result of saturation of the oxidative metabolism pathway; metabolism could not rapidly reduce the high blood concentrations resulting from the gavage exposure, and therefore, most of the PCE was expired.

Buben and O'Flaherty (1985) also investigated the metabolism of PCE in mice. Male Swiss–Cox mice were given PCE in corn oil by gavage five times a week for 6 weeks in doses of 20, 100, 200, 500, 1000, 1500 and 2000 mg/kg per day. Urinary metabolites

Table 3. Schumann Data versus Model Predictions for Mice[a,b]

Quantity	Data	Model predictions
Inhalation of 10 ppm PCE for 6 hr		
Total amount (mg)		
Metabolized + expired	0.4	0.37
% metabolized	88.0 ± 2.3	88.3
% expired	12.0 ± 2.2	11.7
Percent expired over		
intervals (min)		
360–540	7.70 ± 0.51	6.3
540–720	2.26 ± 0.95	2.8
720–1080	1.45 ± 0.53	2.0
1080–1800	0.41 ± 0.17	0.57
Gavage (500 mg/kg)		
Total amount (mg)		
Metabolized + expired	10.77 ± 0.51	12.0
% metabolized	17.40 ± 3.9	18.6
% expired	82.6 ± 4.6	81.4
Percent expired over		
intervals (min)		
0–180	32.3 ± 7.2	41.0
180–360	20.1 ± 3.6	20.0
360–720	26.9 ± 4.2	15.7
720–1440	3.14 ± 2.53	4.5
1440–2160	0.12 ± 0.03	0.17

[a]From Schumann *et al.* (1980).
[b]Body weight = 0.024 kg.

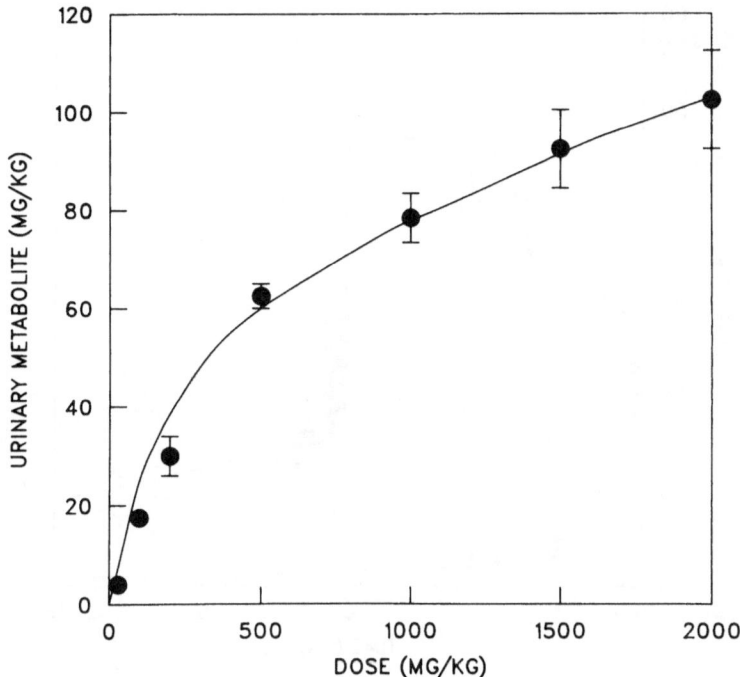

Figure 3. Model predictions of urinary metabolites of PCE as a function of dose. Based on experimental data of Buben and O'Flaherty (1985).

were quantified to estimate the extent of metabolism. The fraction of each dose metabolized decreased with increasing dose, a result consistent with a saturable metabolism pathway. At low doses of PCE about 25% of the dose was detected as urinary metabolites, while at high doses only 5% of the administered dose was metabolized.

Table 3 contains the experimental results of Schumann *et al.* (1980) and the model predictions. In Fig. 3, model predictions (shown as a solid line) are compared with the empirical data (shown as vertical bars) of Buben and O'Flaherty (1985). The graph shows the relationship between PCE metabolism (amount of urinary metabolites (mg/kg) excreted in 24 hr) and dose. The model provides a good fit to both the inhalation data of Schumann *et al.* (1980) and the gavage data of Schumann *et al.* (1980) and Buben and O'Flaherty (1985). This confirms the model's ability to predict mice metabolism of PCE over a wide range of doses, and also for both inhalation and gavage routes of administration.

Humans

Fernandez *et al.* (1976) exposed 24 subjects to concentrations of 100 ppm of PCE for 1 to 8 hr. Figure 4 is the graph of the Fernandez data, showing alveolar concentrations for both 1 and 8 hr exposure durations, against model predictions (solid lines).

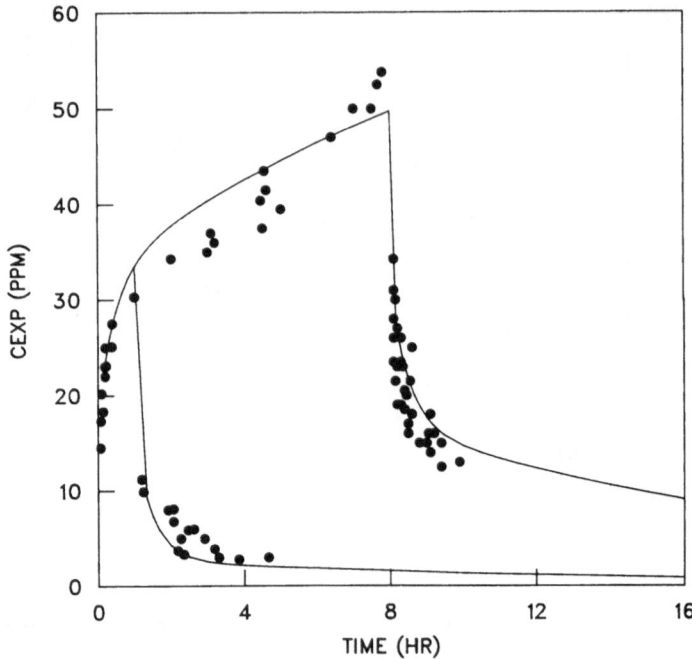

Figure 4. Model predictions of concentrations of PCE in human alveolar air following 100 ppm exposure for varying durations. Empirical data from Fernandez *et al.* (1976).

INTERSPECIES EXTRAPOLATION

One of the fundamental problems in the area of risk assessment is extrapolation of observed experimental results between animal species and man. Lacking detailed information on interspecific differences, it is frequently assumed that experimental results can be extrapolated between species when dosage is standardized as either mg/kg body weight per day (body weight scaling) or mg/m^2 per day (surface area scaling). Several investigators have argued for the efficacy of one or the other of these procedures (Pinkel, 1958; Freireich *et al.*, 1966; Hogan and Hoel, 1982; Crump and Guess, 1980; Hoel, 1979; Crouch and Wilson, 1978).

Metabolic Scaling

Rubner studied the relationship between the body weight of dogs and their metabolic rates. He found that the heat production rate divided by total body surface area (body weight to the two-thirds power) remained constant in dogs of various sizes (Rubner, 1883). These findings established body surface area as a basis for calculating metabolic rates. Unfortunately, the Rubner results were for intraspecific scaling, not interspecific scaling. Kleiber (1932, 1947) and Brody (1945) in examining animals over a size range from mice to elephants determined that metabolic rates actually increase with three-fourths power of body weight. This relationship is now well accepted as the appropriate scaling basis for metabolic rates (Schmidt-Nielsen, 1984; Prothero, 1980; Boxenbaum and Ronfeld, 1983). Subsequent studies (Adolph, 1949) have shown other physiological parameters to scale similarly. Volume rates such as cardiac output and ventilation rates scale with a mass exponent of 3/4 (Stahl, 1967; Calder, 1974; McMahon, 1973; Lindstedt and Calder, 1981; Feldman and McMahon 1983).

Ramsey and Anderson (1984) have suggested that the metabolic parameters V_{max} and K_f can be correlated with the body weight of the particular organism. They proposed scaling laws of the following form:

$$V_{max} = V_{max} \, BW^{0.7}$$

$$K_f = K_{fc} \, BW^{-0.3}$$

and that K_m is constant across species. Since it is known that metabolic rates across species are related to the 3/4 power of body weight (Kleiber, 1961; Holt *et al.*, 1968; and Schmidt-Nielsen, 1970), a more appropriate scaling law is:

$$V_{max} = V_{max} \, BW^{0.75}$$

$$K_f = K_{fc} \, BW^{-0.25}$$

Methylene Chloride

Andersen *et al.* (1987) constructed a physiologically based pharmacokinetic model of methylene chloride (DCM) disposition in 4 mammalian species: mice, rats, hamsters, and humans. The metabolic parameters were found by minimizing the difference between actual data and model predictions. Table 4 presents the metabolic parameters. Notice that K_m is approximately constant across species. A least-squares analysis shows that V_{max} and K_f scale as follows:

$$V_{max} = 6.69 \, BW^{0.65}, \, r = 0.985$$

$$K_f = 1.40 \, BW^{-0.24}, \, r = 0.946$$

Table 4. Kinetic Constants for Methylene Chloride

	Mice	Rats	Hamsters	Humans
Weights (kg)	0.0345	0.233	0.140	70.0
Metabolic constants				
V_{max} (mg/hr)	1.054	1.50	2.047	118.9
K_m (mg/liter)	0.396	0.771	0.649	0.580
K_f (hr^{-1})	4.017	2.21	1.513	0.53

DOSE–ROUTE EXTRAPOLATION

The route of exposure to organic chemicals can significantly affect the quantity of a chemical that reaches a particular target tissue (Angelo *et al.*, 1986; NRC, 1986; Travis, 1987). Pharmacokinetic models provide a tool to quantitatively evaluate the effect of route of administration on dose to the target tissue. This effect must be evaluated on a chemical by chemical basis.

The standard procedures for calculating applied dose following inhalation or ingestion exposures are as follows. For inhalation, the applied dose (mg) is the product of the air concentration (mg/liter) of the chemical, the animal breathing rate (liter/min), and the duration of exposure (min). For drinking water ingestion, the applied dose (mg) is the product of the water concentration (mg/liter) of the chemical, the animal drinking water rate (liter/min), and the duration of exposure (min). In both of these formulas, 100% absorption into the body is assumed, a standard assumption in risk analysis when data to the contrary are lacking.

Travis (1987) applied a pharmacokinetic model for methylene chloride (DCM) (Andersen *et al.*, 1987) to investigate the dose to target tissues following both inhalation and oral administration of DCM in mice. Figure 5 shows model predictions of total metabolized dose to the mouse liver over a 24-hr period. The inhalation exposure was for a duration of six hr and the ingestion exposure for 24 hr. The applied dose for inhalation exposures was calculated using the alveolar ventilation rate as opposed to the minute

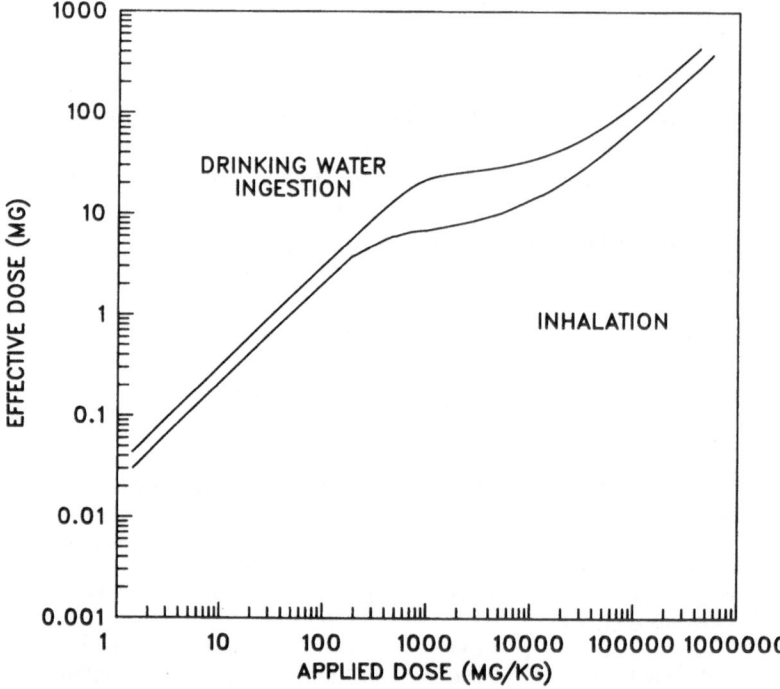

Figure 5. Effective dose (metabolized dose) to the mouse liver from inhalation and oral ingestion of methylene chloride.

volume. Figure 5 indicates fairly good agreement in the effective liver dose for the two routes of administration. The largest difference is a factor of 3 and occurs in the 500 to 10,000 mg/kg applied dose range.

Figure 6 shows model predictions of total metabolized dose to the mouse lung following inhalation and oral administration. As can be seen, the effective lung dose shows greater dependence on the route of administration. The largest difference is a factor of 5 and, in contrast to the liver, occurs in the low applied dose range.

RISK ASSESSMENT

To date, physiologically-based pharmacokinetic models have been used to estimate cancer risk from human exposure to two chemicals: DCM (Andersen *et al.*, 1987) and PCE (Travis *et al.*, 1987b). Anderson *et al.* (1987) obtain a 140- to 170-fold reduction in inhalation risk as a result of using their pharmacokinetic model in the risk assessment process. Application of the pharmacokinetic model for PCE to estimate inhalation cancer risk is discussed in detail below.

Tetrachloroethylene

Tetrachloroethylene has been shown to be carcinogenic in two long-term animal bioassays (NCI, 1977; NTP, 1985). The National Cancer Institute (NCI) studied the

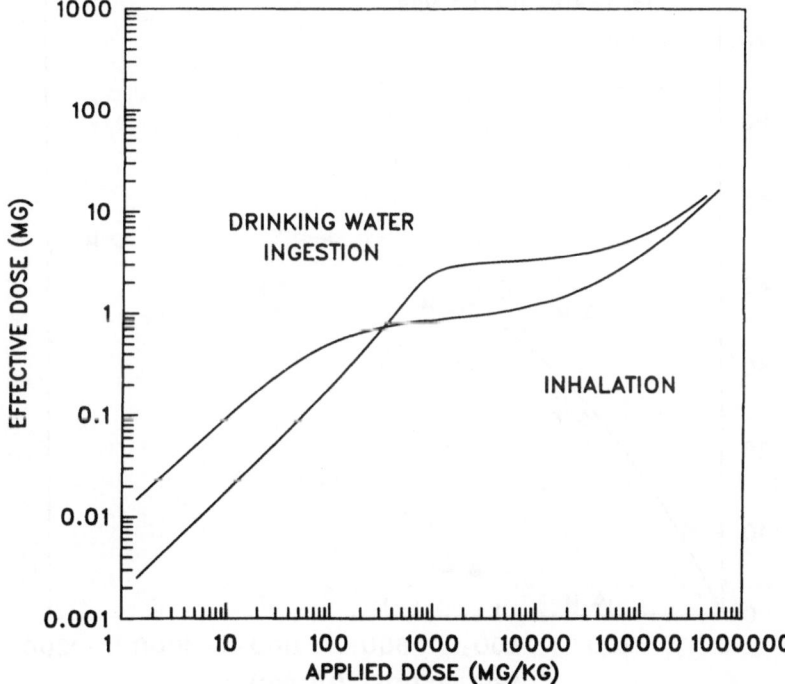

Figure 6. Effective dose (metabolized dose) to the mouse lung from inhalation and oral ingestion of methylene chloride.

response of Osborne–Mendel rats and B6C3F₁ mice exposed to PCE through gavage (NCI, 1977; EPA, 1985). The National Toxicology Program (NTP) studied the response of F344/N rats and B6C3F₁ mice exposed through inhalation. Both studies produced a large increase in hepatocellular carcinomas in mice, but no statistically significant increase in rats.

Using the pharmacokinetic model of Ward *et al.* (1987), Travis *et al.* (1987b) determined the pharmacokinetics of PCE under both of the animal bioassay protocols. They showed that tumor incidence rates were more clearly correlated with the amount of intermediate reactant produced by the nonlinear metabolic pathway of PCE than with either applied dose of the parent compound itself or the metabolite produced via the linear pathway. Figure 7 shows cancer incidence versus applied dose for both the NCI and NTP bioassays. [For the NTP bioassays, applied dose was computed as exposure concentration (mg/m³) × alveolar ventilation rate (m³/hr) × duration of exposure (hr).] The dose response curve was obtained as a least squares fit to the data using the equation $Y = 1 - exp(-q_1d - q_2d^2)$. Figure 8 displays cancer incidence vs. metabolite produced along the nonlinear pathway. The dose response curve was obtained as a least squares fit to the data using the same equation as in Fig. 7. Application of pharmacokinetics has linearized the dose response curve and shown that cancer response across species and routes of admin-

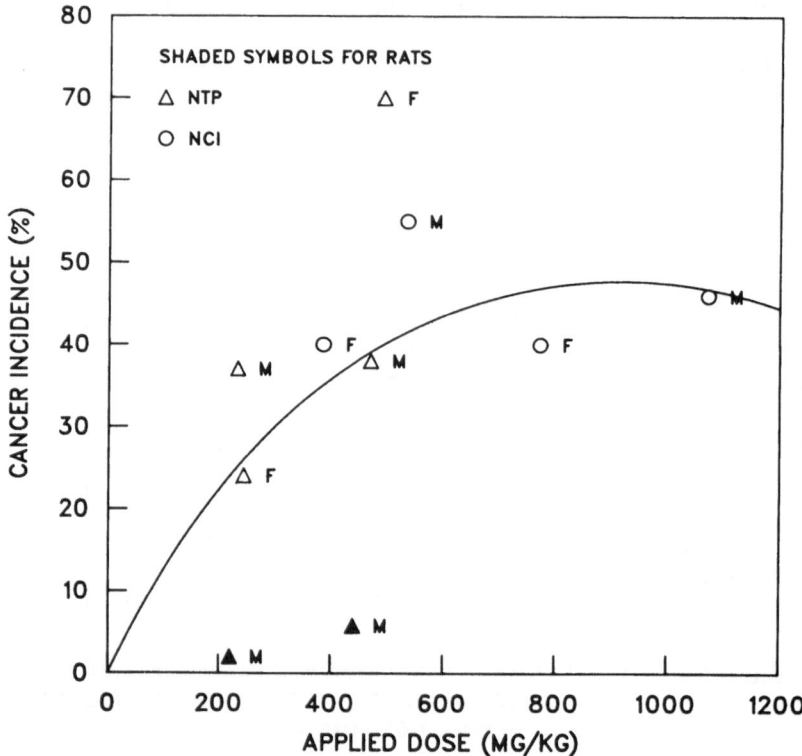

Figure 7. Cancer incidence versus applied dose of tetrachlorethylene for both NCI and NTP bioassays.

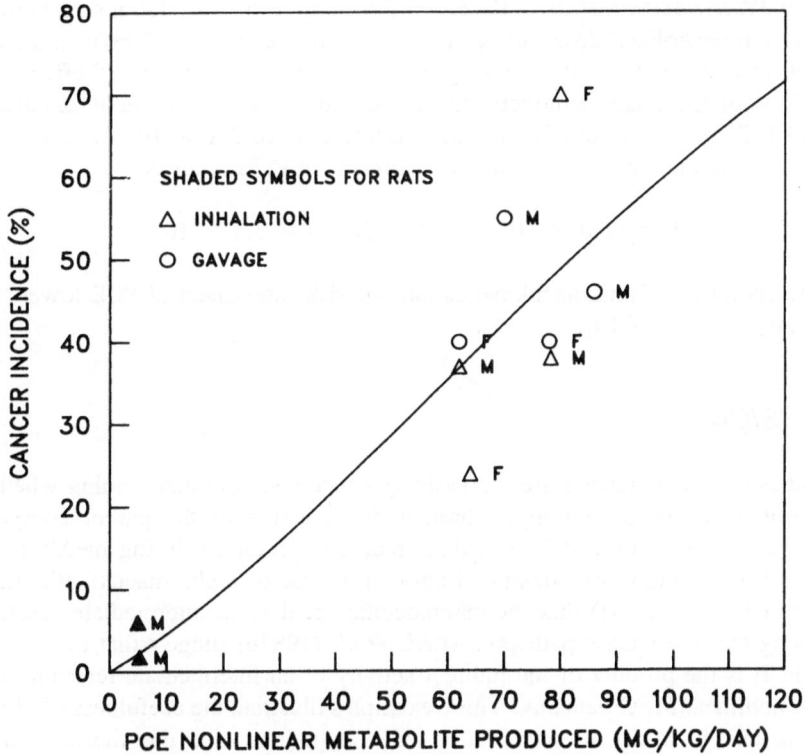

Figure 8. Cancer incidence versus metabolite produced along the nonlinear pathway for both the NCI and NTP bioassays.

istration are consistent. Cancer risk estimates for human exposure to PCE derived with and without pharmacokinetics are compared below.

Without Pharmacokinetics. Based on the dose–response relationship between applied dose and cancer incidence in the NTP bioassay, Travis *et al.* (1987b) estimated q_u to be 2.7×10^{-3} mg/kg per day expressed in terms of administered dose. The administered dose (D) associated with human exposure to 1 μg/m^3 of PCE in air is:

$$D = (1 \ \mu g/m^3) \ (13.4 \ m^3/day) \ (1/70 \ kg) \ (10^{-3} \ mg/\mu g)$$

$$= 1.9 \times 10^{-4} \ mg/kg \ per \ day$$

where 13.4 m^3/day is the daily alveolar ventilation rate of a 70 kg person based on a daily air intake of 20 m^3/day. Thus, the risk (R) to humans associated with 1μg/m^3 of PCE in air is

$$R = (2.7 \times 10^{-3}) \ (1.9 \times 10^{-4}) = 5.1 \times 10^{-7}$$

With Pharmacokinetics.   Based on the dose–response relationship between effective dose (metabolized dose) and cancer incidence (see Fig. 8), Travis *et al.* (1987b) estimated q_u to be 1.0×10^{-2} mg/kg per day expressed in terms of effective dose. Applications of the pharmacokinetic model indicates that a continuous exposure to 1 $\mu g/m^3$ of PCE results in an effective dose to the liver of 3.1×10^{-5} mg/kg per day. Thus, the risk to humans associated with 1 mg/m^3 of PCE in air is

$$R = (1.0 \times 10^{-2})\,(3.1 \times 10^{-5}) = 3.1 \times 10^{-7}$$

Thus, incorporation of pharmacokinetics into the risk assessment of PCE lowers the risk estimates by a factor of 1.6.

DISCUSSION

Studies in carcinogenesis are increasingly concerned with determining whether particular compounds produce tumors through direct action of the parent compound or through the indirect action of intermediate reactants produced during metabolism. Andersen *et al.* (1987) have demonstrated through the use of a pharmacokinetic model for methylene chloride (DCM) that the carcinogenic agent is an intermediate reactant produced along the linear GSH pathway. Travis *et al.* (1987b) suggest that the carcinogenicity of PCE is the product of the indirect activity of an intermediate reactant produced along the nonlinear MFO pathway. These examples illustrate the usefulness of pharmacokinetic models to assist in formulation of a hypothesis for the mechanism of tumorigenicity of a compound. We have also shown that pharmacokinetic models can be used to extrapolate pharmacokinetic responses to a chemical across species, and to investigate the effect of route of administration on dose to target tissue. Since pharmacokinetic models allow for a quantitative extrapolation of exposure data across species and between routes of administration, they provide a tool to quantitatively evaluate assumptions currently used in the risk assessment process. Their use in future risk assessments performed by federal agencies is recommended by the author.

REFERENCES

Adolph, E. F., 1949, Quantitative relations in the physiological constitutions of mammals, *Science* **109:**579–585.

Andersen, M. E., Gargas, M. L., Jones, R. A., and Jenkins, L. J., 1980, Determination of the kinetic constants for metabolism of inhaled toxicants *in vivo* using gas uptake measurements, *Toxicol. Appl. Pharmacol.* **54:**100–116.

Andersen, M. E., Clewell, H. J., III, Gargas, M. L., Smith, F. A., and Reitz, R. H., 1987, Physiologically-based pharmacokinetics and the risk assessment process for methylene chloride, *Toxicol. Appl. Pharmacol.* **87:**185–205.

Angelo, M. J., Pritchard, A. B., Hawkins, D. R., Waller, A. R., and Roberts, A., 1986, The pharmacokinetics of dichloromethane I: Disposition in B6C3F$_1$ mice following intravenous and oral administration, *Food Chem. Toxicol.* **24:**965–974.

Arms, A. D., and Travis, C. C., 1987, Reference physiological parameters in pharmacokinetic modeling (draft of manuscript).

Boxenbaum, H., and Ronfeld, R., 1983, Interspecies pharmacokinetic scaling and the Dedrick plots, *Am. J. Physiol.* **245**:R768–R775.

Brody, S., 1945, *Bioenergetics and Growth: With Special Reference to the Efficiency Complex in Domestic Animals,* Reinhold, New York.

Buben, J. A., and O'Flaherty, E. J., 1985, Delineation of the role of metabolism in the hepatotoxicity of trichloroethylene and perchloroethylene: a dose–effect study, *Toxicol. Appl. Pharmacol.* **78**:105–122.

Calder, W. A., 1974, Consequences of body size for Avian energetics, in: *Avian Energetics* (R. A. Paynter, ed.), pp. 86–151, Nuttall Ornithological Club, Cambridge.

Crouch, E. A. C., and Wilson, R., 1978, Interspecies comparison of carcinogenic potency, *J. Toxicol. Environ. Health* **5**:1095–1118.

Crump, K. S., and Guess, H. A., 1980, *Drinking Water and Cancer: Review of Recent Findings and Assessment of Risks,* Science Research Systems Inc., Ruston, Louisiana. CEQ Contract No. EQ10AC018.

Dedrick, R. L., 1973, Animal scale-up, *J. Pharmacokinet. Biopharm.* **1**:435–461.

Environmental Protection Agency (EPA), 1985, *Health Assessment Document for Tetrachloroethylene (Perchloroethylene),* U. S. EPA, Office of Research and Development, Office of Health and Environmental Assessment, Environmental Criteria and Assessment Office, Pub. No. EPA/600/8-82/005F (July, 1985).

Feldman, H. A., and McMahon, T. A., 1983, The 3/4 mass exponent for energy metabolism is not a statistical artifact, *Respir. Physiol.* **52**:149–163.

Fernandez, J., Guberan, E., and Caperos, J., 1976, Experimental human exposures to tetrachloroethylene vapor and elimination in breath after inhalation, *Am. Ind. Hyg. Assoc. J.* **37**:143–150.

Filser, J. G., and Bolt, H. M., 1979, Pharmacokinetics of halogenated ethylenes in rats, *Arch. Toxicol.* **3**:201–210.

Freireich, E. J., Gehan, E. A., Rall, D. P., Schmidt, L. H., and Skipper, H. E., 1966, Quantitative comparison of toxicity of anticancer agents in mouse, rat, hamster, dog, monkey, and man, *Cancer Chem. Reports* **50**(4):219–244.

Gargas, M. L., Clewell, H. J., III, and Andersen, M. E., 1986, Metabolism of inhaled dihalomethanes *in vivo:* Differentiation of kinetic constants for two independent pathways, *Toxicol. Appl. Pharmacol.* **82**:211–223.

Hoel, D. G., 1979, Low-dose and species to species extrapolation for chemically induced carcinogenesis, in: *Banbury Report No. 1: Assessing Chemical Mutagens: The Risk to Humans,* (V. McElheny, ed.), pp. 135–145, Cold Spring Harbor Laboratory, Cold Spring Harbor, New York.

Hogan, M., and Hoel, D. G., 1982, Extrapolation to man, in: *Principles of Toxicology* (A. W. Hayes, ed.), pp. 711–731, Raven Press, New York.

Holt, J. P., Rhode, E. A., and Kines, H., 1968, Ventricular volumes and body weight in mammals, *Am. J. Physiol.* **215**(3):704–715.

International Agency for Research on Cancer (IARC), 1979, *Monographs on the Evaluation of the Carcinogenic Risk of Chemicals to Humans, IARC* **20**:491–494.

Kleiber, M., 1932, Body size and metabolism, *Hilgardia* **6**:315–353.

Kleiber, M., 1947, Body size and metabolic rate, *Physiol. Rev.* **27**(4):511–541.

Kleiber, M., 1961, *The Fire of Life.* Wiley, New York.

Lindstedt, S. L., and Calder, W. A., 1981, Body size and physiological time, and longevity of homeothermic animals, *Q. Rev. Biol.* **56**:1–16.

McMahon, T., 1973, Size and shape in biology, *Science* **179**:1201–1204.

National Cancer Institute (NCI), 1977, *Bioassay of Tetrachloroethylene for Possible Carcinogenicity,* U. S. Department of Health, Education, and Welfare, Public Health Service, National Institutes of Health, DHEW Pub. No. (NIH) 77-813.

National Research Council (NRC), 1986, *Drinking Water and Health* (Richard D. Thomas, ed.), Safe Drinking Water Committee. Board on Toxicology and Environmental Health Hazards, Commission on Life Sciences. National Academy Press, Washington, D. C.

National Toxicology Program (NTP), 1985, *NTP Technical Report on the Toxicology and Carcinogenesis of Tetrachloroethylene (Perchloroethylene (CAS 127-18-4) in F344/N rats and B6C3F₁ mice (Inhalation studies).* U. S. Department of Health and Human Services, Public Health Service, National Institutes of Health NTP TR 311, NIH Pub. No. 85-2567 (August, 1985).

Pinkel, D., 1958, The use of body surface area as a criterion of drug dosage in cancer chemotherapy, *Cancer Res.* **18**(1):853–856.

Prothero, J., 1980, Scaling of blood parameters in mammals, *Comp. Biochem. Physiol.* **67**(A):649–657.

Ramsey, J. C., and Andersen, M. E., 1984, A physiologically-based description of the inhalation pharmacokinetics of styrene in rats and humans, *Toxicol. Appl. Pharmacol.* **73:**159–175.

Ramsey, J. C., Young, J. D., Karbowski, R., Chenoweth, M. B., McCarty, L. P., and Braun, W. H., 1980, Pharmacokinetics of inhaled styrene in human volunteers, *Toxicol. Appl. Pharmacol.* **53:**54–63.

Reitz, R. H., Fox, T. R., Ramsey, J. C., Quast, J. P., Langvardt, P. W., and Watanabe, P. G., 1982, Pharmacokinetics and macromolecular interactions of ethylene dichloride in rats after inhalation or gavage, *Toxicol. Appl. Pharmacol.* **62:**190–204.

Rubner, M., 1883, Ueber den Einsluss der Kopergross Stoff- und Kraftwechsel, *Z. Biol.* **19:**535.

Sato, A., and Nakajima, T., 1979, Partition coefficients of some aromatic hydrocarbons and ketones in water, blood and oil, *Br. J. Ind. Med.* **36:**231–234.

Schmidt-Nielsen, K., 1970, Energy metabolism, body size, and the problem of scaling, *Fed. Proc.* **29**(4)**:**1524–1532.

Schmidt-Nielsen, K., 1984, *Scaling: Why is Animal Size So Important?* Cambridge University Press, Cambridge.

Schumann, A. M., Quast, J. F., and Watanabe, P. G., 1980, The pharmacokinetics and macromolecular interactions of perchloroethylene in mice and rats as related to oncogenicity, *Toxicol. Appl. Pharmacol.* **55:**207–219.

Stahl, W. R., 1967, Scaling of respiratory variables in mammals, *J. Appl. Physiol.* **22:**453–460.

Travis, C. C., 1987, Interspecies and dose–route extrapolations, in: *Proceedings of the National Academy of Science Workshop on Pharmacokinetics*. Safe Drinking Water Committee, Subcommittee on Pharmacokinetics, Board on Environmental Studies and Toxicology, National Research Council.

Travis, C. C., Killman, R. R., Quillen, J. L., and Ward, R. C., 1987a, Pharmacokinetics of methyl chloroform, (manuscript submitted).

Travis, C. C., Killman, R. R., and Quillen, J. L., 1987b, Cancer risk of human exposure to tetrachloroethylene, (draft of manuscript).

Ward, R. C., Travis, C. C., Hetrick, D. M., Andersen, M. E., and Gargas, M. L., 1987, Pharmacokinetics of tetrachloroethylene, *Toxicol. Appl. Pharmacol.* (in press).

Young, J. D., Ramsey, J. C., Blau, G. E., Karbowski, R. J., Nitschke, K. D., Slauter, R. W., and Braun, W. H., 1979, Pharmacokinetics of inhaled or intraperitoneally administered styrene in rats, in: *Toxicology and Occupational Medicine: Proceedings of the Tenth Inter-American Conference on Toxicology and Occupational Medicine* (W. B. Deichmann, organizer), pp. 297–310, Elsevier/North-Holland, New York.

IV

Special Issues in Risk Assessment

8

Biologically-Based Models to Predict Cancer Risk

Gail Charnley and Todd W. Thorslund

Mathematical dose–response models are currently used to extrapolate cancer risk from the high dose levels used in laboratory bioassays to the low, environmental dose levels to which humans are generally exposed. These models are empirical in nature and lack a biological basis. It has long been recognized that the accuracy with which a mathematical model predicts cancer risks at low doses is dependent upon the validity of the underlying biological paradigm on which it is based. A model that is chosen because it provides a "best fit" to tumor data observed at high doses may greatly over- or underestimate risk at low doses. Historically, regulatory agencies have had to use the available models in the absence of more appropriate alternatives; however, this is no longer the case. Our understanding of the mechanisms of carcinogenesis has advanced to a point where use of a biologically-based cancer model is now feasible.

This chapter describes the emerging consensus on the mechanisms of carcinogenesis and how mathematical models can take such mechanisms into account when used to predict cancer risk at low doses. Two examples are given in which biologically-based models are used to predict cancer risk for specific chemicals.

MECHANISMS OF CARCINOGENESIS

Animal experiments involving different tumor sites, such as skin, liver, breast, and bladder, have permitted the identification and characterization of two primary stages of carcinogenesis, initiation and promotion, both of which are influenced by cell proliferation.

Gail Charnley and Todd W. Thorslund • Clement Associates, Inc., Fairfax, Virginia 22031.

The initiation phase is characterized by an irreversible alteration in the genetic expression of a cell that produces a heritable change in the cell's phenotype. Berenblum and Shubik's (1947) early skin painting studies demonstrated that exposure to an initiating agent produced changes in tissue that persisted for many months following termination of exposure. Experiments with radiation and chemically induced mutagenesis have indicated that at least one round of cell proliferation is required before the mutational change becomes permanent and cannot be repaired (Borek and Sachs, 1968; Kakunaga, 1974). Because of these characteristics, many believe that initiation involves a mutational event in a cell's DNA. A second mutational change is thought to be necessary before a partially transformed cell becomes fully malignant (Land *et al.*, 1983). The actual mechanisms involved in these cellular events are unknown, but it is hypothesized that they involve oncogenes (Hennings *et al.*, 1983).

The promotion phase is less well characterized. Many believe that it involves differential selection of initiated cells (e.g., an increased rate of cell division or increased resistance to terminal differentiation) followed by clonal expansion of these selected cells. This phase is thought to involve epigenetic changes such as modifications in cell-to-cell communication through gap junctions (Trosko *et al.*, 1983). Many researchers emphasize the importance in the cancer process of the clonal expansion of preneoplastic cells. They note that increasing the number of cells that are one mutational change away from being fully malignant will increase the likelihood that malignant tumors will develop.

The kinetics of cell proliferation appear to be an important aspect of both the initiation and promotion phases of the carcinogenic process (Farber, 1984).

TWO-STAGE MATHEMATICAL MODELS

Various investigators have postulated mathematical models that are consistent with a number of the experimental findings discussed in the previous section. Notable among these is that of Armitage and Doll (1957), who proposed that a cell can be transformed into a premalignant cell as a result of chemical exposure and that the premalignant cell proliferates at a constant rate, producing a clone of exponentially growing preneoplastic cells. A preneoplastic cell can then be transformed into a cancerous cell, which may ultimately develop into a tumor.

A mathematical model has been developed by Moolgavkar and Venzon (1979) and Moolgavkar and Knudson (1981) that is based on a two-stage theory for carcinogenesis. This model is depicted in Fig. 1. According to the model, the population of cells at risk are proliferating cells, often referred to as stem cells. Stem cells are those from which most other cells in an organ arise. A cell can differentiate and leave the pool of proliferating cells and no longer be susceptible to heritable alterations of its DNA. A normal, susceptible stem cell may do one of several things. It may divide into two daughter stem cells, terminally differentiate, die, or undergo mutation at a critical site that results in formation of a preneoplastic or intermediate cell. A preneoplastic cell has undergone one of the changes necessary to become a cancer cell but is not yet cancerous. The preneoplastic cell may, in turn, divide into two daughter preneoplastic cells, differentiate, die, or undergo further mutation at another critical site to produce a cancerous cell. The cancerous cell will, after a sufficient length of time, divide into enough cells that it

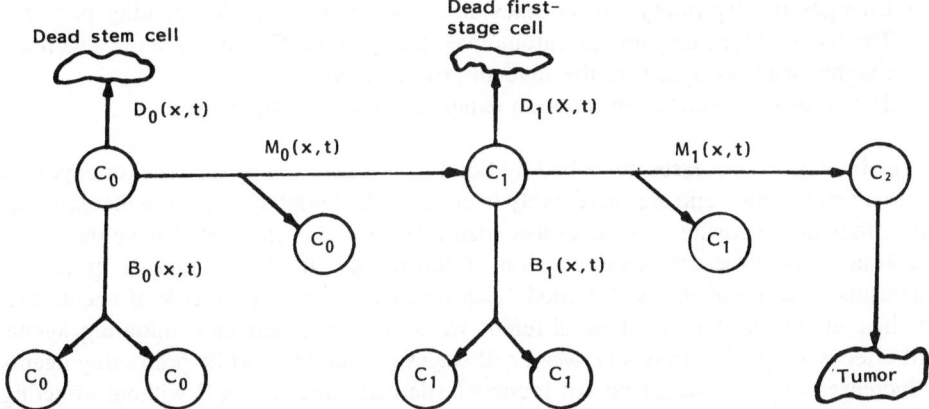

Figure 1. General biological structure underlying exposure- and time-dependent M-V-K model. C_0 is a normal, susceptible stem cell; C_1 is a preneoplastic, first-stage cell, which can proliferate into a premalignant clone; C_2 is a cancerous cell that will eventually develop into a detectable tumor; $D_0(x,t)$, $B_0(x,t)$, and $M_0(x,t)$ are the exposure- and time-dependent death, birth, and transition or mutation rates for the normal stem cell; $D_1(x,t)$, $B_1(x,t)$, and $M_1(x,t)$ are the exposure- and time-dependent death, birth, and transition or mutation rates for the first-stage cell; x is the exposure level, which is assumed to be constant over time; t is the age of the subject.

becomes a detectable tumor. All of these processes can be described mathematically by postulating specific rates for the cell changes. Moolgavkar and Knudson (1981) showed that to a close approximation, the age-specific tumor rate at time t for their two-stage model may be expressed as:

$$I(t) = M_0 M_1 \int_0^t C_0(v) \, exp \, [(B - D) \, (t - v)] \, dv \qquad (1)$$

where $I(t)$ is the age-specific cancer incidence at age t, M_0 is the transition rate from stem to preoplastic cell, M_1 is the transition rate from preneoplastic to cancerous cell, $C_0(v)$ is the number of susceptible stem cells per individual target organ at age v, B is the birth rate or rate of cell proliferation of preneoplastic cells, and D is the death rate of preneoplastic cells.

Essentially, the equation describes the progression from a normal stem cell to a cancerous cell under the assumptions of the two-stage model. This model is a combination of deterministic and stochastic components. The numbers of preneoplastic and fully malignant cells at any time are assumed to be random variables that are dependent upon these event rates, while the number of normal cells at risk of transformation at time t, denoted by $C_0(t)$, is assumed to be deterministic and known.

Using this carcinogenesis model, Moolgavkar and Knudson (1981) successfully described or explained such phenomena as:

- Genetic predisposition to cancer.
- Patterns in childhood cancer rates.
- Hormonally influenced changes in breast cancer rates.

- Changes in respiratory cancer rates associated with variable smoking patterns.
- The fact that for many human carcinomas, the age-specific incidence rates increase roughly with the fourth to the seventh power of age.
- The results of initiation-promotion experiments for multiple agents.

The biological processes described by Eq. 1 can be affected by the level of exposure to carcinogenic agents, and are more likely to occur as the length of exposure increases; as a result, they are exposure- and time-dependent. Thorslund *et al.* (1987) have described an exposure- and time-dependent version of the model. In the context of biological mechanisms of carcinogenesis, the model can be used to predict the risk of agents that exert their effects in a number of different ways. Mutation-inducing initiating agents would affect the transition rates between cell stages (M_0 or M_1), while promoting agents may increase the proliferation rate of preneoplastic cells (increasing B without affecting D). Cocarcinogens may increase the proliferation rate of normal stem cells (C_0), thereby increasing the size of the target for initiating agents. Inhibitors could remove cells from the populations of susceptible stem or preneoplastic cells through toxicity (e.g., increasing D without affecting B) or by inducing differentiation. Within the context of the model, the following observations can be explained:

- Tumor rates at very high experimental doses are often lower than at lower doses, even after adjusting for differential mortality, as a result of high-dose toxicity to stem and preneoplastic cells.
- Exposure to multiple carcinogens can give antagonistic, additive, multiplicative, or super-multiplicative tumor rate responses by affecting different model parameters.
- Such a response to combined agents appears to be dose-dependent because some responses such as increased stem cell proliferation may both occur and have an impact on tumor rates only at high doses.
- Some preneoplastic, benign cell masses that may be precursors of tumors will regress and disappear upon cessation of exposure as a result of a decline in the birth rate and no change in the death rate of such cells.

APPLICATIONS OF THE TWO-STAGE MODEL

Specific forms of the biologically-based two-stage model can be postulated for individual or combinations of carcinogenic agents. Tumor dose response data and any available supplemental information such as rates of DNA adduct formation and increased cell proliferation can be used to estimate the parameters in the models. The nature of the specific dose–response relationships that result will differ for chemicals that have different mechanisms of action such as genotoxic and nongenotoxic agents (e.g., promoters). This section gives examples of how the two-stage model can be applied to agents that are thought to have different biological mechanisms.

Genotoxic Agent: Benzo[a]pyrene

Benzo[a]pyrene (B[a]P) is a carcinogenic polycyclic aromatic hydrocarbon that occurs ubiquitously in air and soil as a product of combustion. B[a]P can be metabolically activated to form derivatives that can react with DNA (Sims and Grover, 1974; Gelboin, 1980; Weinstein *et al.*, 1978). If B[a]P-DNA adducts occur at critical sites that control the regulation of a cell's growth or differentiation, mutations may occur that can lead to cell transformation and ultimately, cancer. Because the experimental evidence (Lee and O'Neil, 1971) strongly suggests that B[a]P is a genotoxic agent acting in at least two sites on DNA, the two-stage model is a useful approach for estimating the cancer risk associated with exposure to B[a]P. Without intermediary experimental information about cell stages and differences in exposure over time, however, it is not possible to estimate the individual background and exposure-induced mutation rates for preneoplastic and transformed cells using tumor rate data from a standard animal carcinogenesis bioassay, nor can the relative transition rates that correspond to each stage be identified. What can be estimated from bioassay data are two exposure-induced relative transition rates and a background transition rate. In the absence of information to the contrary, the assumption can be made that the transition rates from normal to preneoplastic and preneoplastic to cancerous cells are equally likely. If these transition rates are linear functions of dose (which is likely at low doses) and the growth rate of preneoplastic cells is independent of exposure level, the probability that a tumor will develop by time t as a result of exposure to a level of genotoxic agent x can be expressed as:

$$P(x,t) = 1 - exp\{-M(1 + Sx)^2 \, [exp \, (Gt) - 1 - Gt]/G^2\} \tag{2}$$

where M is the background tumor-rate parameter, S is the exposure-dependent transition rate between cell stages, G is $B - D$ and is the exposure-dependent growth rate of preneoplastic cells, and t is the the time (or age) at which risk is evaluated. The level of x at the target tissue is assumed to be directly related to the administered dose.

A chronic study of B[a]P by Thyssen *et al.* (1981) provided clearcut evidence of a does–response relationship between inhaled B[a]P and tumorigenesis. In this experiment, Syrian golden hamsters were exposed throughout their lives to B[a]P by means of a sodium chloride aerosol for 4.5 hr per day, 7 days per week, for 10 weeks, and then for 3 hr per day thereafter. Respiratory tract tumors were induced in the nasal cavity, larynx, and trachea. The dose–response relationship obtained for these tumors is shown in Table 1.

Using the average survival time as the length of observation, the two-stage model (Eq. 2) was fitted to the observed data; cancer risk at the end of the average lifetime of each exposure group can be obtained for B[a]P from the following equation:

$$P(x,t) = 1 - exp \, [-0.000115(1 + 0.312x)^2][exp(0.57t) - 1 - 0.057t]$$

Table 1 shows that the number of tumors predicted by the equation is quite similar to the

Table 1. Data Used to Estimate Dose–Response Relationship between Inhaled B[a]P and Respiratory Tract Tumors[a]

Exposure rate (x) (mg B[a]P/m^3 air)	Average survival time (weeks)	Number of exposed animals	Number of respiratory tract tumors	
			Predicted	Observed
0	96.4	27	0.73	0
2.2	95.2	27	1.88	0
9.5	96.4	26	9.06	9
46.5	59.5	25	12.59	13

[a]From Thyssen *et al.* (1981).

number observed. If the time of observation (average survival) had been assumed to be constant between exposure groups, Eq. 2 reduces to the simplified quadratic form:

$$P(x) = 1 - exp - A(1 + Sx)^2 \qquad (3)$$

where A is the background transition rate between cell stages. Substituting the control group survival time of 96.4 weeks into the numerical form of the equation yields:

$$P(x) = 1 - exp\ [-0.0272\ (1 + 0.312x)^2] $$

Nongenotoxic Agent: Diethylhexyl Phthalate

Diethylhexyl phthalate (DEHP) is a widely-used plasticizer that has been shown to increase the rate of liver tumors in the $B6C3F_1$ strain of mouse, which has a high spontaneous liver tumor rate (NTP, 1983). DEHP increases the rate of cell proliferation in the mouse liver (Smith-Oliver *et al.*, 1985), and in light of its lack of mutagenic and initiating activity in most *in vitro* and animal models (NAS, 1985), it may be hypothesized to exert its carcinogenic activity by increasing the number of mitotic divisions in the liver. Increasing the number of mitotic divisions increases the likelihood that cells with a neoplastic phenotype may be expressed (Peraino *et al.*, 1983). The likelihood of developing a tumor under these assumptions is proportional to the number of susceptible cells times the rate of cell proliferation. The rate of cell proliferation can be measured by an autoradiographically determined [^{3}H]thymidine labeling index. This relative index may be denoted as $r(x)$. As a first approximation, the number of susceptible cells may be taken to be proportional to the organ weight. Thus, the effects of an agent on the total number of mitotic divisions of a susceptible cell in an organ at time t may be expressed as:

$$C_0(x,t) = vW_0(x,t)r(x,t) \qquad (4)$$

where $W_0(x,t)$ and $r(x,t)$ are the organ weight and labeling index, given exposure at level x for a duration of time t, and v is the number of susceptible cells per unit of weight. As a first approximation, the proliferating cells are assumed to be at equilibrium for each exposure level. This assumption is expressed mathematically as $C_0(x) = vW_0(x)r(x)$. Treating all other parameters as fixed constants, substituting Eq. 4 into Eq. 1, and integrating gives the following expression for the age-specific death rate:

$$I(x,t) = vM_0M_1W_0(x)r(x) \, [exp(B - D) \, t - 1]/(B - D) \tag{5}$$

The risk by age t in the absence of competing mortality is

$$P(x,t) = 1 - exp - \int_0^t I(x,v)dv \tag{6}$$

Substituting Eq. 5 into Eq. 6 and integrating yields the result

$$P(x,t) = 1 - exp - \{[vM_0M_1W_0(x)r(x)][(exp \, Gt) - 1 - Gt]/G^2\} \tag{7}$$

where $G = B - D$, which is the net growth rate of preneoplastic cells.

An implicit assumption in this derivation is that any increase in the birth rate of the preneoplastic cells caused by an agent is matched by an increase in the overall death rate, so that the net growth rate, G, remains stable.

In the absence of time-to-tumor data, the response at the end of a bioassay may be expressed as

$$P(x) = 1 - exp - MR(x) \tag{8}$$

where $R(x)$, the relative increase in total mitotic activity, equals $W_0(x)r(x)/W_0(0)r(0)$, and M, a combination of unknown parameters that can be estimated with a minimal amount of bioassay data, equals $vM_0M_1W_0(0)r(0)[(exp \, Gt) - 1 - Gt]/G^2$.

Table 2 shows the National Toxicology Program's (NTP) carcinogenesis bioassay data on DEHP (NTP, 1983). These data can be used to test the hypothesis that the carcinogenesis rate is proportional to the number of mitotic divisions. A limited amount of data currently exists concerning liver proliferation as a response to the ingestion of DEHP. Butterworth and his colleagues (Smith-Oliver *et al.*, 1985; B. E. Butterworth, personal communication) measured the labeling index and liver weights in rats exposed to 6000 parts per million (ppm) DEHP in their diets. The labeling index increased initially and

Table 2. Tumor Incidence in B6C3F₁ Mice Fed DEHP[a]

Exposure (ppm)	Relative liver weight [$R(x)$]	Observed tumor rates[b]	Predicted tumor rate[c]
0	1	14/50	17.4/50
3000	—[d]	25/48	—
6000	1.73	29/50	26.1/50

[a]From NTP (1983).
[b]Hepatocellular carcinomas or adenomas.
[c]$P(x) = 1 - exp - 0.426R(x)$
[d]Liver weight information not available at this exposure level.

then returned to normal after 28 days. During the same 28-day period, the relative increase in liver weight was 1.73, which remained stable over time. The underlying hypothesis that the total number of mitotic divisions of the susceptible cells in the liver is proportional to the cancer rate can be tested using the control and 6000 ppm exposure groups. After an equilibrium in liver weight is reached at 28 days, the total number of mitotic divisions is proportional to this weight. For $x = 6000$ ppm, it follows that $R(x)$ is approximately 1.73. Using the control and 6000 ppm exposure groups and Eq. 8, the maximum likelihood estimate of the unknown parameter is $M = 0.426$. On the basis of this value, the expected cancer rates are computed and shown in Table 2. The observed results are consistent with the hypothesis that the cancer rate is proportional to the total number of mitotic divisions of susceptible cells in the liver, however, more complete data are required for further substantiation.

CONCLUSIONS

A mathematical dose response model for estimating cancer risk has been developed that is predicated on some knowledge of the biological mechanisms of carcinogenesis. The model can account for agents that act by genotoxic or nongenotoxic mechanisms as well as cocarcinogens or inhibitors of carcinogenesis by incorporating parameters that depend on mutation rates as well as cell proliferation rates, both of which play important roles in the process. As a result, it may be possible to estimate parameters in the model for a particular agent or mixture of agents using experimental information from bioassays other than chronic carcinogenicity tests if the latter is unavailable. Furthermore, knowledge of differences in mutation or cell proliferation rates between species would lead to more meaningful inter-species extrapolations than the surface area or body weight adjustments currently used.

REFERENCES

Armitage, P., and Doll, R., 1957, A two-stage theory of carcinogenesis in relation to the age distribution of human cancer, *Br. J. Cancer* **11**:161–169.

Berenblum, I., and Shubik, P., 1947, A new, quantitative approach to the study of the stages of chemical carcinogenesis in the mouse's skin, *Br. J. Cancer* **1**:383–391.

Borek, C., and Sachs, L., 1968, The number of cell generations required to fix the transformed state, *Proc. Natl. Acad. Sci. USA* **59**:83–85.

Farber, E., 1984, The multistep nature of cancer development, *Cancer Res.* **44**:4217–4223.

Gelboin, H. W., 1980, Benzo[a]pyrene metabolism, activation, and carcinogenesis: Role and regulation of mixed-function oxidases and related enzymes, *Physiol. Rev.* **60**:1107–1166.

Hennings, H., Shores, R., Wenk, M. L., Spangler, E. F., Tarone, R., and Yuspa, S. H., 1983, Malignant conversion of mouse skin tumors is increased by tumor initiators and unaffected by tumor parameters, *Nature* **304**:67–69.

Kakunaga, T., 1974, Requirement for cell replication in the fixation and expression of the transformed state in mouse cells treated with 4-nitroquinoline-1-oxide, *Int. J. Cancer* **14**:736–742.

Klein, G., and Klein, E., 1985, Evaluation of tumors and the impact of molecular oncology, *Nature* **315**:190–195.

Land, H., Parada, L. F., and Weinberg, R. A., 1983, Cellular oncogenes and multistep carcinogenesis, *Science* **222:**771–777.

Lee, P. N., and O'Neil, J. A., 1971, The effect both of time and dose applied on tumor incidence rate in benzpyrene skin painting experiments, *Br. J. Cancer* **25:**759–770.

Moolgavkar, S. H., and Venzon, D. J., 1979, Two-event models for carcinogenesis: incidence curves for childhood and adult tumors, *Math. Biosci.* **47:**55–77.

Moolgavkar, S. H., and Knudson, A. G., Jr., 1981, Mutation and cancer: A model for human carcinogenesis, *J. Natl. Cancer Inst.* **66:**1037–1052.

National Academy of Sciences (NAS), 1985, *Drinking Water and Health,* Vol. 6, pp. 53–74, National Academy Press, Washington, D.C.

National Toxicology Program (NTP), 1983, *Carcinogenesis Bioassay of di(2-ethylhexyl)phthalate (CAS No. 117-81-7) in F344 rates and B6C3F1 Mice (Feed Study),* NTP Technical Report Series No. 217, NIH Publication No. 82-1773, U.S. Department of Health and Human Services, Washington, D.C.

Peraino, C., Richards, W. L., and Stevens, F. J., 1983, Multistage hepatocarcinogenesis, in: *Mechanisms of Tumor Promotion, Vol. 1: Tumor Promotion in Internal Organs* (T. J. Slaga, ed.), pp. 1–53, CRC Press, Boca Raton, Florida.

Sims, P., and Grover, P. L., 1974, Epoxides in polycyclic aromatic hydrocarbon metabolism and carcinogenesis, *Adv. Cancer Res.* **20:**165–274.

Smith-Oliver, T., Loury, D., and Butterworth, B. E., 1985, Measurement of DNA repair and cell proliferation in hepatocytes from mice treated with di(2-ethylhexyl)phthalate (DEHP), *Environ. Mutagen.* **7** (Suppl. 3)**:**71 (abstr).

Thorslund, T. W., Brown, C. C., and Charnley, G., 1987, The use of biologically motivated mathematical models to predict the actual cancer risk associated with environmental exposure to a carcinogen, *J. Risk Anal.* (in press).

Thyssen, J., Althoff, J., Kimmerle, G., and Mohr, U., 1981, Inhalation studies with benzo[a]pyrene in Syrian golden hamsters, *J. Natl. Cancer Inst.* **66:**575–577.

Trosko, J. E., Chang, C., and Medcalf, A., 1983, Mechanisms of tumor promotion: Potential role of intercellular communication, *Cancer Invest.* **1:**511–526.

Weinstein, I. B., Jeffrey, A. M., Leffler, S., Pulkrabek, P., Yamasaki, H., and Grunberger, D., 1978, Interactions between polycyclic aromatic hydrocarbons and cellular macromolecules, in: *Polycyclic Hydrocarbons and Cancer, Vol. 2: Molecular and Cell Biology* (P. O. P. Ts'o and H. V. Gelboin, eds.), pp. 3–26, Academic Press, New York.

9

Animal Extrapolation and the Challenge of Human Interindividual Variation

Edward J. Calabrese

Introduction

There are a number of biological factors which may enhance one's susceptibility to experience adverse health effects from exposure to toxic substances, including carcinogens. These include one's age, sex, genetic composition, nutritional status, and preexisting disease conditions (Calabrese, 1978, 1984, 1985, 1986; Propping, 1978).

The extent or magnitude to which predisposing factors enhance susceptibility to toxic substances is known only to a limited extent. The conventional wisdom employed in regulatory toxicology has been to assume that most toxic substances can be accounted for by a factor of 10 (NAS, 1977).

This position was supported in part by Dourson and Stara (1983) who reviewed the response of rodents to acute toxicity for a large number of agents. They found that a 10-fold decrease in dose would reduce the median exposure for an LD_{50} to below the general range expected to result in death from 92% of the individual compounds studied. Since these slopes were obtained with laboratory rats, it is expected that they would have less variation in response to toxic substances than the highly outbred and more heterogeneous human population. Thus, human heterogeneity in response to toxic agents would be expected to be much greater than that in widely used, highly inbred rodent model strains. Given the limited capacity for highly inbred rodent strains to accurately predict the range of human responses, the determination of the extent of interindividual variation among humans in response to toxic agents is an important factor that needs to be documented. This information is necessary to establish the biological basis of the uncertainty (safety)

Edward J. Calabrese • Environmental Science Program, Division of Public Health, University of Massachusetts, Amherst, Massachusetts 01003.

factor of 10 currently recommended for human species variation by the National Academy of Sciences (NAS, 1977) and used by the Environmental Protection Agency (EPA, 1976) in establishing acceptable exposure standards for noncarcinogens. Unfortunately, when the use of such an uncertainty factor has been recommended (NAS, 1977), it has not been accompanied by supportive documentation. Similarly, the problem of human heterogeneity with respect to responses to carcinogenic agents becomes evident when one realizes that prediction of human cancer risk, using quantitative risk assessment biomathematical models applied to bioassay data, assumes that the human distribution of sensitivities will be described by the inbred animal model response. Thus, current approaches for predicting human cancer risks from animal studies do not address the occurrence of human heterogeneity.

This chapter will examine the range of human responses with respect to the degree of variation in xenobiotic metabolism and other relevant end points associated with susceptibility to carcinogenic agents. These data will establish the magnitude of the range of human variation to a number of variables thought to affect susceptibility to cancer-causing agents. A similar examination of animal model variation will be made and then compared to the human response. This comparison will permit an assessment of where the range of human responses lie with respect to various animal responses.

VARIATION IN RESPONSE TO SELECTED XENOBIOTICS

Acetylation

Human. Certain aromatic amines are known to be animal and human carcinogens. These substances tend to be metabolized by acetylation. Within the human population there are both fast and slow acetylators which occupy roughly equal proportions (i.e., 50% : 50%) among Causasians and Blacks in the United States (Calabrese, 1984). Assessment of the acetylation rate of about a dozen aromatic amines by humans revealed a variation of from 3.7- to 13-fold between slow and fast acetylators (Glowinski *et al.*, 1978).

Animal. In 1973, Lower and Bryan (1973) assessed the relative capability of *N*-acetyltransferase enzyme systems from liver cytosol of various mammalian species (i.e. hamsters, guinea pigs, mice, and rats) to carry out *N*-acetylation of three carcinogens: 2-aminofluorene (2-AF), 4-aminobiphenyl, and 2-aminonaphthalene. Relative to the rat, which is arbitrarily given 1 as a value, the enzymatic activity of the mouse is 8, the guinea pig is 12, and the hamster is 18. In contrast, dog cytosol was incapable of carrying out detectable *N*-acetylation of any of the three carcinogenic arylamines studied.

Unlike the above-mentioned species, it is well-known that rabbits and humans display a genetic polymorphism with respect to *N*-acetyltransferase activity towards isoniazid (INH) and several other arylamine drugs, including sulfapyridine, hydralazine, and procainamide. In the case of INH, slow acetylator humans are known to be at increased risk for developing peripheral neuropathies (Devadatta, 1960) while fast acetylators are at increased risk of developing hepatitis (Mitchell *et al.*, 1976). Lower *et al.* (1979) have developed the hypothesis that acetylator phenotype is a risk factor in the development of arylamine-induced bladder cancer in humans. They presented evidence that the *N*-hydroxylated nonacetylated metabolite of the arylamine is the bladder carcinogen. Thus, one's risk may be a function of the capacity to acetylate and deacetylate arylamines following *N*-hydroxylation.

As a result of the recognition that both rabbits and humans display a genetic polymorphism with respect to acetylation, it has been speculated that the rabbit may be an effective predictive animal model for population-based responses. In a direct comparison partially addressing this issue, Glowinski *et al.* (1978) compared the rates of acetylation in both fast and slow acetylator phenotypes in rabbits and humans for seven agents including five arylamine carcinogens [a-naphthylamine, benzidine, β-naphthylamine, 2-AF, and methylene bis(*o*-chloroaniline) (MOCA)]. In general, it was found that the fast acetylator rabbit displayed a rate of activity of from 10- to 50-fold greater than the fast acetylator human. As for the slow acetylator rabbit, its activities range from 1/190 to 1/580 of the fast rabbit acetylator. However, its activity levels were generally in the range displayed by both fast and slow human acetylators, depending on the substrate. For example, the slow acetylator rabbit was very similar to the slow human acetylator for 2-AF (0.013 vs. 0.021 μmole/mg per hr) and benzidine (0.016 vs 0.019 μmole/mg per hr) but more closely comparable to the human fast acetylator for β-naphthylamine (0.28 vs. 0.23 μmole/mg per hr).

The net result of such comparisons is that the rat (Sprague–Dawley (SD) female) and the slow acetylator New Zealand rabbit (both sexes) displayed *N*-acetylator activity for several substrates thought to be carcinogens in the range of both human fast and slow acetylators. In general, the hamster, guinea pig, and mouse displayed acetylation activity which was markedly greater than that displayed by the human fast acetylator.

Deacetylation

The capacity to deacetylate carcinogenic arylacetamides has been shown by Lower and Bryan (1973) to be a significant risk factor affecting the occurrence of bladder cancer in the dog. This hypothesis is derived from observations indicating that the *N*-hydroxy-nonacetylated metabolite is believed to be the carcinogenic agent. Thus, as a result of the ability of the dog to *N*-hydroxylate the aromatic amines but its poor ability to acetylate such compounds, the dog displayed an increased risk of bladder cancer. Similarly, with exposure to carcinogenic arylacetamides, the dog expressed an enhanced risk to bladder cancer from the capacity to *N*-hydroxylate the agent and then to deacetylate it. It is important to recognize that while nonacetylated arylamines which have been *N*-hydroxylated are likely candidates for bladder carcinogens, the *N*-hydroxylated acetylated arylamines are likely candidates for liver carcinogens. Thus, it is seen that enzymes carrying out the *N*-acetylation and deacetylation of arylamines and arylacetamides, respectively, seem to play a role as a determinant of susceptibility to liver and bladder cancer.

The relative capacity of the animal model to acetylate and deacetylate is then an important variable with respect to arylamine induced cancer. In the rat and mouse, the ratio of *N*-acetyltransferase to deacetylase activity is very high relative to the dog. This may provide rodents with some protection against bladder cancer but not for heptatocarcinogenesis (Lower and Bryan, 1973, 1976).

In terms of humans, little is known about the range of variation with respect to deacetylation. However, *in vivo* studies with acetanilide indicate that humans (and rabbits) in contrast to dogs are poor deacetylators of acetylated aromatic amines (Williams, 1959).

Given the greater ability of humans to acetylate than the dog and the lower human capacity to deacetylate aromatic amines, it is likely that humans, especially the fast acetylator phenotypes, would be at considerably lower risk of developing an arylamine bladder cancer than dogs. Finally, it has been recently shown that rat interstrain differences exist with respect to hepatic *N*-acetyltransferases with the magnitude of difference between rapid and slow acetylators similar to that in humans. These new findings appear to be of potential value in more successfully addressing the issue of human heterogenicity for this risk factor (Bond *et al.*, 1986).

Debrisoquine Oxidation

Human.   Among humans, interindividual variations exist with respect to the oxidation of carbon centers in several drugs including debrisoquine, guanoxan, and phenacetin. With respect to debrisoquine, it has been suggested by Mbanebo *et al.* (1980) that at least two alleles occur in the population that affect the oxidation of this antihypertensive drug. The two alleles have been designated D^H (extensive hydroxylation of debrisoquine) and D^L (low hydroxylation). Persons who display homozygosity for the D^L allele show a significantly reduced capacity to metabolize the drug and excrete it, for the most part, unchanged. Those persons homozygous for the D^L allele make up what is called by Mbanebo *et al.* (1980) the poor metabolizing (PM) phenotype. Individuals who are designated as genotypically homozygous D^H or heterozygous are known to readily hydroxylate debrisoquine, and they constitute what is called the extensive metabolizing (EM) phenotype. The quotient, percent dose eliminated as unchanged debrisoquine/percent dose excreted as 4-hydroxydebrisoquine in the urine after a single 10-mg oral dose, is bimodally distributed and referred to as the "metabolic ratio." The EM phenotype exhibits metabolic ratios in the range of 0.01–10.0, while the PM phenotype displays metabolic ratios in the range of 18–200. If one considered the extreme range of values given for the metabolic ratios of 0.01 to 200, a difference of 20,000-fold metabolic variation is seen in humans. However, it should be pointed out that the majority (75–85%) of persons tested fall within a 10-fold range (Idle and Smith, 1979).

Animal.   Al-Dabbagh *et al.* (1980) noted marked interstrain differences with respect to the metabolic ratio of debrisoquine and phenacetin in rat strains. The DA rat displayed a metabolic ratio for debrisoquine of 4.7 while the Lewis rat had a metabolic ratio of 0.29. These values tended to simulate the activity for human poor (PM) and extensive metabolizers (EM), respectively.

Aryl Hydrocarbon Hydroxylase (AHH) Variation

Human.   Interindividual variation of benzo[a]anthracene-induced AHH activity in mitogen-activated human lymphocytes ($N = 300$ people) was about 40-fold (Kouri *et al.*, 1984). Harris *et al.* (1984) reported that interindividual differences in AHH activities also occur in other tissues, including several hundred-fold in the placenta and less than 20-fold in the skin, kidney, and bronchus. With respect to hepatic variation of AHH, Pelkonen *et al.* (1975) reported a variation of 16-fold based on samples from patients with various types of diseases, including cholelithiasis, icterus, cancer, liver injury, and others.

Animal. Pelkonen *et al.* (1975) assessed the level of AHH activity in livers from adult humans, different strains of rats (noninbred SD, inbred SD, DA, Fischer, and Wister), guinea pigs, and rabbits. Based on mean values, the activity of AHH for humans was about 30–60% that of the male rat liver depending on the strain of rat. No sex differences occur for humans while the female rat displayed about 20–40% that of the male rat liver. Interestingly, the range of human values was from approximately 20 to 320 pmole/g of liver per min with the mean being 100 units. This places the human lower range in the vicinity of the female inbred rat which has activity from about 15–20. However, the upper range of human activity is in the activity zone of the male rat. Therefore, the upper and lower tails of the human distribution appear to be in the range of activity of the animal model.

Consideration of rabbits yielded a generally similar but somewhat lower (~60 units) activity than humans along with no sex difference. Interestingly, rabbits, like humans, are also highly outbred. This may have contributed to the nearly six-fold range in rabbit AHH activity (Pelkonen *et al.*, 1975). With respect to the C3H mouse strain, the activity for males and females are about three-fold that of the male inbred SD rat. This places the C3H mouse in the approximate range of 350–450 activity units with a small standard deviation (Oesch, 1973).

While it is instructive to see such comparisons, it is important not to lose sight of the fact that we are concerned with the total bioactivation–detoxification balance in the liver and elsewhere.

Carcinogen Binding to DNA

Human. Many chemical carcinogens are DNA-reactive or genotoxic. Either the parent molecule (activation-independent carcinogens) or a metabolite (activation-dependent carcinogens) are electrophilic reactants that can interact with the nucleophilic centers of biological macromolecules such as DNA to form DNA adducts. This is considered to be an initiation step in the multistage carcinogenic process, since the formation of DNA adducts may lead to mutations if the damage is not repaired (Williams and Weisburger, 1986).

Trachea/bronchus. Benzo[a]pyrene (B[a]P) binding to DNA in cultured human bronchial tissue was found to vary from one- to 150-fold, with $N = 19$ subjects. The range of variation is reduced to about nine-fold for 80% of the group studied (Harris *et al.*, 1984).

Colon. Benzo[a]pyrene binding to DNA in cultured human colonic tissue has been found to vary over an approximately 30-fold range with an $N = 63$. Approximately 90% of the individuals were within a 15-fold range (Harris *et al.*, 1984). However, Autrup *et al.* (1978) found a 100-fold variation in the binding of BP to human colonic tissue among 32 individuals. Approximately 80% of those studied were within a factor of 10.

Esophagus. Benzo[a]pyrene binding to DNA in cultured human esophageal tissue varied over a 20-fold range; however, only six subjects were employed (Harris *et al.*, 1984).

Animal

Trachea/bronchus. While only limited direct animal model comparisons with humans have been conducted, Autrup *et al.* (1980b) found that the Syrian golden hamster displayed on average about 2.5 times as much *in vitro* binding of B[a]P to tracheal DNA as did the human. The human variation ranged from 3–17 units or a nearly six-fold range of variation. Little variation occurred for the hamster (26–27 units). Mouse (DBA) and rat (CD) trachea averaged 9.25 with a narrow range of variation of 9–11 units. In partial contrast to the previous study, Daniel *et al.* (1983) revealed a similar binding capacity of B[a]P to DNA between the human and hamster with the rat, dog, and monkey showing progressively lower binding in studies conducted using tissue explants.

Colon. In 1980, Autrup *et al.* (1980a) evaluated the capacity of three carcinogens [aflatoxin (AFB), B[a]P, and dimethylhydrazine (DMH)] to bind to the DNA of cultured rat (male CD, 4–5 weeks old) and human colonic tissue (nontumorous). They found that the mean level for binding of AFB and DMH to colonic DNA was significantly higher ($P < 0.01$) in the rat than human by 8.3-fold and two-fold, respectively. No statistically significant differences were found to occur for B[a]P binding. Of great interest is that the human colonic DNA displayed wide interindividual variation in binding levels for all three carcinogens: AFB (70-fold, 24 cases), B[a]P (130-fold, 103 cases), and DMH (80-fold, 66 cases). In contrast, the standard deviation of the rat with respect to a percentage of the mean value for AFB, B[a]P, and DMH were 1.5%, 8.2%, and 2.3%, respectively. For humans the comparable values were 126%, 99%, and 103%.

DISCUSSION

The previous information has indicated that there is extensive variation in the human population to biochemical parameters which are believed to be associated with important phases of the process of carcinogenesis, including bioactivation and deactivation components. It is not possible to make very confident generalizations about the extent of this heterogeneity in the human population nor about the distribution of any such range.

Even in the face of such a general inability to describe the extent of human hetero-geneic responses to carcinogenic agents, it is clear from the data that human variation in response is generally much greater than observed in commonly used animal species. Yet, there is almost never a reference to which segment of the human population the model is thought to be related. Given the absence of any specific comment on that issue it is generally assumed that the model represents the population mean. The present analysis has provided a number of examples which try to guide us beyond that generalized approach by providing information on which groups of humans the animal model is likely to extrapolate to. For example, with respect to acetylation, the most appropriate model is different depending on the human phenotype. While it is necessary to combine this information with variations in the ability to *N*-hydroxylate and deacetylate arylamines to much more accurately estimate arylamine-induced cancer risk, nevertheless this type of assessment begins to lay out a new population-based interpretational approach for evaluating the human significance of bioassay data.

The recognition that heterogeneity exists in the human population with respect to the expression of biochemical parameters associated with risk of developing chemically-induced cancer also presents the opportunity to turn the liability of rather large interspecies differences in animal model responses into an asset. For example, it could be that the one animal model may reasonably simulate the response of one segment of the population (e.g., fast acetylator) while another model may best simulate another segment of the population (e.g., slow acetylator). Another approach along these same lines may be to permit the testing agency to select the animal model beforehand in light of the segment of the population that it desires to simulate. Thus, it may be possible to select an animal model that more closely simulates a potential human high risk group. This type of knowledge may be of considerable value in more properly interpreting estimations of cancer risk to humans when performed via the use of biomathematical models.

The approach described here may also be of considerable assistance not only in the development of prospective assessments and in the development of new protocols for testing, but in the reinterpretation of past studies in order to assess their extrapolative relevance. For example, the dog has been used by OSHA in trying to quantitatively assess the bladder cancer risk from exposure to the carcinogenic agent MOCA. Given the observations that MOCA must be N-hydroxylated and not acetylated, it is important to note that the dog is generally considered incapable of acetylating aromatic amines. The fact that the dog has a more favorable deactylase/acetylase ratio than humans with respect to aromatic amines would suggest very strongly that the dog is likely to overestimate human risk. This would even be more so when one considers the high acetylator phenotype.

SUMMARY

The occurrence of human heterogeneity with respect to susceptibility to toxic agents, including carcinogens, is being more broadly recognized. Identification of the causes of differential susceptibility has become a very active area of biomedical/toxicological research. The fact that humans are a highly outbred species and follow a broad variety of dietary patterns and divergent lifestyle orientations all contribute to the highly varied susceptibility to environmental agents. In contrast, the responses of humans to such agents are hoped to be predicted from highly inbred rodent strains that are reared on the same diets with identical environmental conditions. Given this situation, the issue is not whether the models predict human responses but which human we are talking about. This chapter provides an approach for addressing this issue so that more biologically plausible interpretations of cancer bioassay data may occur.

ACKNOWLEDGMENT. Earlier versions of this chapter were presented at the Annual American Pharmaceutical Association Conference, San Francisco, California in April, 1986. It was published in the *Journal of Pharmaceutical Sciences* (October, 1986), and in the conference proceedings of the FDA-sponsored Conference on Interspecies Extrapolation of Carcinogenicity Data, Bethesda, Maryland, January, 1986.

REFERENCES

Al-Dabbagh, S. G., Idle, J. R., and Smith, R. L., 1980, *J. Pharm. Pharmacol.* **33:**161–164.

Autrup, H., Schwartz, R. D., Essigmann, J. M., Smith, L., Trump, B. F., and Harris, C. C., 1980a, *Terat. Carcin. Mutag.* **1:**3–13.

Autrup, H., Wefald, F. C., Jeffrey, A. M., Tate, T., Schwartz, R. D., Trump, B., and Harris, C., 1980b, *Int. J. Can.* **25:**293–300.

Autrup, J., Barrett, L. A., Jackson, F. E., Jeudadon, M. L., Stoner, G., Phelps, P., Trump, B. F., and Harris, C. C., 1978, *Gastroenterology* **74:**1248–1257.

Bond, J. T., Mattano, D. D., and Weber, W. W., 1986, *The Pharmacologists* **28**(3):118 (abst.).

Calabrese, E. J., 1978, *Pollutants and High Risk Groups: The Biological Basis of Enhanced Susceptibility to Environmental and Occupational Pollutants,* Wiley, New York.

Calabrese, E. J., 1984, *Ecogenetics: Genetic Variation in Susceptibility to Environmental Agents,* Wiley, New York.

Calabrese, E. J., 1985, *Toxic Susceptibilities: Male/Female Differences,* Wiley, New York.

Calabrese, E. J., 1986, *Age Differences in Susceptibility to Toxic Agents,* Wiley, New York.

Daniel, F. B., Schut, H. A. J., Sandwisch, D. W., Schenck, K. M., Hoffmann, C. O., Patrick, J. R., and Stoner, G. D., 1983, *Cancer Res.* **43:**4723–4729.

Devadatta, S., Gangadharam, P. R. J., Andrews, R. H., Fox, W., Ramakrishnan, C. V., Selkon, J. B., and Velu, S., 1960, *Bull. WHO* **23:**587–598.

Dourson, M. L., and Stara, J. J., 1983, *Regul. Toxicol. Pharmacol.* **3:**224–238.

Environmental Protection Agency (EPA), 1976, *National Interim Primary Drinking Water Regulations,* EPA, Washington, DC.

Glowinski, I. R., Radtke, H. E., and Weber, W. W., 1978. *Mol. Pharmacol.* **14:**940–949.

Harris, C. C., Autrup, H., Vahakanges, K., and Trump, B. F., 1984, in: *Genetic Variation in Response to Chemical Exposure: Banbury Report 16* (G. S. Omenn and H. V. Gelboin, eds.), pp. 145–153, Cold Spring Harbor Laboratory, New York.

Idle, J. R., and Smith, R. L., 1979, *Drug Metab. Rev.* **9**(2):301–317.

Kouri, R. E., Levine, A. S., Edward, B. K., McLemore, R. L., Vessel, E. S., and Nebert, E. S., 1984, in: *Genetic Variation in Response to Chemical Exposure: Banbury Report 16* (G. S. Omenn and H. V. Gelboin, eds.), pp. 145–153, Cold Spring Harbor Laboratory, New York.

Lower, G. M., Jr., and Bryan, G. T., 1973, *Biochem. Pharm.* **22:**1581–1588.

Lower, G. M., Jr., and Bryan, G. T., 1976, *J. Toxicol. Environ. Health* **1:**421.

Lower, G. M., Jr., Nilsson, T., Nelson, L. E., Wolf, H., Gamsky, T. E., and Bryan, G. T., 1979, *Environ. Health Persp.* **29:**71–79.

Mbanebo, C., Barabunmi, E. A., Mahgoub, A., Sloan, T. P., Idle, J. R., and Smith, R. L., 1980, *Xenobiotica* **10:**811–818.

Mitchell, J. R., Zimmerman, H. J., Ishak, K. G., Thorgeirsson, V. P., Timbrell, J. A., Snodgrass, W. R., and Nelson, S. D., 1976, *Ann. Intern. Med.* **34:**181–192.

National Academy of Sciences (NAS), 1977, *Drinking Water and Human Health, Vol. 1,* pp. 802–803, National Academy Press, Washington, D.C.

Oesch, F., Jerina, D. M., Daly, J. W., and Rice, J. M., 1973, *Chem. Biol. Interact.* **6:**189–202.

Pelkonen, O., Kaltiala, E. H., Karki, N. T., Jalonen, K., and Pyorala, K., 1975, *Xenobiotica* **5:**501–509.

Propping, P., 1978, *Am. J. Med.* **34:**639–662.

Williams, G. M., and Weisburger, J. H., 1986, in: *Cassarett and Doull's Toxicology* (C. D. Klaassen, M. O. Amdur, and J. Doull, eds.), pp. 99–173, MacMillan, New York.

Williams, R. T., 1959, *Detoxification Mechanisms,* p. 438, Wiley, New York.

10

Biological Markers in Risk Assessment

Frederica P. Perera

INTRODUCTION

Traditionally, the field of chemical carcinogenesis has relied upon estimates of administered dose and/or human exposure in constructing dose–response curves and assessing cancer risk. Of far greater relevance to risk is the actual amount of carcinogen that has interracted with target cellular molecules such as DNA, RNA, or protein—the biologically effective dose of the carcinogenic substance.

Laboratory methods are now available to quantify the biologically effective dose of genotoxic carcinogens in cells in culture, laboratory animals, and humans. This recent development can substantially improve human risk assessment by permitting early identification of carcinogenic hazards and estimates of potential risk on the group level. It can also enable us to better extrapolate from quantitative cancer risks in high-dose laboratory experiments or high-exposure epidemiological studies to lower exposure situations in humans. In quantitative risk assessment (QRA), population variability in response to exposure is a key consideration, but one which is usually not accounted for in the process. Biological markers provide a means of assessing the extent of human variation in effective dose, thus providing a potential risk. Biological dosimeters can also allow epidemiology a greater role in risk assessment. Risk assessment is now generally based on animal rather than human data because of the insensitivity of epidemiological methods to small increases in common cancers and because of the lack of reliable estimates of exposure. Not only can markers of biological dose allow epidemiology to become a more timely instrument in qualitative risk assessment but they can significantly increase the power of epidemiological studies to detect a true effect by allowing accurate classification of ''exposed'' versus ''unexposed'' individuals, where the latter have received a significant

Frederica P. Perera • Division of Environmental Science, School of Public Health, Columbia University, New York, New York 10032.

biologically effective dose. At present, available biological markers can and do serve as indicators of carcinogenic hazard; but in most cases considerable work remains to validate them for use in QRA.

This chapter briefly reviews examples of available biological markers and their application to date and discusses major considerations in evaluating biological markers. Finally, it examines the actual and potential role of biological markers in understanding the shape of the low dose–response curve, in extrapolating between species, and in predicting cancer risk.

WHAT ARE BIOLOGICAL MARKERS?

Biological markers of the effective dose of carcinogens are alterations in normal biochemical or molecular processes. These markers not only indicate that exposure has occurred but also that a biological effect has resulted which is relevant to carcinogenesis.

Among the principle biomarkers in current use are carcinogen–DNA and carcinogen–protein adducts. Adducts result from covalent interaction of electrophilic carcinogens with DNA or protein. If unrepaired, DNA adducts can lead to gene mutation and induction of cancer. Protein adducts can serve as a feasible surrogate for those formed with DNA. Various methods are available to measure adducts, including polyclonal and monoclonal antibodies, synchronous fluorescence spectrometry, HPLC and fluorescence spectroscopy, gas chromatography-mass spectrography and postradiolabeling.

Relatively well established cytogenetic methods are available to evaluate chromosomal aberrations, sister chromatid exchange (SCE) and, more recently, micronuclei (MN) in lymphocytes. Point mutations [hypoxanthine-guanine phosphoribosyl transferase (HPRT)] in white blood cells can be detected by autoradiography; and unscheduled DNA synthesis (UDS) by the thymidine incorporation method. (See IARC, 1984; IARC, 1986; Lohman et al., 1984; Tannenbaum and Skipper, 1984, for a review of methods.) Examples of studies which have used these methods to monitor biologically effective dose of carcinogens in humans are summarized in Table 1. While results thus far are encouraging because they illustrate the feasibility and sensitivity of the methods in terms of human studies, they are frequently limited by small sample size, lack of appropriate controls, and inadequate data on exposure (Perera, 1987a).

FACTORS EFFECTING THE USEFULNESS OF BIOLOGICAL MARKERS

Relationship to Carcinogenesis

There are four major considerations in evaluating the usefulness of biological markers in risk assessment. First, one must ask whether the biological marker in question reflects a critical step or mechanism in carcinogenesis. For example, DNA adducts are linked to point mutations in that most carcinogens act by electrophilic interaction with DNA bases. Carcinogen–DNA adducts are formed which can, if unrepaired prior to replication or misrepaired, lead to gene mutation. The mutated cell is thus considered to

Table 1. Examples of Human Studies[a]

Endpoint	Sample	Study population	Exposure	Reference
Protein adducts	RBC	Sterilization plant workers, smokers, controls	Ethylene oxide	Calleman *et al.* (1978) Farmer *et al.* (1986) Törnqvist *et al.* (1986)
Protein adducts	RBC	Smokers, non-smokers	4-ABP	Perera *et al.* (1987)
DNA adducts	WBC	Lung cancer patients nonsmokers, roofers, foundry workers, coke oven workers, controls	BP in mixture	Perera *et al.* (1982) Shamsuddin *et al.* (1985) Harris *et al.* (1985)
Antibodies to DNA adducts	WBC	Coke oven workers	BP in mixture	Harris *et al.* (1985)
DNA adducts (excised)	Urine	African outpatients	AFB$_1$	Autrup *et al.* (1983) Groopman *et al.* (1985)
DNA adducts	WBC	Chemotherapy patients, controls	*Cis*-platinum	Reed *et al.* (1986a,b)
DNA adducts	Placenta	Pregnant women Smokers, non-smokers	Cigarette smoke	Everson *et al.* (1986)
Unscheduled DNA synthesis	WBC	Workers, controls	Propylene oxide	Pero *et al.* (1982)
DNA adducts	Buccal mucosa	Betel and tobacco chewers, controls	Betel nut, tobacco	Dunn and Stich (1986)
Chromosomal aberrations	WBC	Workers, controls	Vinyl chloride	Kucerova (1982)
SCE	WBC	Workers, controls	Ethylene oxide	Stolley *et al.* (1984)
Micronuclei	Lymphocytes	Tank cleaners, controls	Organic solvents, heavy metals	Hogstedt *et al.* (1981)
Somatic cell mutation	RBC	Cancer patients	Chemotherapy agents	Jensen *et al.* (1986)
Somatic cell mutation	Lymphocytes	Medical technicians	Radiotherapy	Messing *et al.* (1986)

[a]From Perera *et al.* (1987), as modified

be "initiated" and may become malignant by passing through subsequent stages known as promotion, conversion, and progression (Weinstein *et al.*, 1984; Harris, 1985; Scherer, 1984). Indeed, there is a generally good correlation between the ability of a series of polycyclic aromatic hydrocarbons (PAH) and alkylating agents to form covalent adducts and their carcinogenic potency (Brookes and Lawley, 1964; Lutz, 1979; Pelkonen *et al.*, 1980; Bartsch *et al.*, 1983). Moreover, there is circumstantial evidence linking DNA adducts to oncogene activation. Certain tumors induced experimentally by chemical exposures show oncogenes apparently activated by point mutations (Marshall *et al.*, 1984; Sukumar *et al.*, 1983) and in the case of methyl nitrosourea (MNU)-induced mouse mammary tumors a particular DNA adduct, the O^6 lesion, may have been related to activation of oncogene (Sukumar *et al.*, 1983). While most data point to an early, initiating role for DNA adducts, recent evidence indicates that exposure to electrophilic, initiating carcinogens may also be important in the malignant conversion or progression stages (Hennings *et al.*, 1983; Sherer, 1984).

The biological rationale for measuring carcinogen–protein (usually hemoglobin) adducts is that they are considered to be a potentially useful surrogate for DNA binding. For a number of carcinogens, a proportional relationship has been shown between DNA and protein binding (Farmer, 1984).

Although the mechanistic role of SCEs is not understood, their good empirical correlation with clastogenicity and carcinogenicity provides the primary basis for using them in biomonitoring of humans exposed to mutagenic carcinogens (Sorsa, 1984). Despite the finding that a number of "nongenotoxic" carcinogens or "promoters" also cause SCEs (Perera, 1984), the marker has not been widely used to monitor human exposures to late-stage carcinogens.

Chromosomal aberrations are also induced by a large number of industrial chemicals (IARC, 1986). They are more directly linked to cancer than SCEs in that they constitute a mutation and are evident in a high proportion of human tumors (Mitelman, 1984). In particular, specific chromosomal aberrations are significantly more common in leukemic cells of occupationally exposed patients than in unexposed patients (Mitelman, 1984). Chromosomal abnormalities take on greater significance because large-scale chromosomal damage such as gene rearrangements or gene amplification have been recently associated with activation or certain oncogenes (Weinstein *et al.*, 1984).

The ability to repair DNA adducts is highly variable in the human population (Setlow, 1983); as measured by UDS, human repair capability is an important determinant of cancer risk. UDS can also provide evidence of DNA damage as a result of chemical exposures (Pero, 1982).

From this very brief discussion of the biological support for using these several markers as carcinogen dosimeters it can be seen that the majority apply most directly to chemicals or agents that operate primarily during the initiation phase. Certain carcinogens to which humans have significant exposure such as hormones, dioxin, and di(2-ethylhexyl)phthalate (DEHP), which are not efficient at binding to DNA or inducing gene mutation or chromosomal aberrations, but which appear to act primarily via other mechanisms, will not be amenable to study with these methods. Other dosimeters will have to be found for such substances. This is an important limitation given the recognized contribution of so called nongenotoxic promoting agents to human cancer (Doll and Peto, 1981; Day and Brown, 1980). Despite this drawback, there is considerable agreement that any electrophile occupying DNA space is potentially mutagenic or carcinogenic (Ehrenberg, 1984). Therefore, where we are dealing with carcinogens that damage the genetic material, available biological markers can be very useful in quantifying biologically-effective dose and indicating potential risk. The ability of specific biological dosimeters such as DNA adducts to act as quantitative predictors of either partial risk (gene mutation/initiation) or total cancer risk will be reviewed in detail at the end of the chapter.

Inter- and Intraindividual Variability

Another consideration in evaluating the biological relevance of molecular dosimetry data is the contribution of inter- and intraindividual variability as well as variation over time in the same individual. This factor is of less concern in laboratory animals than in humans given their greater genetic homogeneity and controlled exposure situation. In humans, both inter- and intraindividual variability are significant. For example, with benzo[a]pyrene (B[a]P) the level of DNA adduct formation in cultured human tissues and cells shows as much as a 350-fold variation (Vahakangas *et al.*, 1984). Less than 30% of exposed coke oven workers tested for B[a]P-DNA antibodies in sera had measurable adducts (Shamsuddin *et al.*, 1985). The extent of *cis*-platinum-DNA adduct formation in treated cancer patients also varies widely, with about 50% of subjects forming measurable adducts (Reed *et al.*, 1986). Studies on smokers of 1–2 packs of cigarettes per day show considerable individual variation in formation of B[a]P-DNA and 4-aminobiphenyl (4-ABP), as well as in SCE frequencies (Perera *et al.*, 1987).

With respect to intraindividual variation upon repeat sampling, SCEs in smokers, nonsmokers and exsmokers varied considerably (40–50% average duration) over time. This was not apparently attributable to any changes in level of exposure (Carrano *et al.*, 1986). Significant variation was also seen in levels of B[a]P-DNA in individual smokers over a period of several days (Perera *et al.*, 1987).

Target Tissue Dose

Another aspect of biological relevance of the marker is whether it varies between the target tissue and the tissue or cells monitored. In human dosimetry studies, in contrast to the animal model, a surrogate must generally be found for the target tissue. This is usually supplied by peripheral blood cells or body fluids such as urine. For each carcinogen and each biomarker the relationship between effective dose at both sites (surrogate and target) should be clearly established. Yet this has been done for few carcinogens. Exceptions are B[a]P and *cis*-platinum for which similar levels of DNA adducts have been found in all tissues studied (Stowers and Anderson, 1985; Reed *et al.*, 1986). In the latter study, comparable levels of adducts were reported in white blood cell DNA and other tissue (including tumor) from chemotherapy patients.

In the interest of feasibility of human studies, surrogates for intracellular targets (DNA and chromosomes) have been sought. Protein such as hemoglobin is in theory a useful substitute for DNA. Proportionality between carcinogen binding to DNA and protein has been established for a number of carcinogens, including ethylene oxide (EtO), methyl methanesulfonate (MMS), ethyl methanesulfonate (EMS), vinyl chloride, PAH and several aromatic amines (Ehrenberg *et al.*, 1983; Murthy *et al.*, 1984). In rodents administered *trans*-4-dimethylaminostilbene and 2-acetylaminofluorene (AAF), binding to hemoglobin was also proportional to DNA binding (Newmann, 1980; Pereira *et al.*, 1981). However, such a relationship cannot be assumed but must be determined for each carcinogen of interest.

Relationship to Exposure Source

A major consideration in evaluating various markers is the degree to which they reflect the exposure source of concern. Researchers have observed substantial variation in "background" levels of biological markers in so-called "unexposed controls." These backgrounds can be significant, as seen in studies of EtO-hemoglobin adducts in non-smokers (Farmer *et al.*, 1984; Wright, 1983; Törnqvist *et al.*, 1986), in B[a]P–DNA adducts in nonsmokers (Perera *et al.*, 1987; Everson *et al.*, 1986), in 4-ABP hemoglobin adducts in nonsmokers (Bryant *et al.*, 1986; Perera *et al.*, 1987); and in nonchewers of betel nut (Dunn and Stich, 1986). Thus a major problem in biological dosimetry in humans, as opposed to experimental animals, is identifying truly unexposed controls (Poirier and Beland, 1986). Few carcinogens derive from single sources; therefore human studies of carcinogens such as PAH, nitrosamines, and aromatic amines are complicated by their pervasiveness in the food supply, ambient air, workplace or tobacco smoke. Even EtO is found not only in certain working environments but in cigarette smoke and ambient air as well. Thus in every human study reported so far, the mean values of DNA or protein adducts for the controls were significantly greater than zero; and in most cases the range of adducts in controls overlapped with those seen in the exposed groups. (Poirier and Beland, 1986; Umbenhauer *et al.*, 1985; Perera *et al.*, 1987; Farmer *et al.*, 1986).

Relationship to Past Exposure

Another problem is that in retrospective studies, ideally, one would like a permanent indicator of exposure that occurred 10–30 years in the past. Such markers do not exist; thus one must select situations in which exposure has not changed significantly over time or one must estimate the fraction of lesions that reflect past periods of exposure. For prospective studies such assumptions are not needed, but it is essential to understand the lifetime of the marker being measured. For hemoglobin adducts this is on the order of four months; for DNA adducts and chromosomal abnormalities it is days to years depending on the compound and cell type being assayed.

Low-Dose Sensitivity

An additional consideration in validating markers is their ability to detect low-level doses of carcinogens. This is critical given the generally low levels of human exposures and the concern on the part of regulators about cancer risks as low as one excess case per million persons exposed. Methods to measure DNA and protein adducts can detect as little as one adduct per 10^7–10^{10} nucleotides and less than 10 picograms of adduct per gram of protein respectively. These detection levels are considered adequate for human studies (Perera and Weinstein, 1982; Tannenbaum and Skipper, 1984). This sensitivity also is considerably higher than that of chromosomal aberrations, SCEs, or MN (Dahlem, 1986). In general, chemical-specific markers are more sensitive than generic methods such as UDS, point mutations, and cytogenetic assays. However, given that most human exposures are to complex mixtures, generic methods are invaluable as a total dosimeter, but should be matched with chemical-specific methods to tease apart the contribution of the various chemical components.

BIOLOGICAL MARKERS AND QUANTITATIVE RISK ASSESSMENT

Turning now to three major issues in risk assessment—high-to-low dose extrapolation, interspecies extrapolation, and ability of markers to provide estimates of human cancer risk—it is helpful to review the available data provided to date regarding DNA and protein adducts as the best developed examples.

Extrapolation from High to Low Dose in Animals

Interspecies extrapolation is the cornerstone of QRA. While use of a multistage model that assumes additivity on background and hence is linear at low dose is considered the most reasonable approach to extrapolation (EPA, 1986; Perera, 1987b); there are many uncertainties as to the true dose–response relationship. There have been several attempts to compare biologically effective dose (DNA, RNA, or protein adducts) at high-(observed tumorigenic) and low-exposure levels in order to determine whether linearity is a valid assumption. In most of these studies a constant ratio was observed between administered dose and macromolecular binding in experimental animals exposed to single administrations of diverse carcinogens over a wide dose range. Some cases included dosages comparable to levels of human exposure. These include: *trans*-4-dimethylaminostilbene, N-nitrosodimethylamine, aflatoxin B_1(AFB$_1$) (Neumann, 1984a), B[a]P metabolites (Dunn, 1983), 4-ABP, various methylating and ethylating agents, (Wogan and Gorelick, 1985; Poirier and Beland, 1986), EMS, dimethylnitrosamine (DMN) (Pegg and Perry, 1981), various PAH metabolites (Stowers and Anderson, 1985), and sterigmatocystin (Reddy *et al.*, 1985) (Fig. 1). These results were in contrast to a short-term exposure study of formaldehyde in which nonlinearity in total [^{14}C]formalde-

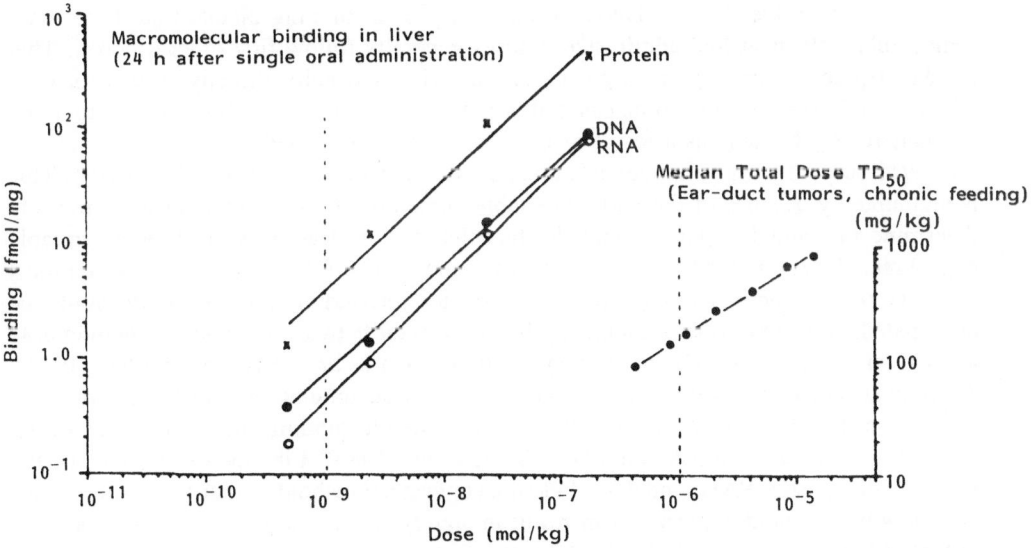

Figure 1. Dose–responses of *trans*-4-acetylaminostilbene in rats. From Neumann (1984).

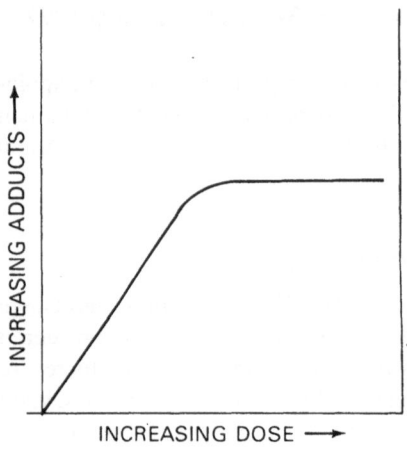

Figure 2. Characteristic dose–response in chronic or multiple dose studies.

hyde incorporation into DNA was reported (Casanova-Schmitz, 1984). However, in this latter study adducts were not isolated or identified.

Chronic administration or multiple dose studies with various methylating and ethylating agents, diethylnitrosamine (DEN), 2-AAF, AFB_1, 4(N-methyl-N-nitrosamino)-1-(3-pyridyl)-1-butanone (or NNK), MMS, and 4-ABP have observed linearity at the low dose with a plateau at higher dosages (Fig. 2) (Poirier and Beland, 1986).

Similarly, protein adduct formation was proportionally related to administered dose of EtO, MMS, 4-ABP, *trans*-4-dimethylaminostilbene, and chloroform. Only for dimethylnitrosamine was the observed dose–response nonlinear (Wogan and Gorelick, 1985).

Thus, extensive data on DNA, RNA, and protein binding dictate that these macromolecular effects at low administered doses generally follow first order kinetics. That is, the degree of binding in target organs *in vivo* is usually directly proportional to administered dose, even in some cases at very low levels similar to those which might be encountered by humans as a result of environmental contamination.

With respect to most human data on adducts, a clear dose–response is not seen. This is undoubtedly because of the widely variable human response, the inability to precisely determine individual exposure, and the fact that one is dealing with chronic, variable exposures. However, for EtO and propylene oxide (unlike PAH and 4-ABP, which must be metabolically activated and for which greater interindividual variability would be anticipated), a proportional relationship has been seen between carcinogen–hemoglobin adducts in humans and estimated exposure (Calleman *et al.*, 1978; van Stittert, 1984). There is also evidence from clinical studies of steady accumulation of *cis*-platinum-DNA adducts in the 50% subset of patients with measurable binding; the cumulative dose–response was linear in those individuals (Reed *et al.*, 1986). Like the experimental data, human data on EtO, PAH, and 4-ABP do not suggest a threshold; rather they indicate that very low background exposures can result in significant levels of adducts in some individuals (Poirier and Beland, 1986; Dahlem, 1986).

Interspecies Extrapolation

This brings us to the difficulties in extrapolating from laboratory animals to humans, and the absolute necessity of obtaining direct information on biologically-effective dose in humans rather than relying solely on pharmacokinetic data in animals. For example, acute studies of putative DNA-protein cross-links in the nasal epithelium of rats observed at tumorigenic and lower levels of formaldehyde were recently proposed as a basis for concluding nonlinearity in carcinogenic response at low dose (Starr and Buck, 1984). However, this interpretation was considered premature by several expert panels (Expert Panel, 1986; Report, 1986); and by the Occupational Safety and Health Administration (OSHA, 1986). The critics cautioned *inter alia* that the adducts were not well characterized and that the acute model is not necessarily relevant to the human exposure situation. In addition, extrapolation is hindered by human variability and background exposures already challenging detoxification and repair systems.

Human variability in response is in fact a significant factor in risk prediction. Given the greater than 100-fold interindividual variation in DNA binding (Harris *et al.*, 1982; Vahakangas *et al.*, 1984) and the severalfold variability in DNA repair (Setlow, 1983), individual variation is considerably wider in the outbred human species than in inbred rats (Harris, 1985). Another factor missing in the animal model is the wide individual variation in humans with respect to the diversity and magnitude of exposures—not only to the chemical of interest but to other chemicals, agents, or lifestyle factors that damage DNA, contribute to later stages of carcinogenesis, or interact with the chemical exposure of concern. Very little human data are available regarding interactions between lifestyle and environmental factors which could lead to higher or lower levels of adducts in humans. However, a synergistic relationship has been observed between alcohol and smoking in the production of SCEs in humans (Obe, 1986).

Perhaps one of the main contributions that biological dosimeters can now make to risk assessment is in providing information about the shape of the human population response curve and the proportion of high versus low responders to carcinogenic exposures. This in turn gives a better idea about the size of the population at greater potential risk (the sensitive subpopulation or "outliers") which is essential to regulators. Society has frequently chosen, as for example in controling air pollution, to set standards which protect the most sensitive individuals.

Usefulness in Risk Assessment

Finally, a key question regarding DNA adducts is whether they can serve as qualitative or quantitative predictors of risk of cancer in humans. A large and growing literature suggests that DNA adducts can qualitatively indicate a hazard to humans and, for certain chemicals, quantitatively indicate risk.

Results of studies in cells in culture and experimental animals suggest that where the critical DNA adduct has been determined and quantified, there is a good correlation between levels of that DNA adduct and the frequency of induced mutations. The ratio of adducts to mutations seems to be fairly similar across several systems as well as within classes of chemicals. For example, with a number of alkylating agents a constant relationship was seen between [O^6]ethylguanine formed in DNA and frequencies of mutation induction in cells *in vitro* (van Zeeland, *et al.*, 1985). The ratio of [O^6]ethylguanine adducts to HPRT mutations in V79 cells (11 : 1) was similar to that observed between [O^6]alkyl-guanine adducts and sex-linked recessive lethal mutations in *Drosophila* exposed to alkylating agents (Vogel, 1986; Vogel *et al.*, 1986; van Zeeland 1986). Studies of various nitrated pyrenes in *Salmonella* and Chinese hamster ovary (CHO) cells also show a correlation between the extent of DNA adduct formation and mutation induction (Heflich *et al.*, 1985; 1986).

With respect to the quantitative relationship between DNA adducts and carcinogenicity, there is a good correlation between the ability of a wide range of chemical classes to form covalent DNA adducts and their carcinogenic potency (Brookes and Lawley, 1964; Wigley *et al.*, 1979; Lutz, 1979; Bartsch *et al.*, 1983). A proportional relationship has also been seen between the frequency of *in vitro* cell transformation and the number of B[a]P-DNA adducts formed (Poirier, 1984). In many, but not all, studies a correlation exists between the ability of a susceptible species to form persistent DNA adducts at the target organ and cancer induction (see Wogan and Gorelick, 1985 for review).

There is increasing evidence that persistence and rate of repair prior to cell replication are important determinants of the carcinogenic effects of adducts (Swenberg *et al.*, 1985; Maher and McCormick, 1986; Wogan and Gorelick, 1985) as are specific characteristics of the adduct formed (e.g., location in the tissue, cell type, and site on the genome) (Kriek *et al.*, 1984; Poirier, 1984).

The above discussion illustrates the complexity of the relationship of DNA and protein adducts to mutation and cancer. However, adducts can provide valuable information about potential risk and, in certain cases where critical adducts have been identified and can be measured at the target site or a surrogate, more precise quantitative risk assessment can be derived.

A QUANTITATIVE EXAMPLE

The "parallelogram" approach based on biological dosimetry (specifically adduct) data has been used to a limited extent to predict human risk. The best developed example of prediction of human cancer risk based on human and experimental data is that of EtO. Briefly, this was done as follows: the tissue dose (the actual concentration of the reactive electrophile within the tissue) of EtO was assumed to be directly proportional to the extent of both DNA and protein binding in humans, as had been demonstrated in mice exposed to EtO. The *in vivo* tissue dose (mol/hr) of EtO that produced the same mutagenic response in experimental systems as 1 rad of low-LET radiation in the low dose–response region was calculated and termed the "rad equivalent." Measurements of EtO-hemoglobin binding in sterilizer plant workers were then used to estimate their tissue dose of EtO in terms of rad equivalents (Tables 2 and 3). This rad equivalent measure allowed a calculation of the excess risk of leukemia in the workers (Ehrenberg *et al.*, 1974; Calleman *et al.*, 1978; Calleman, 1984; Neumann, 1984b). The resultant prediction of increased risk of cancer in this cohort was subsequently borne out by epidemiological studies (Hogstedt, 1986).

Table 2. Ethylene Oxide: Experiments With Laboratory Mammals[a,b]

	Values for mouse (for calculations see below)
1. EtO in ambient air Exposure level: L_1 (1–10^2 ppm) Exposure dose: D_1 (1–10^3 ppm hr)	$k_{12} = \alpha_{12} \times 2.2 \times 10^{-6}$ mole (kg bw)$^{-1}$ (ppm hr)$^{-1}$ $\alpha_{12} \approx 1$
2. (a) Amount absorbed through inhalation from step 1. $dL_2^0 = k_{12}L_1 dt$ (b) EtO injected i.p. Pharmacological dose: L_2^0	$k_{13} = 0.58 \times 10^{-6}$ M hr (ppm hr)^1 $k_{23} = 0.22$ hr $\left(= \bar{t}_{ret} = \dfrac{1}{\lambda_3} \right)$ $\lambda_3 = 4.6$ hr^{-1}
3. Tissue dose: D_3 Determined from degree of alkylation of Hb-His $D_3 = k_{23}L_2^0 \ (= \bar{t}_{ret}L_2^0)$ (Eq. 4)	$k_{34} \approx 1$ (liver, gonads and other organs)
4. Target dose: D_4 Determined from degree of alkylation of Gua-N-7 in DNA (and of proteins)	$k_{45} = k_{n-2} = 1.4 \times 10^{-2}$ M^{-1} hr^{-1} (from submammalian systems and reaction kinetic data)
5. Molecular dose $= L_5^0 = \dfrac{[\text{R} - \text{DNA}_c]}{[\text{DNA}_c]}$	$k_{56} = 1 \times 10^7$ rad-equ $\left(\dfrac{\text{mole R} - \text{DNA}_c}{\text{mole DNA}_c} \right)^{-1}_a$ (from submammalian systems)
6. (a) Response (b) Dose equivalent for risk estimation D_{6b}	Dose equivalent in acceptable agreement with biological responses; but better data for biological endpoints desirable.

[a]Mouse.
[b]From Ehrenberg *et al* (1983)

While the results with EtO are generally encouraging, this may be a somewhat special case because EtO is a stable electrophile that distributes evenly between tissues, in contrast to substances such as vinyl chloride and dimethylnitrosamine, which require metabolism and thus produce less stable intermediates (Neumann, 1984b).

At present, in few cases do we have any comparative data on adducts in humans and laboratory animals with chronic exposure. While this situation should improve rapidly for individual substances, human exposures frequently involve complex mixtures which are

Table 3. Ethylene Oxide: Man[a]

1.	Exposure level (ppm) and its variation ($L_1(t)$) estimated; $D_1 = \int_t L_1(t)dt$
	$k_{12} = \alpha_{12} \times$ respiration rate/kg bw
	$\alpha_{12} \simeq 1$ (as found in animal experiments)
2.	$k_{23} = k_{13}/k_{23} = 0.1\text{--}0.2$ hr ($\lambda = 10\text{--}5$ hr^{-1})
3.	D_3 determined in persons with known D_1
4.	$D_4 \simeq D_3$ as in animal experiments
5.	$L_5^0 \simeq k_{n-2}D_4$ as in laboratory organisms
	k_{35} assumed to be same as in mouse experiments
6b.	D_{6b} per unit D_1 estimated to
	$k_{16b} = D_{6b}/D_1 = 1 \times 10^{-2}$ rad-equivalents (ppm hr)$^{-1}$

[a]From Ehrenberg *et al* (1983).

rarely tested in laboratory animals. In addition, human studies are generally carried out in worker populations, smokers, chemotherapy patients, or accidental situations where exposures are far higher than those encountered by the general population. Thus, risk assessment will still frequently necessitate low-dose extrapolation with its underlying assumptions.

Based upon this review, a reasonable assumption regarding low dose–response to carcinogens in humans continues to be one of linearity. According to Ehrenberg *et al.* (1986), cancer risk should be expected to depend on dose in the same way as initiation (mutation) because in the human situation initiators present at low levels are able to interact with promotive conditions already at hand. In addition, genetic changes operating at later stages of carcinogenesis can be expected to contribute to risk in the same dose–dependent fashion.

CONCLUSION

Biological markers are not a panacea to quantitative risk assessment but can provide valuable handles on the relationship between exposure, effective dose, and tumor induction. Considerable research is needed before these methods can realize their full potential. Prospective animal and human studies (ideally including case-control studies nested within prospective cohort studies) are essential in this regard as are comparative studies at low doses in both species. A number of methods appear to be adequately sensitive for this task so that a major effort should be made to understand their biological significance regarding cancer, as well as their relevance to the exposure of concern.

REFERENCES

Autrup, H., Bradley, K. A., Shamsuddin, A. K. M., Wakhisi, J., and Wasunna, A., 1983, Detection of putative adduct with fluorescence characteristics identical to 2,3-dihydro-2-(7-guanyl)-3-hydroxyaflatoxin B in human urine collected in Murang'a District, Kenya, *Carcinogenesis* 4:1193–1195.

Bartsch, H., Terracini, B., Malaveille, C., Tomatis, L., Wahrendorf, J., Brun, G., Dodet, B., 1983, Quantitative comparisons of carcinogenicity, mutagenicity and electrophilicity of 10 direct-acting alkylating agents and the initial 0:7-alkylguanine ratio in DNA with carcinogenic potency in rodents, *Mutat. Res.* 110:181–219.

Brookes, P., and Lawley, P. D., 1964, Evidence for the binding of polynuclear aromatic hydrocarbons to the nucleic acids of mouse skin: Relation between carcinogenic power of hydrocarbons and their binding to DNA, *Nature* 202:781–784.

Bryant, M. S., Skipper, P. L., Tannenbaum, S. R., and Maclure, M., 1987, Hemoglobin adducts of 4-aminobiphenyl in smokers and nonsmokers, *Cancer Res.* 47:602–608.

Calleman, C. J., 1984, *Hemoglobin as a Dose Monitor and Its Application to the Risk Estimation of Ethylene Oxide*, Ph.D. thesis, Department of Radiobiology, University of Stockholm, Stockholm.

Calleman, C. J., Ehrenberg, L., Jansson, B., Osterman-Golkar, S., Segerback, D., Svensson, K., and Wachtmeister, C. A., 1978, Monitoring and risk assessment by means of alkyl groups in hemoglobin in persons occupationally exposed to ethylene oxide, *J. Environ. Pathol. Toxicol.* 2:427–442.

Carrano, A. V., Ashworth, L. K., Minkler, J. L., and Moore, D. H., II, 1986, Variation in baseline SCE frequencies in humans, in: *Genetic Toxicity of Environmental Chemicals, Part B: Genetic Effects and Applied Mutagenesis* (C. Ramel, B. Lambert, and J. Magnusson, eds.), pp. 309–314, Alan R. Liss, New York.

Casanova-Schmitz, M., Starr, T. B., and Heck, H. D'A, 1984, Differentiation between metabolic incorporation and covalent binding in the labeling of macromolecules in the rat nasal mucosa and bone from inhaled [^{14}C]- and [^{3}H]formaldehyde, *Toxicol. Appl. Pharmacol.* 76:26–44.

Dahlem Proceedings, 1987, in: *Mechanisms of Cellular Toxicity* (B. Fowler, ed.), Dahlem, Springer-Verlag, Berlin (in press).

Day, N. E., and Brown, C. C., 1980, Multistage models and primary prevention of cancer, *J. Natl. Cancer Inst.* 64:977–989.

Doll, R., and Peto, R. (eds.), 1981, *The Causes of Cancer*, Oxford Press, New York.

Dunn, B. P., 1983, Wide-range linear dose–response curve for DNA binding of orally administered benzo[a]pyrene in mice, *Cancer Res.* 43:2654–2658.

Dunn, B. P., and Stich, H. F., 1986, ^{32}P postlabeling analysis of aromatic DNA adducts in human oral mucosal cells, *Carcinogenesis* 7:1115–1120.

Ehrenberg, L., 1984, Covalent binding of genotoxic agents to proteins and nucleic acids, in: *IARC 1984*, pp. 107–114.

Ehrenberg, L., Hiesche, K. D., Osterman-Golkar, S., and Wennberg, I., 1974, Evaluation of genetic risks of alkylating agents: Tissue dose in the mouse from air contaminated with ethylene oxide, *Mutat. Res.* 24:83–103.

Ehrenberg, L., Moustacchi, E., Osterman-Golkar, S., and Ekman, G., 1983, Dosimetry of genotoxic agents and dose–response relationship of their effects, *Mutat. Res.* 123:121–182.

Ehrenberg, L., Osterman-Golkar, S., and Törnqvist, M., 1986, Macromolecule adducts, target dose, and risk assessment, in: *Genetic Toxicology of Environmental Chemicals Part B: Genetic Effects and Applied Mutagenesis* (C. Ramel, B. Lambert, and J. Magnusson, eds.), pp. 253–260, Alan R. Liss, New York.

Environmental Protection Agency (EPA), 1986, Guidelines for carcinogen risk assessment, *Fed. Regist.* 51:33992–34003.

Everson, R. B., Randerath, E., Santella, R. M., Cefalo, R. C., Avitts, T. A., and Randerath, K., 1986, Detection of smoking-related covalent DNA adducts in human placenta, *Science* 231:54–57.

Expert Panel 1986, *Expert Review of Pharmacokinetic Data: Formaldehyde, Final Evaluation Report*, Prepared for EPA under Program No. 1415 for Work Assignment No. 07, Contract No. 68-02-4228, Jan. 2.

Farmer, P. B., Bailey, E., and Campbell, J. B., 1984, Use of alkylated proteins in the monitoring of exposure to alkylating agents, in: *IARC 1984*, pp. 189–198.

Farmer, P. B., Bailey, E., Gorf, S. M., Törnqvist, M., Osterman-Golkar, S., Kautiainen, A., and Lewis Enright, D. P., 1986, Monitoring human exposure to ethylene oxide by the determination of hemoglobin adducts using gas chromatography–mass spectrometry, *Carcinogenesis* 7:637–640.

Groopman, J. D., Donahue, P. R., Zhu, J., Chen, J., and Wogan, G. N., 1985, Aflatoxin metabolism in humans: Detection of metabolites and nucleic acid adducts in urine by affinity chromatography, *Proc. Natl. Acad. Sci. USA* 82:6492–6496.

Harris, C. C., 1985, Future directions in the use of DNA adducts as internal dosimeters for monitoring human exposure to environmental mutagens and carcinogens. *Environ. Health Perspect.* 62:185–191.

Harris, C. C., Trump, B. F., Grafstrom, R., and Autrup, H., 1982, Differences in metabolism of chemical carcinogens in cultured human epithelial tissues and cells, *J. Cell. Biochem.* 18:285–94.

Harris, C. C., Vahakangas, K., Newman, M. J., Trivers, G. E., Shamsuddin, A., Sinopoli, N., Mann, D. L., and Wright, W. E., 1985, Detection of benzo[a]pyrene diol epoxide-DNA adducts in peripheral blood lymphocytes and antibodies to the adducts in serum from coke oven workers, *Proc. Natl. Acad. Sci. USA* **82:**6672–6676.

Heflich, R. H., Fifer, E. K., Djuric, Z., and Beland, F. A., 1985, DNA adduct formation and mutation induction by nitropyrenes in *Salmonella* and Chinese hamster ovary cells: Relationships with nitroreduction and acetylation, *Environ. Health Perspect.* **62:**135–143.

Heflich, R. H., Fifer, E. K., Djuric, Z., and Beland, F. A., 1986, Mutation induction and DNA adduct formation by 1,8-dinitropyrene in Chinese hamster ovary cells, in: *Genetic Toxicology of Environmental Chemicals, Part A: Basic Principles and Mechanisms of Action* (C. Ramel, B. Lambert, and J. Magnusson, eds.), pp. 265–273, Alan R. Liss, New York.

Hennings, H., Shores, R., Wenk, M. L., Spangler, E. F., Tarone, R., and Yuspa, S. H., 1983, Malignant conversion of mouse skin tumors is increased by tumor initiators and unaffected by tumor promoters, *Nature* **304:**67–69.

Hogstedt, C., 1986, Future perspectives, needs and expectations of biological monitoring of exposure to genotoxicants in prevention of occupational disease, in: *Monitoring of Occupational Genotoxicants: Progress in Clinical and Biological Research,* Vol. 207 (M. Sorsa and H. Norppa, eds.), pp. 231–243, Alan R. Liss, New York.

Hogstedt, B., Gullberg, B., Mark-Vendel, E., Mitelman, F., and Skerkving, S., 1981, Increased frequency of lymphocyte micronuclei in workers producing reinforced polyester resin with low exposure to styrene, *Scand. J. Work Environ. Health* **49:**271–276.

IARC 1984, *International Seminar on Methods of Monitoring Human Exposure to Carcinogenic and Mutagenic Agents* (A. Berlin, M. Draper, K. Hemminki, and H. Vainio eds.), IARC Scientific Publications #59, Lyon.

IARC 1986, Monitoring of Humans with Exposures to Carcinogens, Mutagens and Epidemiological Applications, in: *Cancer Occurrence, Causes and Control* (L. Tomatis *et al.,* eds.), IARC Scientific Publications Series, Section 6.3, Lyon.

Jensen, R. H., Langlois, R. G., Bigbee, W. L., 1986, Determination of somatic mutations in human erythrocytes by flow cytometry, in: *Genotoxic Toxicology of Environmental Chemicals, Part B: Genetic Effects and Applied Mutagenesis* (C. Ramel, B. Lambert, and J. Magnusson, eds.), pp. 177–184, Alan R. Liss, New York.

Kriek, E., Engelse, L. D., Scherer, E., and Westra, J. G., 1984, Formation of DNA modifications by chemical carcinogens: Identification, localization and quantification, *Biochim. Biophys. Acta* **738:**181–201.

Kucerova, M., 1982, Chromosomal aberrations induced in occupationally exposed persons, in: *Mutagenicity: New Horizons in Genetic Toxicology* (J. A. Heddle, ed.), pp. 241–266, Academic Press, New York.

Lohman, P. H. M., Lauwerys, R., Sorsa, M., 1984, Methods of monitoring human exposure to carcinogenic and mutagenic agents, in: *IARC 1984,* pp. 423–427.

Lutz, W. K., 1979, *In vivo* covalent binding of organic chemicals to DNA as a quantitative indicator in the process of chemical carcinogenesis, *Mutat. Res.* **65:**289–356.

Maher, V., and McCormick, J. J., 1986, Role of DNA lesions and DNA repair in mutagenesis by carcinogens in diploid human fibroblasts, in: *Genetic Toxicology of Environmental Chemicals, Part A: Basic Principles and Mechanisms of Action* (C. Ramel, B. Lambert, and J. Magnusson, eds.), pp. 245–253, Alan R. Liss, New York.

Marshall, C. J., Vousden, K. H., and Phillips, D. H., 1984, Activation of c-Ha-*ras*-1 proto oncogene by *in vitro* modification with the chemical carcinogen, benzo[a]pyrene diol-epoxide, *Nature* **310:**586–589.

Messing, K., Seifert, A. M., and Bradley, W. E. C., 1986, *In vivo* mutant frequency of technicians professionally exposed to ionizing radiation, in: *Monitoring of Occupational Genotoxicants* (M. Sorsa and H. Norppa, eds.), pp. 87–97, Alan R. Liss, New York.

Mitelman, F., 1984, Chromosomal changes in cancer in relation to exposure to carcinogenic agents, in: *IARC 1984,* pp. 351–360.

Murthy, M. S. S., Calleman, C. J., Osterman-Golkar, S., Segerback, D., and Svensson, K., 1984, Relationships between ethylation of hemoglobin, ethylation of DNA and administered amount of ethyl methanesulfonate in the mouse, *Mutat. Res.* **127:**1–8.

Neumann, H.-G., 1980, Dose relationships in the primary lesion of strong electrophilic carcinogens, *Arch. Toxicol.* **3** (Suppl.):69–77.

Neumann, H.-G., 1983, Role of extent and persistence of DNA modifications in chemical carcinogenesis by aromatic amines, *Rec. Results Cancer Res.* **84:**77–89.

Neumann, H.-G., 1984a, Dosimetry and dose–response relationships, in: *Monitoring Human Exposure to Carcinogenic and Mutagenic Agents* (A. Berlin, M. Draper, K. Hemminki, and H. Vainio, eds.), IARC Scientific Publications No. 59, Lyon.

Neumann, H.-G., 1984b, Analysis of hemoglobin as a dose monitor for alkylating and arylating agents, *Arch. Toxicol.* **56:**1–6.

Occupational Safety and Health Administration (OSHA), 1985, Occupational exposure to formaldehyde, *Fed. Regist.* **50:**50412–50499.

Pegg, A. E., and Perry, W., 1981, Alkylation of nucleic acids and metabolism of small doses of di-methylnitrosamine in the rat, *Cancer Res.* **41:**3128–3132.

Pelkonen, O., Vahakangas, K., and Nebert, D. W., 1980, Binding of polycyclic aromatic hydrocarbons to DNA: Comparison with mutagenesis and tumorigenesis, *J. Toxicol. Environ. Health.* **6:**1009–1020.

Pereira, M. A., Lin, L.-H. C., and Chang, L. W., 1981, Dose dependency of 2-acetylaminofluorene binding to liver DNA and hemoglobin in mice and rats, *Toxicol. Appl. Pharmacol.* **60:**472–478.

Perera, F., 1987a, Molecular cancer epidemiology: A new tool in cancer prevention, *J. Natl. Cancer Inst.* **78:**887–898.

Perera, F., 1987b, Quantitative risk assessment and cost-benefit analysis for carcinogens at EPA: A critique, *J. Public Health Pol.* **8:**202–221.

Perera, F., and Weinstein, I. B., 1982, Molecular epidemiology and carcinogen-DNA adduct detection: New approaches to studies of human cancer causation, *J. Chronic Dis.* **35:**581–600.

Perera, F. P., 1984, The genotoxic/epigenetic distinction: Relevance to cancer policy, *Environ. Res.* **43:**175–191.

Perera, F. P., Santella, R. M., Brenner, D., Poirier, M. C., Munshi, A. A., Fischman, H. K., and van Ryzin, J., 1987, DNA adducts, protein adducts and sister chromatid exchange in cigarette smokers and non-smokers, *J. Natl. Cancer Inst.* **79:**449–456.

Pero, R. W., Bryngelsson, T., Widegren, B., Hogstedt, B., and Welinder, H., 1982, A reduced capacity for unscheduled DNA synthesis in lymphocytes from individuals exposed to propylene oxide and ethylene oxide, *Mutat. Res.* **104:**193–200.

Poirier, M. C., 1984, The use of carcinogen-DNA adduct antisera for quantitation and localization of genomic damage in animal models and the human population, *Environ. Mutagen.* **6:**879–887.

Poirier, M. C., and Beland, F. A., 1986, Determination of carcinogen-induced macromolecular adducts in animals and humans, in: *Progress in Experimental Tumor Research,* Vol. 31 (in press).

Reddy, M. V., Irwin, T. R., and Randerath, E., 1985, Formation and persistence of sterigmatocystin-DNA adducts in rat liver determined via P-postlabeling analysis, *Mutat. Res.* **152:**85–96.

Reed, E., Ozols, R. F., Fasy, T., Yuspa, S. H., and Poirier, M. C., 1986a, Biomonitoring of cisplatin-DNA adducts in cancer patients receiving cisplatin chemotherapy, in: *Genetic Toxicology of Environmental Chemicals, Part B: Genetic Effects and Applied Mutagenesis* (C. Ramel, B. Lambert, and J. Magnusson, eds.), pp. 247–252, Alan R. Liss, New York.

Reed, E., Yuspa, S. H., Zwelling, L. A., Ozols, R. F., Poirier, M. C., 1986b, Quantitation of *cis*-diam-minedichloro-platinum II (cis-platin)-DNA-intrastrand adducts in testicular and ovarian cancer patients receiving cisplatin chemotherapy, *J. Clin. Invest.* **77:**545–550.

Report, 1986, Report of the Formaldehyde Panel of the Workshop on the Contribution of Airborne Pollutants to Respiratory Cancer, Snowbird, Utah, July 13–18, *Environ. Health Perspect.* **70:**3–83.

Scherer, E., 1984, Neoplastic progression in experimental hepatocarcinogenesis, *Biochim. Biophys. Acta* **738:**219–236.

Setlow, R. B., 1983, Variations in DNA repair among humans, in: *Human Carcinogenesis* (C. C. Harris and H. Autrup, eds.), pp. 231–254, Academic Press, New York.

Shamsuddin, A. K. M., Sinopoli, N. T., Hemminki, K., Boesch, R. R., and Harris, C. C., 1985, Detection of benzo[a]pyrene-DNA adducts in human white blood cells, *Cancer Res.* **45:**66–68.

Starr, T. B., and Buck, R. D., 1984, The importance of delivered dose in estimating low-dose cancer risk from inhalation exposure to formaldehyde, *Fund. Appl. Toxicol.* **4:**740–753.

Stolley, P., Soper, K., Galloway, S., Nichols, W., Norman, S., and Wolman, S., 1984, Sister chromatid exchanges in association with occupational exposure to ethylene oxide, *Mutat. Res.* **129:**89–102.

Stowers, S. J., and Anderson, M. W., 1985, Formation and persistence of benzo[a]pyrene metabolite-DNA adducts, *Environ. Health Perspect.* **62:**31–39.

Sukumar, S., Notario, V., Martin-Zanca, D., and Barbacid, M., 1983, Induction of mammary carcinomas in rats by nitrosomethylurea involves malignant activation of Ha-ras-1 locus by single point mutations, *Nature* **306:**658–661.

Sukumar, S., Pulciani, S., Doniger, J., DiPaolo, J. A., Evans, C. H., Zbar, B., and Barbacid, M., 1984, A transforming *ras* gene in tumorigenic guinea pig cell lines initiated by diverse chemical carcinogens, *Science* **223:**1197–1199.

Swenberg, J. A., Richardson, F. C., Boucheron, J. A., and Dryoff, M. C., 1985, Relationships between DNA adduct formation and carcinogenesis, *Environ. Health Perspect.* **62:**177–183.

Törnqvist, M., Osterman-Golkar, S., Kautiainen, A., Jensen, S., Farmer, P. B., and Ehrenberg, L., 1986, Tissue doses of ethylene oxide in cigarette smokers determined from adduct levels in hemoglobin, *Carcinogenesis* **7:**1519–1521.

Umbenhauer, D., Wild, C. P., Montesano, R., Saffhill, R., Boyle, J. M., Huh, N., Kirstein, U., Thomale, J., Rajewsky, M. F., and Lu, S. H., 1985, O-methyldeoxy-guanosine in oesophageal DNA among individuals at high risk of oesopageal cancer, *Int. J. Cancer* **36:**661–665.

Vahakangas, K., Autrup, H., and Harris, C. C., 1984, Interindividual variation in carcinogen metabolism, DNA damage and repair, in: *IARC 1984,* pp. 85–98.

van Zeeland, A. A., 1986, *DNA Adducts Workshop,* Banbury Conference Center, Cold Spring Harbor Laboratory, New York, Sept. 30–Oct. 2.

van Zeeland, A. A., Mohn, G. R., Neuhauser-Klaus, A., and Ehling, U. H., 1985, Quantitative comparison of genetic effects of ethylating agents on the basis of DNA adduct formation. Use of O-ethylguanine as molecular dosimeter for extrapolation from cells in culture to the mouse, *Environ. Health Perspect.* **62:**163–169.

Vogel, E. W., 1986, *DNA Adducts Workshop,* Banbury Conference Center, Cold Spring Harbor Laboratory, New York, Sept. 30–Oct. 2.

Vogel, E. W., Nivard, M. J. M., Raaymakers-Jansen Verplanke, C. A., van Zeeland, A. A., and Zijlstra, J. A., 1986, Alkylation-induced mutagenesis in higher eukaryotic systems: Significance of DNA modifications and DNA repair with regard to genetic endpoints, in: *Genetic Toxicology of Environmental Chemicals, Part A: Basic Principles and Mechanisms of Action* (C. Ramel, B. Lambert, and J. Magnusson, eds.), pp. 219–228, Alan R. Liss, New York.

Weinstein, I. B., Gattoni-Celli, S., Kirschmeier, P., Lambert, M., Hsiao, W., Backer, J., and Jeffrey, A., 1984, Multistage carcinogenesis involves multiple genes and multiple mechanisms, in: *Cancer Cells 1: The Transformed Phenotype,* pp. 229–237, Cold Spring Harbor Laboratory, New York.

Wigley, C. B., Newbold, R. F., Amos, J., and Brookes, P., 1979, Cell-mediated mutagenesis in cultured Chinese hamster cells by polycyclic hydrocarbons: Mutagenicity and DNA reaction related to carcinogenicity in a series of compounds, *Int. J. Cancer* **23:**691–696.

Wogan, G. N., and Gorelick, N. J., 1985, Chemical and biochemical dosimetry of exposure to genotoxic chemicals, *Environ. Health Perspect.* **62:**5–18.

Wright, A. S., 1983, Molecular dosimetry techniques in human risk assessment: An industrial perspective, in: *Developments in the Science and Practice of Toxicology* (A. W. Hayes, R. C. Schnell, and T. S. Miya, eds.), pp. 311–318, Elsevier, Amsterdam.

V

Risk Management

11

Managing Environmental Risks

Lester B. Lave

THE 1960s ENVIRONMENTAL–CONSUMERIST MOVEMENT

A world with acute health problems, economic depression, war or the threat of nuclear annihilation, and high injury rates is not one where environmental issues are likely to be the focus of attention. Only when short-term health problems are under control, income is at a high level, and other immediate threats such as war are viewed as being under control is the environment likely to emerge as a major social concern (Lave, 1980a). The late 1960s was such a time in the United States and in much of the developed world. Spectacular progress had been made in lowering the infant mortality rate and vanquishing infectious disease. Trauma was viewed as basically being under control, due in part to the creation of the National Highway Transportation Safety Administration and Occupational Safety and Health Administration (OSHA). The perceived threat of nuclear war had receded far from the preoccupation of the early 1950s. Per capita income had increased steadily in the post-war period and fears of a deep depression had evaporated with the steady performance of the economy over two and a half decades. In short, immediate, high-level concerns had been satisfied and other issues might emerge to take their place.

Into this situation, Rachel Carson (1962), and later Ralph Nader (1965), introduced the public to new environmental and safety threats. Environmentalism and consumerism caught the public's conscience and emerged as issues that would play a large, often dominant, role for the next decade. The public wanted a cleaner, safer environment, a safer work place, and safer products. For a nation that had photographed the Earth from space and sent men to the moon, all goals seemed achievable, and the public was impatient with anyone who enumerated the difficulties.

At the end of the 1960s, environmental problems were viewed as obvious. One could

Lester B. Lave • Graduate School of Industrial Administration, Carnegie-Mellon University, Pittsburgh, Pennsylvania 15213.

see and smell the air and water pollution, see the effects of pesticides on the reproductive abilities of hawks and in mothers' breast milk, and it was obvious that toxic chemicals were causing problems, especially when they were dumped into the environment as waste. I grew up in Los Angeles where the smog problem was all too apparent and everyone suffered discomforts from its manifestations, such as eye irritation. When I moved to Pittsburgh in 1963, there were different kinds of air pollution and water pollution, but they were equally apparent.

By the late 1960s, air and water pollution ceased to be viewed as a necessary evil associated with economic prosperity. Instead, it was just an evil that an activist federal government and U.S. technology could eliminate, if only the nation shook off its lethargy and focused its attention.

1960s LEGISLATIVE SOLUTIONS

The solutions to the environmental and safety problems were viewed as obvious. Discharges of waste into rivers and lakes could be seen by anyone who cared to look; these were to be eliminated by 1985. Air pollution from automobiles and factories was obvious and these emissions were to be stopped (or abated by 90–95%) by 1976. Toxic chemicals were to be banned; only benign pesticides would be permitted and toxic chemicals could not be manufactured. When waste dumps emerged as a major issue, the solution was to control future dumping so that it would not create problems and to clean up existing hazardous dumps. If there were any costs, the polluter would pay.

Congress responded to the public demands by enacting simple legislation. According to the Clean Air Act of 1970, the Environmental Protection Agency (EPA) was to set primary air quality standards that "protected the most sensitive group in the population with an ample margin of safety." The Occupational Safety and Health Act directed OSHA to set standards to assure "that no employee will suffer material impairment of health or functional capacity even if such employee has regular exposure to the hazard . . . for the period of his working life." The Clean Water Act of 1972 declared the goal of "eliminating all discharges into waterways."

Congress believed that there were thresholds for the injurious effects of air pollution and required that air be cleaned at least to this standard by 1976. They required that emissions from automobiles be reduced 90–95% by 1975, and large enough reductions be made in emissions from factories, electricity generation plants, and other stationary sources to eliminate any health effects. Congress seemed unwilling to take seriously the notion that this environmental cleanup might be costly or even technologically infeasible in the time frame specified.

EVALUATION OF HEALTH, SAFETY, AND ENVIRONMENTAL REGULATION

Two decades have elapsed since the first of this environmental–safety legislation. The goals have not been achieved and there is no indication the goals will be achieved in the near term (Council on Environmental Quality, 1980; Simon and Kahn, 1984). This is not to say there has been no progress. The progress in many areas has been notable, although it falls far short of the goals.

The legislation and resulting regulations have been found to be expensive and disruptive, and to have increased the pace of closing old factories and exporting some jobs (Lave, 1980a; Weidenbaum and de Fina, 1978; Mendeloff, 1979; Crandall, 1983). The enforcement of the regulations has been burdensome. These results should surprise no one, since the legislation and regulations were never designed to be efficient or effective. The Administrator of EPA interprets the Clean Air Act to bar him from taking account of the cost of abatement in setting primary air quality standards. There is no explicit benefit–cost test in any of this legislation. Only when it was clear to Congress that chemicals were inherently harmful, as with pesticides, did Congress instruct the agencies to weigh risks against benefits in setting standards. Furthermore, Congress viewed the environmental movement as a welcome vehicle for pork barrel and giving economic relief to depressed regions (Ackerman and Hassler, 1981; Crandall, 1983; Peltzman, 1983; Pashigian, 1985). For example, Congress appropriated huge amounts of money for municipal sewage treatment plants, some of which were built but never operated. Congress has used the Clean Air Act to impede industry relocation to other regions and to rescue coal mines in the East. Such actions were not designed to achieve environmental clean-up efficiently or effectively; rather the environment was merely a convenient vehicle for "politics as usual."

However, by 1980 people had had enough of the disruption, red tape, and ineffective programs; a major theme of the 1980 presidential campaign was "getting the government off our backs." Ann Gorsuch-Burford and James Watt set about the dismantling of many aspects of environmental policy in 1981 (Lash *et al.*, 1984). Because they saw the problem as regulations to improve health, safety and the environment, rather than as achieving the public's goals efficiently and effectively, these "regulationphobes" proved to be liabilities to the Reagan administration and were replaced quickly.

THE ENVIRONMENTAL AGENDA IN 1987

From the viewpoint of 1987, a few themes have become clear. The first is that the public still desires a clean, safe environment and a lowering of risks. Public desires have been manifested in opinion surveys and in the demand for legislation. The Reagan administration has refused to take the lead in formulating an environmental agenda and so Congress has filled the void. For example, the Clean Water Act of 1987 was passed over a presidential veto. Progress has been set back a decade, because the rhetoric has focused on whether one is for a clean environment, rather than on how to achieve environmental goals effectively and efficiently.

It is also clear that the goals in the initial acts have not been achieved and are not achievable, at least in the short term. The levels of suspended particles and sulfur oxides have been reduced significantly, but the ozone problem is worse. Most sewage is treated, but disposal of toxic wastes has proven a more difficult problem and the levels of carcinogens in water do not appear to have been reduced.

A large scholarly literature has investigated the regulatory agencies and found them to be inefficient and ineffective. If the goals were abating pollution quickly and cheaply, they have not succeeded. Examining the amount of abatement achieved per dollar expended reveals that the agencies have been inefficient. Political scientists point out that a large number of purposes were being served by the regulatory agencies, and that efficiency and effectiveness were not dominant or even important goals to Congress or the agencies (Melnick, 1983; Wilson, 1980).

REGULATORY REFORM

Thus, there is general agreement on the need for reform (American Bar Association, 1979; American Enterprise Institute, 1979; Lave, 1981). A large number of reforms have been suggested. One was to depoliticize the agencies and put them under the stewardship of neutral professionals. The hope is that these professionals will determine what is technically possible and then achieve it efficiently. Since it is unlikely that the solution chosen by engineers would be the same one chosen by economists, there are two variants of this proposal. The first would rid the agency of political appointees and economists, instructing the scientists and engineers to make reasonable decisions. The second would be to put the economists in charge and do what President Reagan's Executive Order 12291 requires: Choose the alternative with the highest benefit–cost ratio. Few people want a coldly professional specification and enforcement of standards; they want agencies to take account of the particular circumstances in each case. That is, people want the agencies to be "political" and responsive.

A second reform is to give the agencies more staff and larger budgets. With more resources they could improve the scientific basis, better review the scientific evidence, and formulate and evaluate more options. However, one of the criticisms of the agencies is that they are paralyzed by red tape. There are so many approvals required and so many offices to check with that promulgating a regulation takes years and thousands of professional days. Increasing the size of the staff is likely to add to red tape, not solve the difficulties.

A third reform is to simplify procedures and get regulations promulgated with less public review and staff work. However, this means giving up some of the procedural reviews that have served to protect the public or industry at one time or another. No one is anxious to loosen control over the agencies.

A fourth reform is essentially to complicate procedures by mandating Congressional or judicial review of new regulations. The legislative veto would give one house, or even a committee power to overturn a regulation, thus adding another step to the process. Judicial review would instruct the courts not to defer to the agencies, but rather to review the wisdom of a regulation as well as whether the agency followed correct procedures and acted within its statute. The Supreme Court has declared the legislative veto to be unconstitutional, and the courts react with horror at the notion that they would have to scrutinize the substance of each regulation. A vast increase in the capacity of federal courts would be required, and there is no reason to believe that federal judges would have the technical expertise to understand and review the substance of regulations.

A fifth reform is to limit judicial challenges to regulation. In this view, the process would be faster and more efficient if court challenges were more difficult than at present. However, as with simplifying procedures, this proposal would mean less protection for those who believe that the environment is not getting clean enough or that the regulations are too stringent.

James Watt, Ann Gorsuch-Burford, and others wanted to deregulate; i.e., they wanted to let environmental issues be handled by the private sector or by states. This is the sixth reform. In the jargon of economics, environmental problems are caused by "externalities," and market forces cannot deal with these issues. Many environmental problems spill across the boundaries of a city, county, or state, and there would have to be so much negotiation among political jurisdictions that the federal government appears to be a better place of making rules.

A seventh reform has grown more popular during the Reagan administration. Distrusting EPA, Congress has enacted legislation that requires EPA to do specific things by specific dates. These "list and hammer" provisions are designed to force EPA to take action. However, they are likely to prevent an intelligent administrator from carrying out a reasonable program and are unlikely to force a recalcitrant administrator to do what Congress wants. The provisions are terribly specific, but they do not help to clarify the goals.

In short, there are no end of critics and suggestions for reform, but none of them seems to satisfy all interested parties. I think the idea of depoliticizing the agencies is nonsense, since environmental decisions are inherently political. The agency needs to be better administered, not to have more staff or budget.

The principal problem is that Congress has not specified workable goals for the agencies. Congress has failed to give realistic guidance to the agencies because the public has not settled on realistic goals. Thus, the agencies are slow and inefficient because the nation is attempting to figure out what it wants in the course of implementing environmental programs. None of the suggested reforms are likely to do much good until the public becomes clearer about what it wants from these health, safety, and environmental programs. Thus, the most helpful steps would be to help crystallize public desires, rather than to "reform" agencies that do not really know what they are to do.

THE ROLE OF RISK ANALYSIS IN RISK MANAGEMENT

Risk management can be described in terms of a sequence of steps (Lave, 1982). As shown in Fig. 1, the first step is identifying potential hazards. For example, a new

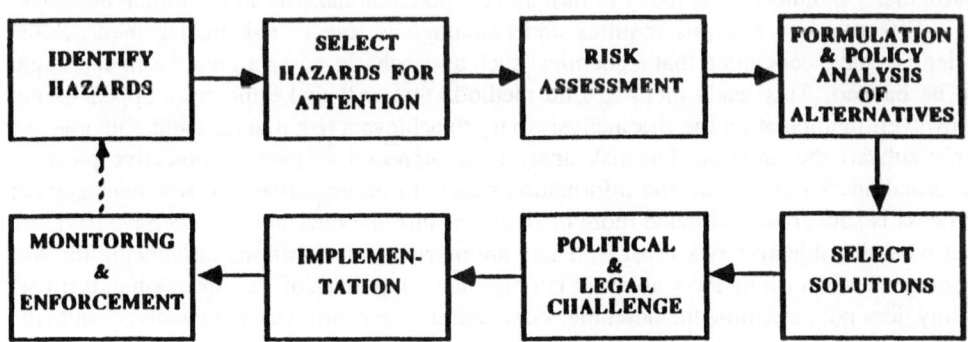

Figure 1. Hazard management.

chemical may be a potential hazard. Because there are so many potential hazards, the next step is prioritization and some of the potential hazards receive attention, while others are ignored. For example, if the new chemical is structurally similar to one that is a carcinogen, it might receive attention. Or, if most of the U.S. population will come into contact with a chemical, it might receive attention.

The third step is risk analysis, consisting of determining the nature of the hazard (e.g., carcinogenicity), estimating the dose–response relationship, the size of the population to be exposed and the level of exposure, the estimated probability of harm and expected number of people harmed, along with their uncertainties. For example, in 1978 when the Food and Drug Administration (FDA) and Congress were concerned with saccharin, the hazard of concern was bladder cancer and the dose–response relationship was estimated from long-term bioassays with rats. Perhaps 100,000,000 people were regularly exposed at levels that could be estimated. The National Research Council risk analysis indicated that up to 2000 bladder cancers per year might result from saccharin use and also that the uncertainty was large, because *no* bladder cancers might result from human saccharin use (NRC, 1979).

On the basis of the risk analysis, a decision must be made whether the risks are trivial, intermediate, or significant; this is the fourth step. This analysis is needed in setting priorities to decide which hazards get immediate attention, which are put aside, and which receive deliberate attention.

The fifth step is defining the range of regulatory options (including no action) and analyzing each. For saccharin, these options included (1) banning the substance, (2) banning it in foods while permitting it to be sold as an "over the counter" drug, (3) labeling foods with saccharin and requiring that posters be present in any place the saccharin is sold warning of the dangers, or (4) doing nothing. Congress and FDA decided on the fourth option.

Inevitably, every major regulation is challenged in court and in Congress, the sixth stage. Some groups think the regulation is too stringent and others think it is too lax. They search for places where the agency did not follow the Administrative Procedures Act or try to convince the courts to examine the substance of the decision. They try to convince Congress that the regulation is a bad one that is not in the public interest. Each challenge can take many years.

Whatever emerges from this challenge has to be implemented, the seventh step. Implementation requires the eighth step, monitoring and enforcement. The entire process, particularly monitoring, is likely to turn up new potential hazards and reinitiate the cycle.

Effective risk analysis requires understanding its role in risk management. Some scientists have concluded that a chemical such as saccharin poses a great harm and ought to be banned. This leads them to find methods that will make the risks appear large. However, manipulating the risk analysis to try to achieve a risk management outcome can only subvert the process. The risk analysis is supposed to give an objective piece of information. To the extent the information ceases to be objective, the risk management process is subverted and made more difficult because the decision makers have to figure out what the objective risk level is. There are myriad considerations influencing the risk management decision. Risk analysis is only one component of that decision and it certainly does not determine the outcome. For example, saccharin was not banned despite the evidence that it is an animal carcinogen. Some chemicals are banned, despite the fact that only very limited, somewhat inconclusive evidence is available (or because there are more innocuous substitutes available, e.g., cyclamate). The risk analysis must be as scientific and objective as possible, and not be influenced by the possible regulatory decisions and the risk analyst's feeling about what is the proper decision.

THE OUTCOME OF CURRENT RISK SITUATIONS

One of the most important aspects of risk management is understanding whether the environment is getting safer or becoming more hazardous, and knowing what the major current risks are. It makes little sense to ignore large hazards that could easily be fixed and to focus on minuscule hazards that are nearly impossible to remedy. One important observation is that life expectancy in the United States and in most of the world has been rising steadily in the 20th century. As part of this increase, infant mortality has fallen and life has become safer for most people. Thus, it is clear that in some overall sense, risk management has improved during the last 87 years.

Wildavsky (1979) argues that this lowering of risks is not accidental, but is associated with increases in per capita income. In his words, "richer is safer." Certainly there is a close relationship across countries between life expectancy and the level of income. However, there is nothing in Wildavsky's analysis to suggest that the risk reduction is automatic or can be achieved without thought and sacrifice. Rather, Wildavsky warns against sacrificing economic progress to achieve risk reduction; this is the wrong tradeoff and is inherently doomed to fail. Wildavsky also warns against a general belief that economic progress has increased risk or is generally detrimental.

Popular discussion is loose and fuzzy in talking about risks. A toxic chemical is said to cause "death" (Shelling, 1968; Zeckhauser and Shepard, 1976). In fact, death is inevitable for all people; the concern is with premature death or disability. Similarly, a premature death in someone who would have died of other causes within a few days is less of a social loss than a premature death that shortens life by three-fourths of a century. One discussion proposes the right measure to be "quality adjusted life-years" to account for pain and disability as well as premature death (Zeckhauser and Shepard, 1976).

Table 1 shows Cohen's (1985) calculations of the reduction in life expectancy in the United States due to a range of causes. Since almost half of deaths are due to heart disease, it is not surprising that eliminating heart disease would add the greatest increase in life expectancy (2100 days). The second item is due to statistics that show that unmarried people have shortened life expectancies due to a variety of causes. It appears astonishing that being unmarried costs 2000 days of life expectancy.

Cigarette smoking costs 1600 days of life expectancy due to increased heart disease, increased cancer, and respiratory diseases. All cancers account for 980 days of life expectancy lost; the estimate is smaller than one might think because the incidence of cancer is much higher among the elderly so that little life expectancy would be gained by eliminating the disease.

One inference from the table is that hazards associated with environmental chemicals appear to be small. Indeed, Doll and Peto (1981) have estimated that perhaps 2–4% of cancers are associated with environmental chemicals. I cannot help wondering whether

Table 1. Estimated Life Expectancy Reduction from
Risks and Activities

Activity or risk	Days LER
Heart disease	2100
Being unmarried	2000
Cigarette smoking	1600
Cancer	980
Being 30 lb overweight	900
Grade school dropout	800
Unskilled laborer	700
Stroke	520
Vietnam army duty	400
Mining or construction work (due to accidents only)	300
Motor vehicle accidents	200
Pneumonia, influenza	130
Homicide	90
Drowning	40
Poison + suffocation + asphyxiation	37
Energy production and use	25
Diet drinks	2
Hurricanes, tornadoes	1
Airline crashes	1
All-nuclear electricity	0.04–2[a]
Harrisburg area residents (from TMI accident)	0.001
Radioactive waste burial ground leaks, risk to nearest neighbors	0.0001
Sky-Lab fall	0.00000002

[a]The lower number is the estimate of government-sponsored scientists, and the higher number is the
  estimate of nuclear critics.

society is focusing its attention on the wrong hazards. One popular exposé (Whelan, 1985) argues that some people have deliberately misled the public.

Figure 2 and Table 2 from Milvy (1987) are a summary of agency decisions about what to regulate and what the risks are after regulation. The total number of premature deaths prevented by these regulatory actions seems small compared to what might have been achieved by devoting these resources to other hazards. With current information about the role of diet and other habits on heart disease and cancer, it seems clear that much life expectancy could be gained by convincing people to eat a healthy diet, give up tobacco, and engage in other healthful habits (NCI, 1987). Such a program would have much more effect on life expectancy than the actions of the regulatory agencies.

In particular, there has been a spectacular decline in the cardiovascular disease death rate in the United States during the past decade and a half. The decline is ascribed to screening for hypertension and effective medication for treating it, to more effective medical care, but principally to changes in diet and exercise (Levy, 1981). A similar decline in the cancer mortality rate might be achieved by more effective medical intervention, but more importantly through smoking cessation and changes in diet (NCI, 1987).

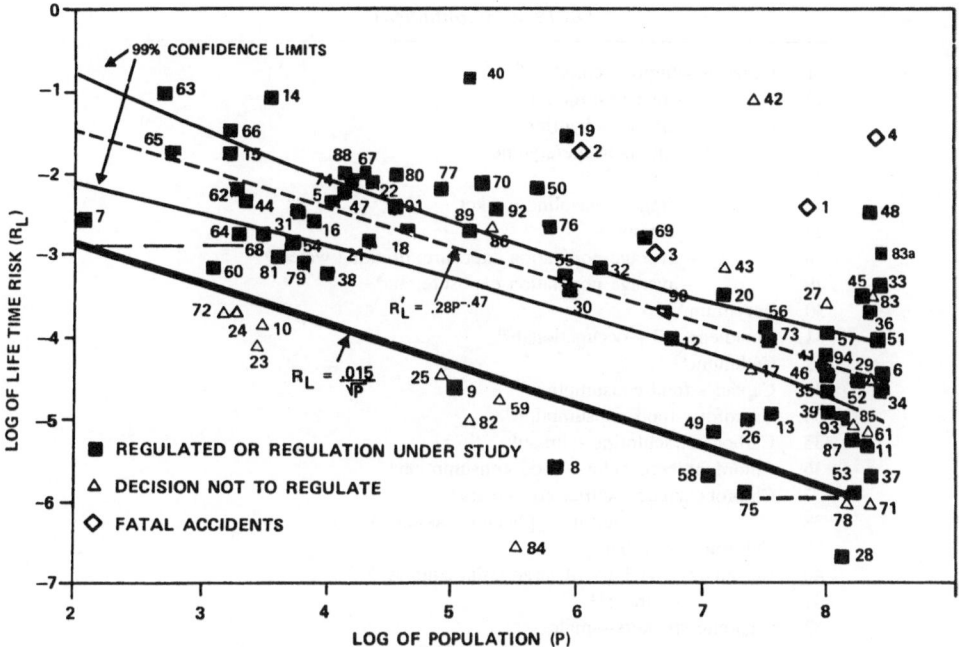

Figure 2. Effect of individual risk and exposed population on agency decisions to regulate. Adapted from Milvy (1987).

Table 2. Key to Figure 2[a,b]

1.	Accident, fatal—private sector 1982
2.	—mining
3.	—finance, insurance, and real estate, 47 years (18–65)
4.	—all, 1982 rate for 70 years
5.	Acrylonitrile[8]
6.	Alachlor—dietary[17]
7.	—flaggers[17]
8.	—farmers[17]
9.	—ground applicators[17]
10.	Amitraz—apple and pear sprayers[4]
11.	—apple and pear consumers[4]
12.	—apple, dietary[9]
13.	—pears, dietary[9]
14.	Arsenic—copper smelters: high[9]
15.	—copper smelters: low[9]
16.	—glass manufacturing[9]
17.	—Inorganic, neighboring population average exposure[4,9]
18.	—maximum exposure[4]
19.	Asbestos—occupational[9]
20.	—school; students and teachers[10]

(continued)

Table 2. (*Continued*)

21. Benzene—fugitive emission[9]
22.   —coke by-product[7,9]
23.   —maleic anhydride[9]
24.   —ethylbenzene/styrene[9]
25.   —storage[9]
26.   —Stage II gasoline market[7]
27.   —urban[6]
28.   —average population exposure: drinking water[26]
29.   —average population exposure: air[4]
30. Beryllium[3]
31. Butadiene,1,3—occupational[20]
32. Cadmium[11]
33. Captan—food consumption[18]
34. Captofol—food consumption[19]
35. Carbon tetrachloride—urban[6]
36. Chlordane/heptachlor—food consumption[4]
37. Chlorobenzilate—citrus consumers[4]
38.   —citrus applicators (assumed)[4]
39. Chloroform—urban[6]
40. Chromium—vicinity of large point sources[11,15]
41.   —urban[11]
42. Cigarette smokers—male
43. Coke ovens—average exposure for U.S. population at risk[4]
44.   —occupational[4]
45. Daminozide—food consumption[22]
46. 1,2-dichloroethane—urban[6]
47. Ethylene dibromide—occupational[9]
48.   —immediate postregulatory dietary[9]
49. Ethylene dichloride[1]
50. Ethylene oxide[11]
51. Folpet—food consumption[23]
52. Formaldehyde—urban ambient[9]
53.   —production use release[9]
54.   —resin manufacturing workers[9]
55.   —apparel workers[9]
56.   —mobile homes[10]
57.   —non-urea/formaldehyde homes[10]
58. Lindane—shelf paper[3]
59.   —livestock applicators[3]
60.   —pecan applicators[3]
61.   —food[3]
62.   —indirect occupational exposure[9]
63.   —direct occupational exposure[9]
64.   —non-production workers (occupational)[9]
65.   —manufacturing workers[9]
66.   —processing workers[9]
67.   —all workers: OTS-based[9]
68.   —all workers: TLV-based[9]
69. Nickel[11]
70. Nitrosamines—occupational exposure from metal-working fluids[21]

Table 2. (*Continued*)

71. NTA— public drinking water[4]
72.   —fomulators (occupational)[4]
73. PCB—dietary fish[10]
74. Pentachlorophenol—applicators/workers[25]
75.   —air[2]
76. Radiation, ionizing—all workers in medicine and industry[12]
77.   —power reactor workers[12]
78.   —coal-fired boilers[16]
79. Radionuclides—DOE facilities[16]
80.   —uranium mines[16]
81.   —elemental phosphorus plants[16]
82.   —phosphate industry[16]
83. Radon—drinking water[5]
83a.   —indoor[27]
84. Styrene monomer—occupational[2]
85. Tetrachloroethylene—urban population[14]
86.   —dry cleaners[14]
87. Trichloroethylene—urban air[14]
88. Uranium mill tailings—inactive sites[9]
89.   —active sites[9]
90. Vinyl chloride—average exposure for population: air[4]
91.   —maximum exposure (occupational)[4]
92.   —workers (occupational)[11]
93.   —average exposure to population: water[26]
94. Volatile synthetic organic compounds[24]

[a]The values provided in the references to this table reflect current state-of-the-art estimates of risk and population at risk. They are subject to revision and improvement, and their inherent limitations should be borne in mind.
[b]See pp. 155–156 for references to table

THE PRESSURE FOR RISK ASSESSMENT

The role that risk analysis should play in the risk management process is easily understood. As a result, risk managers want these analyses in making decisions. In addition to the demand stemming from good sense, there are a number of other sources of pressure to do risk analysis. The first is administrative edict. Each president since Richard Nixon has required that the benefits of proposed regulations be estimated in order to ensure the regulation will be effective and will accomplish the objective at low cost. In particular, Ronald Reagan issued Executive Order 12292 in February 1981 requiring that the benefits and costs of each major regulation be assessed. Quantifying benefits of a health or safety regulation requires a risk analysis. Thus, the executive order requires risk analysis of health and safety regulations.

The second source of pressure comes from the Supreme Court (1980). In the "Benzene Case" the court vacated an OSHA regulation on the common law principle that "the law does not concern itself with trivia" and that OSHA had not concluded that benzene at the current standard posed a "significant" risk. Without such a finding, no regulation could take place. To find that a risk is significant, it must be quantified. This means that the Supreme Court was essentially requiring risk analysis before regulation could begin. However, getting consensus on what are significant and "de minimis" risks has not been possible (Byrd and Lave, 1987).

A third source of pressure comes from Congress, the media, and the public. People are wary of hearing that a chemical may cause a hazard. There are more potential hazards than society can hope to deal with. Instead, decision makers need to know the magnitude of the threat, which requires risk assessment.

The fourth source of pressure comes from scientists. We understand that there are so many potential hazards that we need to be able to know which get priority. Risk assessment is a means of finding what the most important issues are and which uncertainties have to be resolved. Risk assessment focuses the science by indicating precisely which questions are of greatest interest. Risk assessment shows the difference between the concerns of charlatans or naive scientists and the issues of greatest importance.

HOW TO DO RISK ASSESSMENT

A great deal has been written on how to do risk assessment, which is not my focus here (Lave, 1982; Office of Technology Assessment, 1981; Office of Scientific Technology and Policy, 1984); I want to stress the uncertainties and the need to quantify them. Point estimates tell little of the story, particularly when they are meant to be reasonable upper-bound estimates. Decision makers need to know the sources and quantitative implications of uncertainty. No risk analysis is complete or informative without estimates of the range of uncertainty.

I also want to stress interactions among hazards, such as mixtures of chemicals. The interactions can serve either to dampen the effects of individual chemicals or to increase them.

Complicating risk analysis is the difference between group and individual risk. There are those who are sensitive because of genetic or somatic factors (Omenn, 1982). One cannot assume that individuals are homogeneous.

HOW ACCURATE ARE RISK ESTIMATES?

The procedures for estimating risks are meant to provide "reasonable upper-bound estimates" (Andersen and CAG, 1983). They are meant to be upper bounds, but not to use such extreme assumptions that estimates make no sense. Thus, the point estimate is at the top of the distribution.

In virtually every case, the reasonable lower-bound estimate is zero. For example, for chemicals that are carcinogenic in rodents and for which there is no human evidence of carcinogenicity, it is a reasonable assumption that the chemical may not be a human carcinogen. Even when a chemical is known to be a human carcinogen, the relationship is known to exist at much higher doses than those that people are currently exposed to. A reasonable lower-bound assumption is that there is a threshold and that the risk is zero at this dose. Thus, in virtually every case, the reasonable range of uncertainty extends from zero to the point estimate from risk analysis.

HOW USEFUL ARE THE RISK ESTIMATES?

Given this enormous range of uncertainty, from zero to the point estimate, it is not a trivial question to ask how useful is the estimate. There are several important points. The first is that the risk analysis focuses the debate. It isolates the crucial assumptions and reveals which are the important issues.

An extension of this point is that risk analysis gets away from "black box" science which gives no attention to mechanisms. Instead, risk analysis utilizes the available information about mechanism to determine the shape of the dose–response relationship and determine if there is a threshold. It also isolates who may be most sensitive to the exposure. The risk analysis implicitly sets out a research agenda to resolve the principal difficulties. The risk analysis points analysts toward asking the right questions: What is the population at risk? What are their exposures?

Importantly, risk analysis shifts attention away from the statistical significance of an effect and onto the quantitative significance. Epidemiologists and toxicologists tend to focus on statistical significance in asking whether an association could have arisen by chance. What is more important for decision making is the quantitative importance of the effect, whether it is significant or not. This shift in focus implies a redesign of both epidemiological and toxicological studies to get better estimates of the quantitative importance, rather than focusing on the statistical significance.

SETTING RISK GOALS

The most difficult and important step in risk management is setting goals. A great deal has been written about this and it is not the focus here. However, contributions by Fishhoff *et al.* (1981) and recent work on de minimis and significant risk (Milvy, 1986; Whipple, 1987) are of particular interest.

In the past, much of risk management was regarded as the province of professionals who were to make the technology safe. These professionals generally did not know and did not care to know public concerns. After all, the public did not understand the nature of the risk or the technology and so had little to contribute. This led to addressing concerns that did not bother the public and not addressing concerns that did. The important point is that it is the public that must be satisfied that risk has been properly managed. This means that the public must feel that its concerns are properly addressed and have confidence in the analysis and decisions.

CONCLUSION

The emergence of public concern for health and safety in the late 1960s can be seen as a manifestation of the steady increase in income and steady reduction of other social risks. The management of risk, particularly those from carcinogens, came to occupy a central part of public concern, as well as the time and energy of government and industry. Risk analysis is invaluable in managing environmental risks, as long as it reflects the best available science, rather than arbitrary conventions about dose–response relationships, estimates of potency, etc. Scientists must exclude their values from the risk estimation and can channel them into other steps of the risk management process. Initially, risk assessment won acceptance by making a set of highly conservative assumptions; however, much more is known about mechanisms and arbitrarily conservative assumptions are no longer warranted or helpful.

Risk analysis is still highly uncertain. Enhancing usefulness requires explicit examination of the uncertainty and specification of the reasonable range of possible adverse effects. Basic research is needed on the physiological mechanisms of disease. The greatest progress will result not from more somewhat arbitrary characterizations of the risks of compounds, but from greater understanding that serves to reduce uncertainty and make the risk analysis more powerful.

In the 1980 presidential campaign, popular dissatisfaction was manifested with the federal regulatory agencies. These agencies have been striving to accomplish their goals more efficiently and effectively, with risk analysis playing a more important role. Regulatory reform starts with better understanding of the risks. The pressure for risk analysis is widespread, coming not only from the recognition that it is required for better decisions, but also from presidential order, court decrees, and scientists in search of less arbitrary regulation.

This is not to say that risk assessment is simple or the only way of improving risk management. However, risk assessment has an important role to play in structuring the agenda of basic and applied research and in improving risk management.

REFERENCES

Ackerman, B., and Hassler, W., 1981, *Clean Coal, Dirty Air,* Yale University Press, New Haven.

American Bar Association, 1979, *Federal Regulation: Roads to Reform, Final Report and Recommendations of the Commission on Law and the Economy,* American Bar Association, New York.

American Enterprise Institute, 1979, *Government Regulation: Proposals for Procedural Reform,* American Enterprise Institute, Washington.

Anderson, E., and the Carcinogen Assessment Group (CAG) of the U.S. Environmental Protection Agency, 1983, Quantitative approaches in use to assess cancer risks, *Risk Anal.* 3:277–295.

Byrd, D., and Lave, L., 1987, Significant risk is not the antonym of de minimis risk, in: *De Minimis Risk, Contemporary Issues in Risk Analysis,* Vol. 2 (C. Whipple, ed.), pp. 41–60, Plenum Press, New York.

Carson, R., 1962, *Silent Spring,* Houghton-Mifflin, New York.

Cohen, B., 1985, Risks in our society, in: *Nuclear Energy: A Sensible Alternative* (K. Ott and B. Spinrad, eds.), pp. 317–325, Plenum Press, New York.

Council on Environmental Quality, 1980, *The Global 2000 Report to the President: Entering the 21st Century,* U.S. Government Printing Office, Washington.

Crandall, R., 1983, *Controlling Industrial Pollution: The Economics and Politics of Clean Air,* Brookings Institution, Washington.

Doll, R., and Peto, R., 1981, *The Causes of Cancer,* Oxford University Press, New York.

Fischhoff, B., Lichtenstein, S., Slovic, P., Darby, S., and Keeny, R., 1981, *Acceptable Risk,* Cambridge University Press, Cambridge.

Lash, J., Gillman, K., and Sheridan, D., 1984, *A Season of Spoils: The Story of the Reagan Administration's Attack on the Environment,* Pantheon, New York.

Lave, L., 1980a, Environmental risks, in: *Societal Risk Analysis: How Safe is Safe Enough* (R. Schwing and W. Albers, eds.), Plenum Press, New York.

Lave, L., 1980b, Health, safety, and environmental regulation, in: *Setting National Priorities: Agenda for the 1980s* (J. Pechman, ed.), pp. 131–168, Brookings Institution, Washington.

Lave, L., 1981, *The Strategy of Social Regulation,* Brookings Institution, Washington.

Lave, L., 1982, *Quantitative Risk Assessment in Regulation, Brookings Institution,* Washington.

Levy, R., 1981, The decline in cardiovascular disease mortality, *Ann. Rev. Public Health,* **2**:49–70.

Melnick, R., 1983, *Regulation and the Courts: The Case of the Clean Air Act,* Brookings Institution, Washington.

Mendeloff, J., 1979, *Regulating Safety: An Economic and Political Analysis of Occupational Safety and Health Policy,* MIT Press, Cambridge.

Milvy, P., 1986, A general guideline for management of risk from carcinogens, *Risk Anal.* **6**:69–80.

Milvy, P., 1987, Actual and perceived risks from chemical carcinogens, in: *De Minimis Risk: Contemporary Issues in Risk Analysis,* Vol. 2 (C. Whipple, ed.), pp. 75–86, Plenum Press, New York.

Nader, R., 1965, *Unsafe at Any Speed,* Grossman, New York.

National Cancer Institute (NCI), 1987, *Cancer Goals for 2000,* Department of Health and Human Services, Washington.

National Research Council (NRC), Committee for a Study on Saccharin and Food Safety Policy, 1979, *Food Safety Policy,* National Academy Press, Washington.

Office of Science and Technology Policy, 1984, Chemical carcinogens: Notice of review of the science and its associated principles, *Fed. Regist.* **49**(100):21593–21661, (Books 1 and 2, May 22, 1984).

Office of Technology Assessment, 1981, *Assessment of Technologies of Determining Cancer Risks from the Environment,* U.S. Office of Technology Assessment, Washington.

Omenn, G., 1982, Predictive identification of hypersensitive individuals, *J. Occup. Med.* **24**:369–74.

Pashigian, B., 1985, Environmental regulation: Whose self-interests are being protected? *Econ. Inq.,* **23**:551–584.

Peltzman, S., 1983, *An Economic Interpretation of the History of Congressional Voting in the Twentieth Century,* University of Chicago Press, Chicago.

Shelling, T., 1968, The life you save may be your own, in: *Problems in Public Expenditure Analysis* (S. Chase, ed.), pp. 127–161, Brookings Institution, Washington.

Simon, J., and Kahn, H., 1984, *The Resourceful Earth: A Response to Global 2000,* Blackwell, New York.

Supreme Court of the United States, 1980, *Industrial Union Department, AFL-CIO v. American Petroleum Institute,* 448 U.S. 607.

Weidenbaum, M., and de Fina, R., 1978, *The Cost of Federal Regulation of Economic Activity,* American Enterprise Institute, Washington.

Whelan, E., 1985, *Toxic Terror: The Truth About the Cancer Scare,* Jameson Books, Ottawa, Illinois.

Whipple, C. (ed.), 1987, *De Minimis Risk: Contemporary Issues in Risk Analysis,* Vol. 2, Plenum Press, New York.

Wildavsky, A., 1979, No risk is the highest risk of all, *Am. Sci.* **67**:32–37.

Wilson, J., 1980, *The Politics of Regulation,* Basic Books, New York.

Zeckhauser, R., and Shepard, D., 1976, Where now for saving lives? *Law Contemp. Prob.,* **40**:5–45.

REFERENCES FOR TABLE 2

1. Suta, B., *Assessment of Human Exposures to Atmospheric Ethylene Dichloride,* SRI International (May 1979).

2. EPA, Office of Policy Analysis, *Unit Risk Estimates For Toxic Air Pollution,* Office of Air Quality Planning and Standards, *Maximum Exposure Levels and Population Totals* (1984).

3. EPA, Lindane PD-4 (draft) (August 1983).

4. Anderson, E. L., "Quantitative Approaches in Use to Assess Cancer Risk," *Risk Analysis 3,* No. 4, 277–295 (1983).

5. Cothern, R. C., *et al., Development of Quantitative Estimates of Uncertainty in Environmental Risk Assessment When the Scientific Data Base is Inadequate* (Draft), Office of Drinking Water, EPA, Washington, D.C.

6. Bussard, D., Memorandum dated 3/15/84, EPA, Washington, D.C.

7. Gorman, T., NESHAP briefing paper, OPPE, EPA (1984).

8. Office of Air Quality and Standards, *Need for Regulation of Coke Oven Emissions and Acrylonitrile Under CAA,* briefing paper, EPA, Washington, D.C. (March 1984).

9. Dobkowski, D., Memorandum to A. Jennings dated 4/3/84, Acting Director Statistical Policy Division, EPA, Washington, D.C.

10. Chemical Coordination Staff for the Six Month Air Toxics Study "Acceptable Risk Levels and Federal Regulations . . . ," EPA, Washington, D.C. (May 1984).

11. Haemisegger, E., Jones, A., *et al, The Air Toxics Problem in the United States: An Analysis of Cancer Risks for Selected Pollutants,* EPA (Final Agency Internal Review); Washington, D.C. (May 1985).

12. Kumazawa, S. *et al., Occupational Exposure to Ionizing Radiation in the United States,* EPA, Washington, D.C. (March 1983).

13. Britton, B., *Risk Characteristics for Various Pollutants Regulated or Being Considered by EPA Program Offices,* Chemical and Statistical Policy Division, EPA, Washington, D.C. (1985).

14. Milvy, P., *Estimates of Cancers from Perchloroethylene (PCE) Exposure (4/3/84) and Health Assessment Document for Tetrachloraethylene,* EPA, Washington, D.C. (December 1983).

15. EPA-OHEA, Health Assessment Document for Chromium, 7/83 draft.

16. Office of Radiation Programs, *Background Information; Final Rules for Radionuclides,* 11 (October 23, 1982).

17. EPA, Draft Alachlor PD-1 (12/4/84), 54.

18. EPA, Draft Captan PD-2/3 (2/5/85), 11–68.

19. EPA, Captofol PD-1 (December 1984).

20. EPA, Office of Toxic Substances, *Assessment of Cancer Risk to Workers, Exposure to 1,3-Butadiene in Plants Producing Synthetic Rubber, Plastics and Resins* (November 21, 1984).

21. Preliminary Economic Analysis of Proposed Regulations for the Use of Nitrites in Metalworking Fluids; PHD, Inc. (October 1984).

22. EPA registration standard, 21 (June 1984).

23. EPA, Preliminary Folpet Risk Assessment Briefing Paper for S.I.S., OPP (1985).

24. EPA, Regulatory Impact Analysis, Regulatory Flexibility Analysis and Paperwork Reduction Act Analysis for Proposed Regulations to Control Volatile Synthetic Organic Chemicals (VOCs) in Drinking Water (EPA -570/9-85-004) (Calculated from pages I-5 and IV-8) (May 1985).

25. EPA, Office of Pesticide Programs Position Document 2/3 on Wood Preservatives, 364, 582, 589 (1984).

26. Cothern, R. C., Coniglio, W. A., and Marcus, W. L., *Techniques for the Assessment of the Carcinogenic Risk to the U.S. Population Due to Exposure from Selected Volatile Organic Compounds from Drinking Water Via the Ingestion, Inhalation, and Dermal Routes* (EPA-570/9-85-001) (July 25, 1984). (Calculations based on the multistage model for extrapolation of risk to low dose).

27. Nero, A. V., Jr., "Risk and Policy Implications of Indoor Exposure to [222]Rn Decay Products and Other Air Pollutants." Paper presented at the 1985 Annual Meeting of the Society for Risk Analysis, Alexandria, Va.

12

Acceptable Risk

Chris Whipple

INTRODUCTION

The acceptability of risk is a complex subject. Judgments of acceptability are made at many levels—by individuals, families and other groups, and by the society at large. A risk may be acceptable to the consumer of a product or technology, but those who receive no benefit but some risk from the technology may disagree. A risk which was accepted in prospect may become unacceptable in hindsight.

Traditionally, acceptable risk has been judged in engineering by whether good engineering practice has been followed, both in the application of appropriate design standards and in analysis resulting in engineering decisions where no standards apply precisely. Similarly, the courts rely on tradition-based standards in tort law to define a risk maker's responsibility to avert risk and a risk bearer's right to be free from significant risk impositions. A substantially different perspective holds in welfare economics, where risk is viewed as a social cost, and where acceptability depends to a significant degree on the costs of avoiding risk. Risk can be considered analytically from either perspective: as a matter of costs and benefits, or as a matter of rights and responsibilities.

The useful purpose of such analyses is not to proclaim one risk to be acceptable and another unacceptable. While analysis provides insight into values and trade-offs implicit in alternate social choices, analysis is not generally an acceptable way to make important social choices. Analysis does not define the risk management agenda, however it can help shape the response to evolving public opinion about which risks are too high and about which are of little concern.

A version of this chapter appears as "Approaches to Acceptable Risk" in Y. Haimes and E. Z. Stakhiv, eds., *Risk-Based Decision Making in Water Resources*, pp. 30–45, American Society of Civil Engineers, New York.

Chris Whipple • Electric Power Research Institute, Palo Alto, California 94303.

The long-term historical definition of acceptable risk is briefly described in the following section; a subsequent section reviews comparative and analytical approaches proposed to develop workable definitions of acceptable risk, including publicly-derived risk criteria. Finally, the way in which diverse objectives for risk management become apparent in risk standard setting is described.

A HISTORICAL OVERVIEW

Hammer (1980) describes legal milestones in product liability from ancient times to the present in terms of the broad trends that have occurred; this provides a useful perspective on our current situation. According to Hammer's review, the balance between an individual's right to be free from imposed risks and the right of a producer to make less than perfectly safe products has undergone two basic transitions. The ancient ethic of ''an eye for an eye'' as codified in the Code of Hammurabi established that a person was liable and required to suffer the same injury he caused, whether or not the injury was intentional. The implementation of this rule seems unfair from our present perspective; for example, if a house fell down and killed the son of the owner, the builder's son was put to death. Hammer notes how, with time, the law evolved to permit financial restitution in place of punishment where harm was unintentional. Presumably, such compromises provided for houses that did not fall down for the most part, and also permitted sufficient incentives for people to be builders.

Under the British law that followed the onset of the Industrial Revolution, and on which American law was partially based, this balance of rights and responsibilities was dramatically altered. The need to follow good safety practices and to compensate injured parties was seen as an impediment to progress. Industrial development was regarded as an unmixed blessing much more then than now, and it followed that obstacles to such development, such as claims by injured parties, were not regarded as socially desirable. A major decision in 1842, referred to as the Rule of Privity, established that a seller is liable for injury from his product only to those with whom he has a contract, such as the direct purchaser of the product. Hammer quotes the decision by Lord Arbinger in the landmark case (which involved a driver for the mail service and a coach with a defective wheel): ''Every passenger, or even any person passing along the road, who was injured by the upsetting of the coach, might bring a similar (legal) action. Unless we confine the operation of such contracts as this to the parties who entered into them, the most absurd and outrageous consequences to which I can see no limit would ensue.''

Since the mid-nineteenth century, the law has shifted substantially. Many laws and court decisions have established consumer rights and producer responsibilities, and the Rule of Privity has been eliminated. In particular, in the United States during the 1960s and 1970s, many changes occurred which strengthened a consumer's rights to protection and recovery of damages. Much responsibility for safety was shifted back to the producer; laws and courts extended protection to bystanders and employees as well as to customers, and restricted a producer's ability to avoid responsibility through warnings or contract provisions.

Many other changes in social risk management have occurred in the past several decades. The use of government regulation, in place of and in addition to the tort system, has been one such change. This is due partially to the recognition that many modern risks are not well managed by the trial and error method embodied in tort law. The recent emphasis on risk from a rights perspective, coupled with analytic abilities to measure extremely small risks, has created new areas for tort law that are still being untangled. And the increasing recognition that laws and court decisions intended to help consumers can have perverse effects (such as by reducing the number of producers or insurers) is influencing efforts to find a socially acceptable way to make acceptable risk decisions. It is against this evolving perspective that analytical approaches to determine acceptable risk have emerged.

RISK COMPARISONS

One basic way to consider the acceptability of a risk is to compare it to other risks. Comparisons, in their simplest form, serve as benchmarks for the calibration of intuition. Where the mathematical expression of risk is unfamiliar, as with an annual probability of death of 10^{-6}, a comparison can help; for example, "the risk is twice as great as being struck and killed by lightning," or "the same chance of death as driving 100 miles, on average." While these are perhaps familiar reference points, the use of comparisons for judging the acceptability of risk is controversial. One criticism concerns the comparison of dissimilar risks, as Kirk Smith notes (Smith, 1980):

> . . . a risk assessment procedure must demonstrate the relevance of the comparison. If tonsillectomies, for illustration, are less dangerous per hour than open-heart operations, it doesn't necessarily mean that the latter are too risky or that hospitals should be encouraged to remove more tonsils and to open fewer hearts. Nor does it mean that a particular energy system is acceptable merely because it is less dangerous than a tonsillectomy. The social benefits of these activities are so different that direct comparisons of their risks are nearly meaningless.

A different point of view was expressed by Lord Rothschild in an opinion piece in *The Wall Street Journal* in 1979 (Rothschild, 1979): "There is no point in getting into a panic about the risks of life until you have compared the risks which worry you with those that don't, but perhaps should."

These perspectives are not necessarily in conflict. Smith's point is simply that the existence of a large risk does not excuse a small one when the benefits and other contextual factors are different; Lord Rothschild's point is that social concern and attention to risk should bear some relation to the magnitude of risk.

One source of confusion regarding risk comparisons is that risk can be measured many ways. There are conflicting views among risk analysts regarding the appropriate expression for risk, quite separate from the complex way in which the characteristics of risk correspond to its public perception. Risk analysts frequently describe a risk by its expectation, sometimes referring to this value as societal risk. This measure is appropriate when the primary objective of risk management or of a risk-related decision is to minimize consequences over a large population. But often the risk to individuals or small groups at greatest risk is the measure of interest. The importance of considering both individual and societal risk in risk management is discussed below in greater detail. The question of how to measure and express risk goes beyond individual versus societal risk, as the following examples indicate.

Figure 1 is a typical "risk ladder," used to describe individual risks, and Table 1 provides additional information about current levels of risk. Even within this individual risk framework, the basis for comparison can be disputed. For example, some recreational activities which are quite risky on an hourly basis (e.g., rock climbing) do not stand out on an annual basis because few hours are spent engaged in the activity per year, on average. Although one commonly sees these risks expressed as annual averages, a different perspective is obtained from the hourly basis. In Chauncey Starr's influential paper, the hourly basis was selected because, Starr reasoned, this more closely resembled the decision basis for voluntary, recreational risks (Starr, 1969). On this basis, Starr noted a significant difference between the level of self-imposed risks and involuntary exposures.

Some risks have characteristics which neither expectation nor individual risk measures capture. For example, Figs. 2 and 3, from the Nuclear Regulatory Commission's Reactor Safety Study (NRC, 1975), describe and compare the estimated risks from nuclear power with a number of other risks having catastrophic potential. It has long been argued that a social risk aversion against severe accidents exists. If this is the case then it would be inappropriate to describe a risk distribution with severe consequences by its expectation, or to compare a potentially catastrophic risk with a routine one.

Figure 4 illustrates another kind of comparison. Sometimes referred to as a natural standard or natural baseline comparison, this figure compares pollutant exposures and standards from anthropogenic sources with natural levels. The implied logic, occasionally made explicit (see Adler and Weinberg, 1978), is that since we are indifferent to small variations in natural exposures, we should also be insensitive to man-made exposures

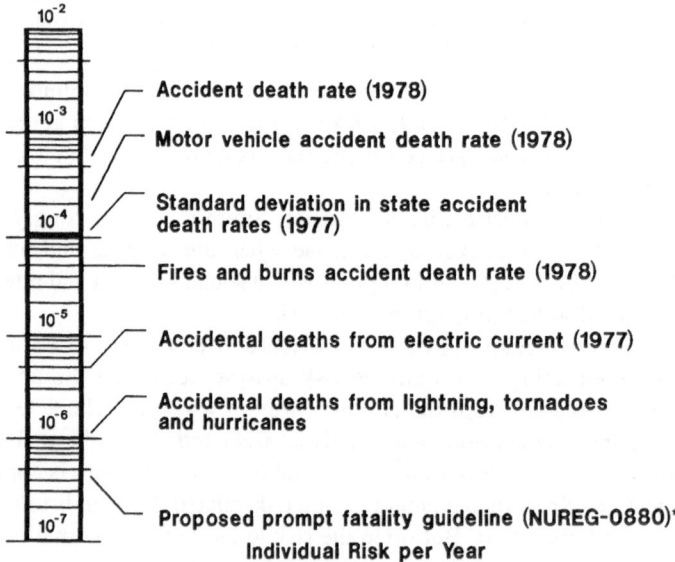

Figure 1. Individual prompt fatality risks: A comparison. Prompt fatality safety goal risk applies to small population of plant neighbors; all other risks are to the entire U. S. population.

Table 1. Risk Acceptability: Current Levels for Individual Fatality Risks

Unacceptable risk
  Short-time risks (e.g., recreational activities)
    Risk usually $< 10^{-6}$/hr
      (If activity continuous, this would be $\sim 10^{-2}$/year risk, equivalent to average population risk from all causes.)
  Occupational risks
    Risk usually $< 10^{-3}$/year
      Logging 1.4×10^{-3}/year
      Coal mining 6.4×10^{-4}/year
      Heavy construction 4.2×10^{-4}/year
      All occupations 1.1×10^{-4}/year (1983)
      Safe occupations 5×10^{-5}/year
  Public risks
    Risk usually $< 10^{-4}$/year for involuntary exposures, such as living below a dam

De minimis risk
  Individual risks below 10^{-6}–10^{-7}/year frequently ignored even if involuntary; e.g. FDA is 10^{-6}/–10^{-8}/lifetime, NRC proposed prompt safety goal is 5×10^{-7}/year

Between unacceptable and de minimis
  Risk decisions guided by cost-effectiveness of proposed risk reductions.

smaller than the natural variance. One limitation of this approach is that many risk exposures of concern have no natural counterpart.

A major difficulty of using risk comparisons as an aid to judging risk acceptability was noted by Kirk Smith in the quotation above: the relevance of the comparison must be established. Even when a relevant comparison can be made, often other factors are

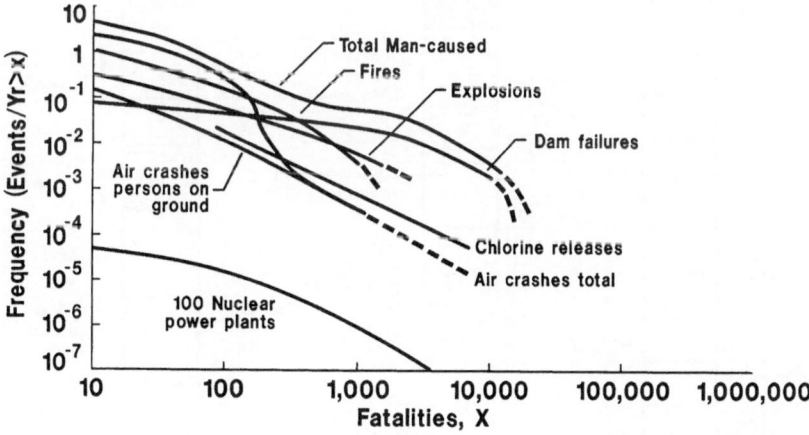

Figure 2. Frequency of man-caused events involving fatalities. Fatalities due to auto accidents are not shown because data is not available for large consequence accidents. From WASH-1400 (1975).

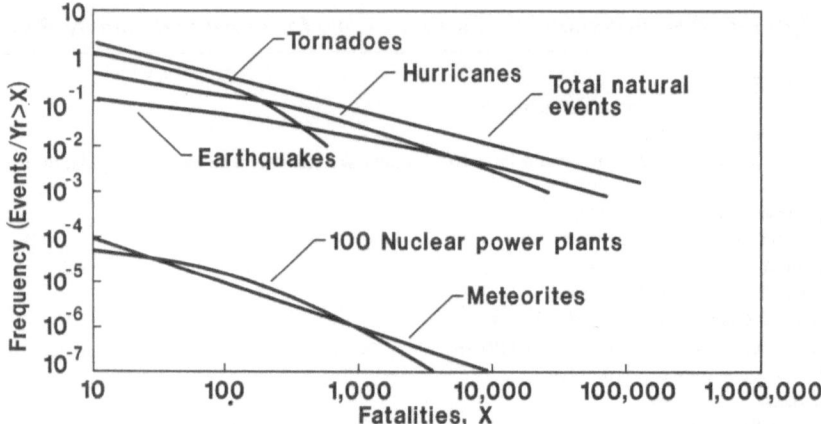

Figure 3. Frequency of natural events involving fatalities. From WASH-1400 (1975).

important to a decision. Decisions which depend solely on a risk comparison are rare. For example, it is frequently noted that commercial air travel is safer than travel by automobile. But this does not mean that one should fly even when it is cheaper and more convenient to drive. Risk may be the dominant consideration in the selection of treatment for a serious medical problem, but cases in which risk is the only decisive factor are rare. Risk is not judged to be acceptable or not, technologies are.

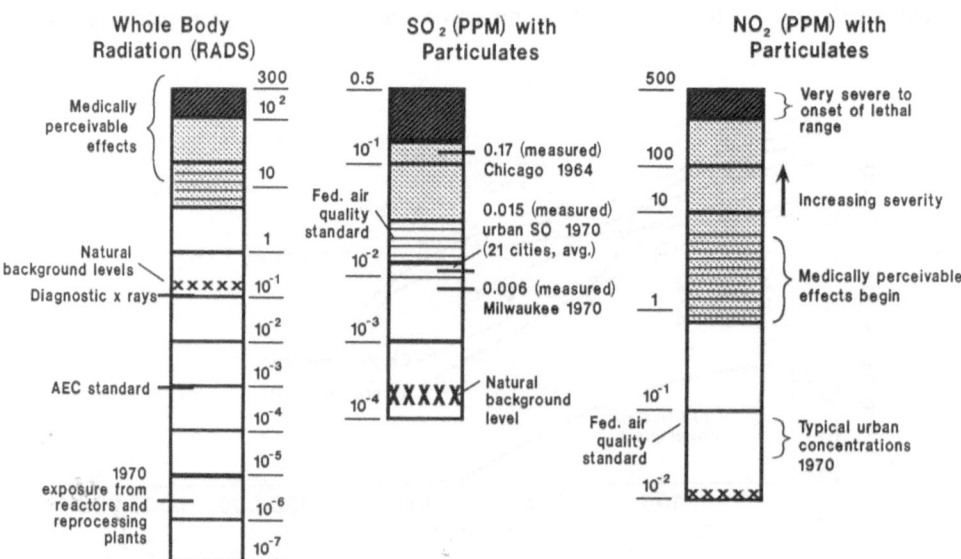

Figure 4. Comparison of pollutant standards, background levels, man-made exposures, and health effects. Neither the units nor factors of 10 on the scales are the same. From WASH-1224 (1974).

INDIVIDUAL AND SOCIETAL RISK

Disagreement regarding the appropriate measures for risk usually reflects differing objectives for risk management. One common question is whether and when it is appropriate to describe a risk as the expected number of consequences per unit time in a population, for example, as deaths per year in the United States, and when one should be more sensitive to levels of individual risk. As the following example illustrates, it is inadequate to rely solely on either risk measure.

Consider a risk of death of 10^{-6} per year to a population of 1000; this produces an expectation of 10^{-3} fatalities per year (or one fatality per 1000 years on average). The same 10^{-6} per year risk to the entire U.S. population produces an expectation of 240 fatalities per year. On the basis of individual risk alone, these two cases are equivalent. But under current policies, the social evaluation of these risks differs significantly. In the case of risk to a small population, it is unlikely that any effort made at risk management on the reasonable basis that to do so would waste resources better applied to larger risks. Conversely, substantial resources would be justified to reduce a risk with 240 expected fatalities. This example illustrates that the population risk is an important consideration when the primary objective of risk management or of a risk-related decision is to minimize consequences over a large population.

But individual risk to the exposed population, and to the subgroups at greatest risk, is also often an important concern. A risk of fatality of 10^{-3} per year to a single individual has an expectation of 10^{-3} fatalities per year—the same as the above case of a 10^{-6} per year fatality risk to a population of 1000. A 10^{-3} per year fatality risk to an individual is rarely accepted; the most hazardous occupations incur risks of about this level, as do cigarette smokers. But for environmental exposures to carcinogens, individual fatality risks of 10^{-3} per year are unacceptably high.

The description of a risk by its expectation or by individual levels of risk is not just an arbitrary question of units. The choice of a measure refers to the rights versus efficiency perspective described above. Individual risk is used where the primary concern is whether individuals are being exposed to inequitably high risks. Expected risk consequences, such as fatalities or disability days, are appropriate when the focus is efficiency, i.e., to minimize social consequences when no individual is at an inequitable level of risk.

ANALYTICAL APPROACHES

The revealed preferences method to determine acceptable risk was suggested by Starr (1969). The approach is based on an interpretation of actual, observable social risk acceptance, generalized to reveal the implied risk-taking values of the observed patterns, applicable to new risk contexts (Fig. 5). Starr's primary conclusion was that risk-taking increased with increasing benefit, subject to the voluntary–involuntary distinction noted above. There are several limitations with this approach. As Starr notes, "this empirical approach provides some interesting insights into accepted social values relative to personal risk. Because this methodology is based on historical data, it does not serve to distinguish what is 'best' for society from what is 'traditionally acceptable.' " Even so, the

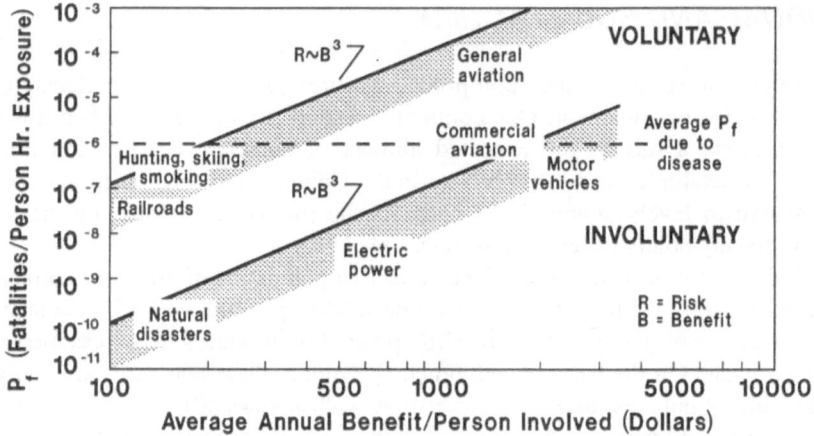

Figure 5. Risk versus benefit, voluntary and involuntary exposure. R, risk; B, benefit.

revealed preferences approach has been useful in illuminating social values toward risk taking.

A common analytical approach to questions of acceptable risk is cost–benefit analysis. While this method provides an accounting framework for project evaluation and comparison, it does not of itself provide insight into the acceptability of risk—values regarding risk taking must be imported into the analysis. The common way in which this has been done is by analyses of willingness-to-pay for risk reduction, typically based on evidence from wage premiums paid to workers in hazardous occupations. This is a revealed preference approach constrained to fit an economic model. A difficulty with such studies is that jobs, like technologies, are not evaluated on risk grounds alone. In particular, high risk jobs are often held by workers with limited alternative employment opportunities and poor education; the degree to which this evidence regarding risk-taking values can be applied to the general population is disputable.

Decision analysis provides another analytic framework useful for evaluating risk decisions. But, as with cost–benefit analysis, the values regarding social risk taking are exogenous to the method. A contribution of the decision analysis to the issue of acceptable risk has been to challenge whether the question is meaningful—whether acceptable technology is not a more relevant perspective than acceptable risk, for example. Decision analysts regard the risk associated with the preferred decision alternative as acceptable. Under this view, which seems to me to be widely held among those who study social values relating to risk concerns, attempts to seek numerical definitions of acceptability are meaningful only in context.

The limited degree to which people understand the level of risk they face, and their lack of detailed knowledge of the availability and costs of methods to reduce that risk, is a limitation in all revealed preferences studies. It is more likely that people act on their perceptions of risk. There is a rich psychological literature on the subject; two points are particularly relevant to the issue of acceptable risk. First, psychological surveys show that subjective rankings of risk differ from expected fatality estimates in a consistent way. Perceived risk rankings are elevated for risks which are highly uncertain and believed to be catastrophic, among other characteristics (Fischhoff *et al.*, 1978). Another persistent pattern in perceived risk is a scale compression, illustrated in Fig. 6 (Lichtenstein *et al.*, 1978). Low probability risks are seen as being relatively more likely than they actually are. In an earlier analysis, Starr and I suggested that this could be one explanation for the heated controversies over low-probability, high-consequence risks (Starr and Whipple, 1980). It appears that some people classify low probability risks as unlikely, while others believe them to be virtually impossible (Fig. 7). The preferred action regarding such risks could depend significantly on this perception.

The analytical approaches to define acceptable risk are logically sound and self-consistent, and make explicit the decision structure, assumptions, and value judgments of the analysis. This can be extremely useful when detailed documentation of a decision is required, or when the same decision is preferred under a wide range on value judgments or analytical assumptions. But applications of analytic approaches to social risk decisions have important limitations. Often, political compromises can best be made when values are not made explicit, and in some cases Congress has established regulatory approaches in which cost–benefit balancing is not permitted. The menu of decision options a competent analyst might develop can be inconsistent with regulatory structure, as when responsibilities to regulate different decision options are distributed to different agencies. Finally, analytic decision methods, applied to public problems, are difficult to apply when facts are in dispute.

SETTING RISK STANDARDS: CRITERIA

Although there are many approaches to regulate risks, a common list of considerations applies. The relative emphasis given to each decision factor shapes to regulatory approach. Important factors are:

- *Risk*. Risk means different things under different laws, just as it means different

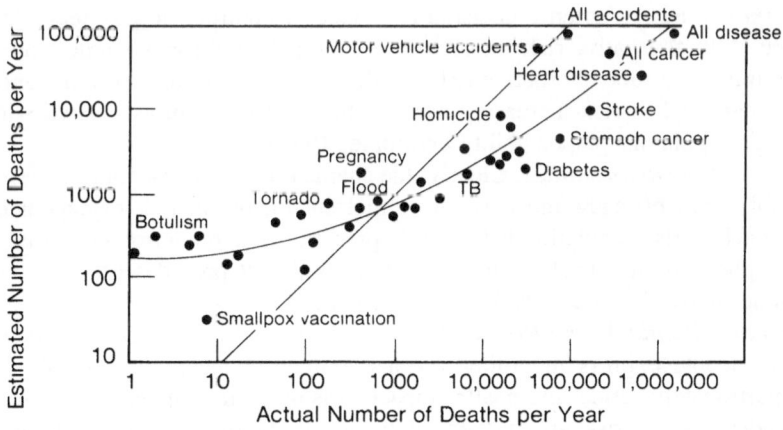

Figure 6. Comparison of perceived risk to actual risk. From Lichtenstein *et al.* (1978).

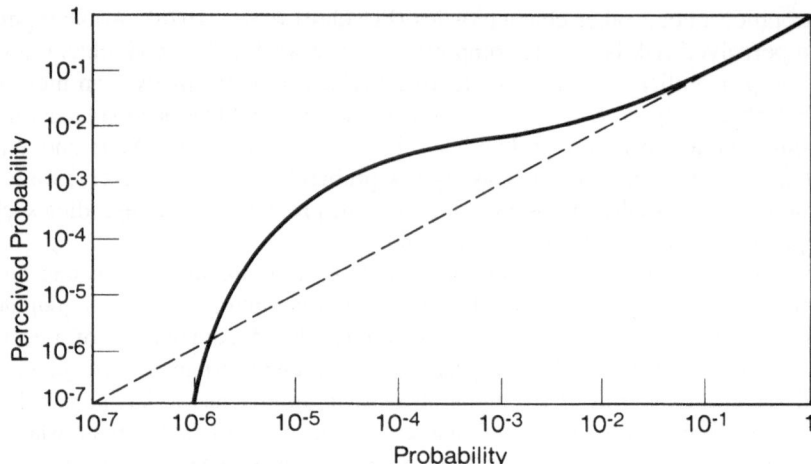

Figure 7. Probability perception.

things to different risk analysts. In some cases, it can refer to the severity of damages without regard to probability (e.g., the Delaney Clause regarding food additives); in other cases it includes consideration of the likelihood of impact. As noted above, risk sometimes refers to individual risk, at other times to anticipated or expected consequences in a population.

- *Benefit.* In the historical usage, benefit refers to the social benefits of technology, against which risks are considered. This is the prevailing usage in cost–benefit studies of water resource issues, where benefits often include new recreational opportunities. However, as decisions come to be made more often on marginal risk control, benefit has come to mean the benefits associated with a risk reduction. Regulatory impact analyses conducted under the Executive Order 12291 generally follow this second definition. The appropriate definition depends upon the scope of the decision at issue.
- *Alternative Risks.* Often a decision to reduce or control one risk requires acceptance of an alternative risk. In such cases, the potential for risk reduction may be determined by such alternative risks. Failure to recognize and examine alternative risks can lead to risk-increasing actions; this is a problem associated with fragmented regulatory responsibility (Whipple, 1985).
- *Risk Control Opportunities.* Clearly, the characteristics of risk control alternatives, notably their efficacy and cost, are important factors in risk management. One approach to risk regulation is to simply prescribe which control alternatives are to be applied. A drawback with this method is that it provides little incentive for finding innovative methods for reducing risk.
- *Statutory, Political, and Practical Considerations.* It is apparent that the concern many people express regarding various sources of technological risk does not proportionately reflect the health impacts arising from that risk. Perceptions and attitudes toward risk are influenced by a variety of risk characteristics (e.g., newness, uncertainty) as well as by the context in which exposures to risk occur.

Statutory requirements and political pressures often reflect these attitudes in the way in which risk management responsibility is defined.

In some cases, the admissible array of decision criteria are limited to risk measures, and other factors such as cost criteria are not legitimately considered. Practical or institutional considerations in implementing a safety standard are also important; these include the political response by interested parties, the time and cost required to reach a decision, its enforceability, the degree to which the agency and its management will be open to criticism, even in hindsight, and the other issues competing for resources and attention.

SETTING RISK STANDARDS: APPROACHES

The list of decision factors relevant to risk decisions, including standard setting, is long; to formally include all these factors in a decision would require elaborate and well-articulated decision criteria, as well as time and money. However, these criteria are not precisely defined; they emerge from a number of laws, policies, and past decisions over a period and are inconsistent, context-dependent, and time-varying. While analysis may be useful in such problems, many decision factors are only considered judgmentally. But while no agency follows a recipe to set standards, there are three basic decision processes that frequently appear. These are cost–benefit or cost-effectiveness methods, risk-based approaches, and technology-based standards. Each is briefly described below in terms of the degree of protection typically provided, the economic efficiency of the approach, its relation to risk substitutions, and the political factors important to its application. A somewhat more detailed version of what follows is available (Whipple, 1984).

Risk standards appear in many forms—as speed limits, as allowable concentrations for a pollutant, as the number of hours per month an airline pilot may fly. Since it is usually necessary to have these standards in measurable units, it is generally not apparent how a standard was set. In fact, standards developed on the basis of available control technologies can be and are justified in cost–benefit or risk-level terms.

- *Cost–Benefit.* Cost–benefit analysis is based on the principle that for any action (in this case, setting a standard), the benefit should exceed risk or cost, and that marginal cost equal marginal benefit. By definition, this approach is economically efficient. However, because risk standards are driven by a marginal cost balance, the residual levels of risk remaining after control vary widely, and may not be considered acceptable or equitable. This approach does not generally focus attention on alternative actions even when they exist, because the major premise of cost–benefit is that a decision can be made given information about benefits and risks. Finally, marginal cost-effectiveness analysis, applied to health and safety decisions, is very difficult to justify politically when there are identified victims (e.g., the Pinto gas tank).
- *Risk-Level Approaches.* A risk-level or safety goal approach generally is based on the objective of ensuring that individual risks are acceptably low—acceptable depends on the specific context. The advantages of this is that predictable risks result, and that innovation in risk control is encouraged. However, such an ap-

proach does not provide for marginal balancing of cost and benefit. Because risk-level approaches are often developed in conjunction with relevant comparisons, the method does encourage the examination of alternatives and their risks. Politically, this approach is defensible on equity grounds, however it places great weight on the credibility of risk estimates.

- *Technology-Based Approaches.* Technology-based approaches have long been used for setting safety standards; good engineering practice, best available control technology, and as low as feasible are examples. In recent applications, these methods have tended toward effective controls (i.e., low-risk residuals), but at a high price. Where accidents are likely to lead to identifiable victims, this approach permits the regulator to claim that the best control technology was applied.

In practice, a blend of these methods is often used. An illustration is provided in the case of principles developed by the International Commission on Radiological Protection (ICRP) for protection from ionizing radiation. The ICRP has three basic principles: (1) Justification of dose, based on the social benefits of the activity giving rise to exposure; (2) limitation of the exposure received by any individual; and (3) optimization, in which exposures to a population are reduced taking the costs of reduction in exposure into account (ICRP, 1977).

The basis for decisions is not always as apparent as in the ICRP criteria, but given a sufficient number of decisions, one can derive criteria that are consistent with past decisions. The historical balance in emphasis between protection of individuals and reduction of expected consequences has been examined (Travis *et al.*, 1987), with surprisingly consistent results indicating that both individual and societal risks have been considered, as have the costs of risk control.

DE MINIMIS RISK

In risk regulation and management, de minimis refers to the general theme that some risks are too small to address. It is easy to show that all organizations with risk management responsibilities use some type of de minimis approach, since risk management resources are always finite, and the supply of very small risks virtually inexhaustible. To cite just one example, the prohibition of carcinogenic food additives under both the Delaney Clause and earlier food safety laws is commonly cited as a "zero risk" policy statement that is as protective as any risk policy on the federal level. Even so, no serious consideration has ever been given to the idea that the Food and Drug Administration should ban food additives which contain a radioactive molecule or two, since that would include virtually all substances.

The de minimis concept, as it has historically been used, derives from the principle *de minimis non curat lex;* "the law does not concern itself with trifles." Under this definition, a de minimis risk is one which is trivial, that is, one which is of no concern to the average person. This view is consistent with the legal concern for individual risks that are too high; it does not derive from a societal or cost–benefit perspective. There is an alternate approach, referred to as Below Regulatory Concern by the Environmental Protection Agency (EPA), which is more closely aligned with the economic perspective on risk. Risks are below regulatory concern if, in comparison to other risk management opportunities, it would be a poor use of available resources to regulate them.

The impetus to establish a consistent de minimis approach to risk regulation has increased in recent years, as technologies for identifying risks have improved. Improvements in analytical chemistry permit the detection of hazardous substances at the part-per-billion or even part-per-trillion level. Only a decade ago such exposures would have been ignored simply because they would have been undetectable. In addition, our view of the nature of low-level risks has shifted. The view that we face rare but potent carcinogens has given way to the view that carcinogens (at least as determined by high-dose animal tests and by inference from *in vitro* bioassays) are fairly commonplace, and significantly varied in their carcinogenic potential.

An impact of the increasing number of candidate substances for regulation and of the apparent need to prioritize regulatory efforts is that case-by-case decision making is seen as too cumbersome. As the regulatory approaches to low-level agents mature, more systematic methods are sought. To regulators, the de minimis approach appears to provide a means of normalizing the process, by providing an alternative to standard setting for substances which pose very low risks. To the scientific community, the de minimis approach may provide a policy solution to questions that lie beyond the reach of scientific resolution. This would reduce the pressures for regulatory agencies and their scientific staffs to produce scientific judgments regarding low-level risks where information is unavailable. A review of de minimis risk, including regulatory applications, has been published (Whipple, 1987).

CONCLUSIONS

The definition of acceptable risk is a political judgment, dependent on context. Analysis can contribute to the process which determines what risk will be accepted in a given situation, but only as an aid to judgment. It is in this role that analytical methods, including cost–benefit approaches and comparisons of risk are helpful to current risk decisions. No analytical approach so far identified has proved practical for dealing with the complex objectives common to risk decisions, although such methods can help explain and defend decisions and can identify weaknesses with judgmentally developed approaches.

Common elements to risk management and the definition of acceptable risk can nonetheless be found. Some levels of risk are apparently too high to be accepted except when self-imposed. When environmental health exposures are thought to produce high individual risks, the usual response is to put health before cost, and to move to correct the situation. The speed with which the EPA banned ethylene dibromide (EDB) reflects this situation. Some small risks are unregulated, apparently because they are de minimis or below regulatory concern. And evidence suggests (Travis *et al.*, 1987) that the definition of a de minimis level can depend on both the level of individual risk and the number of people at risk. Between the limits of unacceptably high risk and de minimis, risk management decisions can depend on cost and other considerations noted above.

REFERENCES

Adler, H. L., and Weinberg, A. M., 1978, An approach to setting radiation standards, *Health Phys.* **34:**710–720.

Fischhoff, B., Slovic, P., Lichtenstein, S., Read, S., and Combs, B., 1978, How safe is safe enough? A psychometric survey of attitudes towards technological risks and benefits, *Policy Sci.* **8:**127–152.

Hammer, W., 1980, *Product Safety Management and Engineering,* Prentice-Hall, Englewood Cliffs, New Jersey.

International Commission on Radiological Protection Publication 26, 1977, *Recommendations of the International Commission on Radiological Protection,* Pergamon Press, New York.

Lichtenstein, S., Slovic, P., Fischhoff, B., Layman, M., and Combs, B., 1978, *J. Exp. Psychol. [Hum. Learn.] Mem.* **4:**551.

Rothschild, N., 1979, "Coming to Grips with Risk," *The Wall Street Journal,* May 13.

Smith, K., 1980, "Risk Analysis: Toward a Standard Method," Presented at the American/European Nuclear Societies' Meeting on Thermal Reactor Safety, Knoxville, April 8–11.

Starr, C., 1969, Social benefit versus technological risk, *Science* **165:**1232.

Starr, C., and Whipple, C., 1980, Risks of risk decisions, *Science* **208:**1114–1119.

Travis, C. C., Richter, S. A., Crouch, E. A. C., Wilson, R., and Klema, E., 1987, Cancer risk management by federal agencies, *Environ. Sci. Techol.* **21:**415–420.

U.S. Atomic Energy Commission, 1974, *Comparative Risk–Cost–Benefit Study of Alternate Sources of Electrical Energy,* WASH 1224, Washington, D.C.

U.S. Nuclear Regulatory Commission, 1975, *Reactor Safety Study: An Assessment of Accident Risks in U.S. Commercial Nuclear Power Plants,* WASH 1400 (NUREG-75/014).

U.S. Nuclear Regulatory Commission, 1983, *Safety Goals for Nuclear Power Plants,* NUREG-0880, Revision 1 for Comment, Washington, D.C.

Whipple, C., 1984, "Risk Approaches in Setting Radiation Standards," Presented at the AIF Conference on Radiation Protection: Standards and Regulatory Issues, Orlando, Oct. 9.

Whipple, C., 1985, Redistributing risk, *Regulation* (May/June).

Whipple, C. (ed.), 1987, *De Minimis Risk,* Plenum Press, New York.

13

Risk Perception

Paul Slovic

In industrialized societies, the question "How safe is safe enough?" has emerged as one of the major policy issues of the 1980s. The frequent discovery of new hazards and the widespread publicity they receive is causing more and more individuals to see themselves as the victims, rather than as the beneficiaries, of technology. These fears and the opposition to technology that they produce have puzzled and frustrated industrialists and regulators and have led numerous observers to argue that the public's apparent pursuit of a "zero-risk society" threatens the nation's political and economic stability. Political Scientist Aaron Wildavsky commented on this state of affairs (Wildavsky, 1979):

> How extraordinary! The richest, longest-lived, best-protected, most resourceful civilization, with the highest degree of insight into its own technology, is on its way to becoming the most frightened.
>
> Is it our environment or ourselves that have changed? Would people like us have had this sort of concern in the past? . . . today, there are risks from numerous small dams far exceeding those from nuclear reactors. Why is the one feared and not the other? Is it just that we are used to the old or are some of us looking differently at essentially the same sorts of experience?

Over the past decade, a small number of researchers have been attempting to answer such questions by examining the opinions that people express when they are asked, in a variety of ways, to evaluate hazardous activities, substances, and technologies. This research has attempted to develop techniques for assessing the complex and subtle opinions that people have about risk. With these techniques, researchers have sought to discover what people mean when they say that something is (or is not) "risky," and to determine what factors underlie those perceptions. If successful, this research should aid policy makers by improving their communication with the lay public, by directing educa-

---

Paul Slovic • Decision Research, Eugene, Oregon 97401.

tional efforts, and by predicting public responses to new hazards, events (such as a good safety record or an accident), and management strategies (such as warning labels, regulations, substitute products). A broad agenda for this research includes the following questions:

1. *What are the determinants of perceived risk?* What are the concepts by which people characterize risks? How are those concepts related to their attitudes and behavior toward different technologies? To what extent are risk perceptions affected by emotional factors? Are they really sensitive, as is often claimed, to perceived controllability of risks and the dread they evoke? How adequate are the methods used to study perceptions of risk?

2. *How accurate are public perceptions?* When laypeople err, is it because they are poorly informed or because they are unable to do better? Are people so poorly informed (and uneducable) that they require paternalistic institutions to protect them? Would they be better off letting technical experts make most of the important decisions? Or do they know enough to be able to make their own decisions in the marketplace? When experts and laypeople disagree about risk, is it always the latter who are in error?

3. *What steps are needed to foster enlightened behavior with regard to risk?* What information do policy makers and the public need? How should such information be presented? What indices or criteria are useful for putting diverse risks in perspective? How can the news media and the schools help to educate people about risk and its management?

4. *What is the role of judgment in technical assessments of risk?* When experts are forced to go beyond hard evidence and rely on educated intuition, do they encounter judgmental difficulties similar to those experienced by laypeople? How well do experts assess the limits of their knowledge? How can technical judgments be improved?

5. *How do people perceive the benefits of risky technologies?* Almost all questions asked about risk perceptions have analogs with benefit perceptions.

6. *What determines the relative acceptability of hazardous technologies?* How are assessments of their various risks and benefits combined subjectively? What role do considerations such as voluntariness, catastrophic potential, and equity play? What risk-benefit considerations motivate people to political action? Are some kinds of risks unacceptable, no matter what benefits they are expected to bring?

7. *What makes a risk analysis "acceptable?"* Some analyses are able to guide society's responses, whereas others only fuel debate. Are these differences due to the specific hazards involved, the political philosophy underlying the analytical methods, the way that the public is involved in the decision-making process, the results of the analysis, or the manner in which the results are communicated? Can policy makers responsibly incorporate social values into risk analysis?

8. *How can polarized social conflict involving risk be reduced?* Can an atmosphere of trust and mutual respect be created among opposing parties? How can we design an environment in which effective, multiway communication, constructive debate, and compromise can take place?

THE PSYCHOMETRIC PARADIGM

One broad strategy for studying perceived risk is to develop a taxonomy for hazards that can be used to understand and predict responses to their risks. A taxonomic scheme might explain, for example, the extreme aversion of people to some hazards, their indifference to others, and the discrepancies between these reactions and the opinions of experts. The most common approach to this goal has employed the "psychometric paradigm" (Fischhoff *et al.*, 1978; Slovic *et al.*, 1984a), which uses psychophysical scaling and multivariate analysis techniques to produce quantitative representations or "cognitive maps" of risk attitudes and perceptions. Within the psychometric paradigm, people make quantitative judgments about the current and desired risk of diverse hazards and the desired level of regulation of each. These judgments are then related to judgments about other properties, such as (1) the status of the hazard on characteristics that have been hypothesized to account for risk perceptions and attitudes (such as voluntariness, dread, knowledge, controllability); (2) the benefits that each hazard provides to society; (3) the number of deaths caused by the hazard in an average year; (4) the number of deaths caused by the hazard in a disastrous year; and (5) the seriousness of each death from a particular hazard relative to a death due to other causes.

The remainder of this chapter briefly reviews some of the results obtained from psychometric studies of risk perception and outlines some of the implications of these results for risk communication and risk management.

REVEALED AND EXPRESSED PREFERENCES

The original impetus for the psychometric paradigm came from the pioneering effort of Starr (1969) to develop a method for weighing technological risks against benefits in order to answer the fundamental question "How safe is safe enough?" His "revealed preference" approach assumed that, by trial and error, society has arrived at an "essentially optimum" balance between the risks and benefits associated with any activity. One may therefore use historical or current risk and benefit data to reveal patterns of "acceptable" risk–benefit tradeoffs. Examining such data for several industries and activities, Starr concluded that (1) acceptability of risk from an activity is roughly proportional to the third power (cube) of the benefits for that activity, and (2) the public will accept risks from voluntary activities, such as skiing, that are roughly 1000 times greater than it would tolerate from involuntary hazards, such as food preservatives, that provide the same level of benefits.

The merits and deficiencies of Starr's approach have been debated at length (see Fischhoff *et al.*, 1981). They will not be elaborated here, except to note that concern about the validity of the many assumptions inherent in the revealed preferences approach stimulated Fischhoff *et al.* (1978) to conduct an analogous psychometric analysis of questionnaire data, resulting in "expressed preferences." In recent years, numerous other studies of expressed preferences have been carried out within the psychometric paradigm (see, for example, Brown and Green, 1980; Gardner *et al.*, 1982; Green, 1980; Green and Brown, 1980; Johnson and Tversky, 1984; Lindell and Earle, 1983; MacGill, 1983;

Renn, 1981; Slovic *et al.* 1980, 1984a; Vlek and Stallen, 1981; von Winterfeldt *et al.*, 1981).

These studies have shown that perceived risk is quantifiable and predictable. Psychometric techniques seem well suited for identifying similarities and differences among groups with regard to risk perceptions and attitudes (Table 1). They have also shown that the concept of "risk" means different things to different people. When experts judge risk, their responses correlate highly with technical estimates of annual fatalities. Laypeople can assess annual fatalities if they are asked to (and produce estimates somewhat like the technical estimates). However, their judgments of risk are sensitive to other factors as well, such as catastrophic potential and threat to future generations, and, as a result, tend to differ from their own (and experts') estimates of annual fatalities.

Another consistent result from psychometric studies of expressed preferences is that people tend to view current risk levels as unacceptably high for most activities. The gap between perceived and desired risk levels suggests that people are not satisfied with the way that market and other regulatory mechanisms have balanced risks and benefits. Across the domain of hazards, there seems to be little systematic relationship between perceived existing risks and benefits. However, studies of expressed preferences do seem to support Starr's claim that people are willing to tolerate higher risks from actitivies seen as highly beneficial. But whereas Starr concluded that voluntariness of exposure was the key mediator of risk acceptance, expressed preference studies have shown that other characteristics such as familiarity, control, catastrophic potential, equity, and level of knowledge also seem to influence the relationship between perceived risk, perceived benefit, and risk acceptance (see Fischhoff *et al.*, 1978; Slovic *et al.*, 1980).

Various models have been advanced to represent the relationships between perceptions, behavior, and these qualitative characteristics of hazards. As we shall see, the picture that emerges from this work is both orderly and complex.

FACTOR-ANALYTIC REPRESENTATIONS

Many of the qualitative risk characteristics are highly correlated with each other, across a wide range of hazards. For example, hazards rated as "voluntary" tend also to be rated as "controllable" and "well-known"; hazards that appear to threaten future generations tend also to be seen as having catastrophic potential, and so on. Investigation of these interrelationships by means of factor analysis has shown that the broader domain of characteristics can be condensed to a small set of higher-order characteristics or factors.

The factor space presented in Fig. 1 has been replicated across groups of laypeople and experts judging large and diverse sets of hazards. The factors in this space reflect the degree to which a risk is understood and the degree to which it evokes a feeling of dread. A third factor, reflecting the number of people exposed to the risk, has been obtained in several studies. Making the set of hazards more or less specific (e.g., partitioning nuclear power into radioactive waste transport, uranium mining, and nuclear reactor accidents) has had little effect on the factor structure or its relationship to risk perceptions (Slovic *et al.*, 1985).

Table 1. Ordering of Perceived Risk for 30 Activities and Technologies[a,b]

	League of Women Voters	College students	Active club members	Experts
Nuclear power	1	1	8	20
Motor vehicles	2	5	3	1
Handguns	3	2	1	4
Smoking	4	3	4	2
Motorcycles	5	6	2	6
Alcoholic beverages	6	7	5	3
General (private) aviation	7	15	11	12
Police work	8	8	7	17
Pesticides	9	4	15	8
Surgery	10	11	9	5
Fire fighting	11	10	6	18
Large construction	12	14	13	13
Hunting	13	18	10	23
Spray cans	14	13	23	26
Mountain climbing	15	22	12	29
Bicycles	16	24	14	15
Commercial aviation	17	16	18	16
Electric power (nonnuclear)	18	19	19	9
Swimming	19	30	17	10
Contraceptives	20	9	22	11
Skiing	21	25	16	30
X rays	22	17	24	7
High school and college football	23	26	21	27
Railroads	24	23	20	19
Food preservatives	25	12	28	14
Food coloring	26	20	30	21
Power mowers	27	28	25	28
Prescription antibiotics	28	21	26	24
Home appliances	29	27	27	22
Vaccinations	30	29	29	25

[a]Ordering is based on the geometric mean risk ratings within each group Rank 1 represents the most risky activity or technology
[b]From Slovic *et al* , (1981)

Research has shown that the risk perceptions and attitudes of laypeople are closely related to the position of a hazard within the factor space. Most important is the factor "dread risk." The higher a hazard's score on this factor (i.e., the further to the right it appears in the space), the higher its perceived risk, the more people want to see its current risks reduced, and the more they want to see strict regulation employed to achieve the desired reduction in risk (Fig. 2). In contrast, perceptions of risk by experts are not closely related to any of the various risk characteristics or factors derived from these characteristics (Slovic *et al.*, 1979). Instead, experts appear to see riskiness as synonymous with expected annual mortality (Slovic *et al.*, 1981). As a result, some conflicts over risk may result from experts and laypeople having different definitions of the concept.

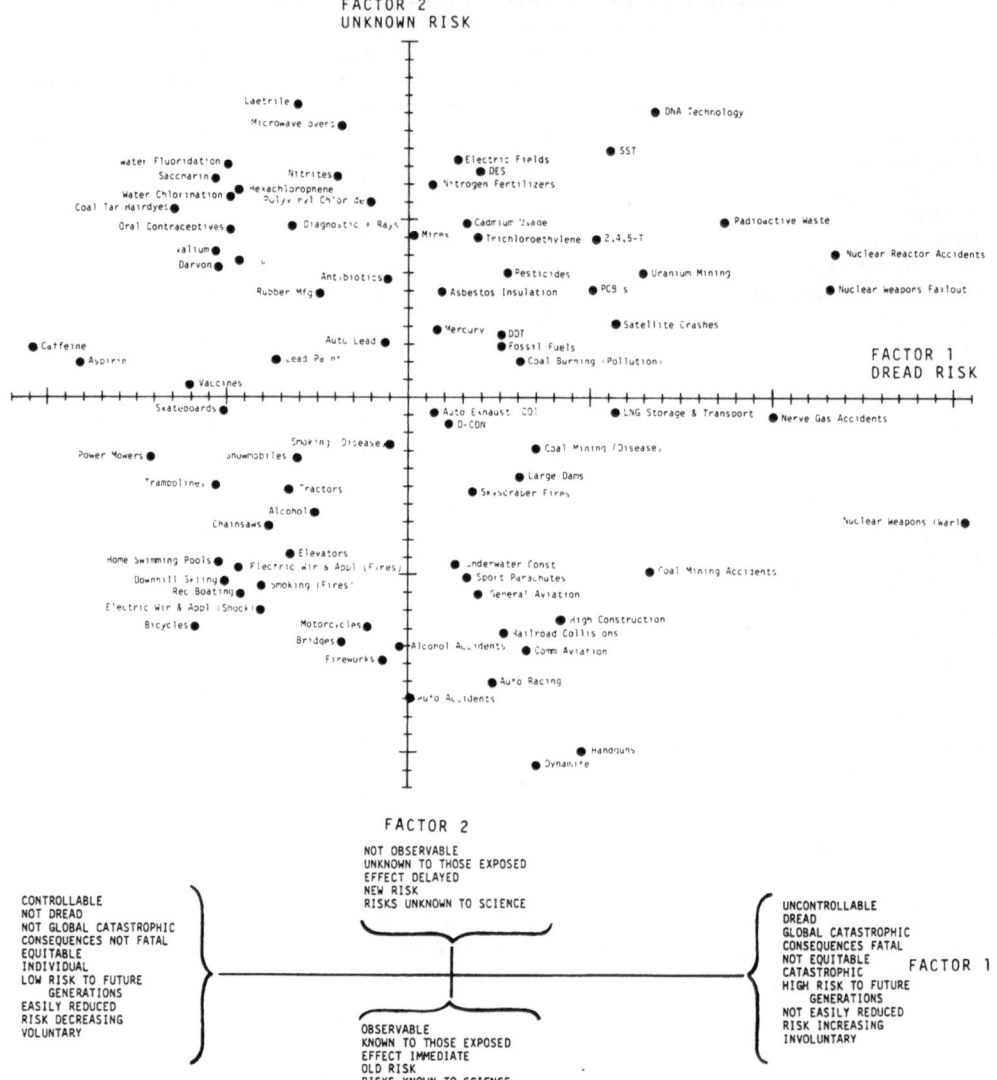

Figure 1. Location of 81 hazards on Factors 1 and 2 derived from the interrelationships among 18 risk characteristics. Each factor is made up of a combination of characteristics, as indicated by the lower diagram. From Slovic *et al.* (1985).

ACCIDENTS AS SIGNALS

Risk analyses typically model the impacts of unfortunate events (e.g., an accident, a discovery of pollution, sabotage, or product tampering) in terms of direct harm to vic-

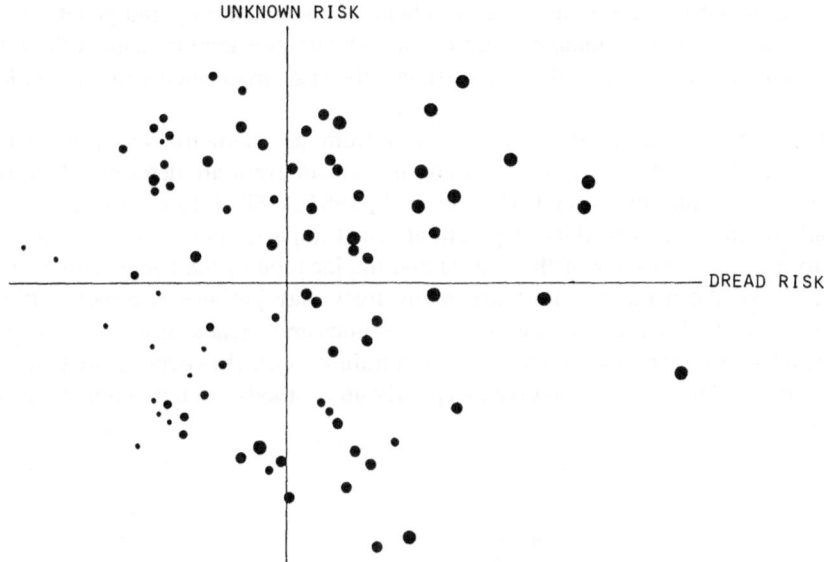

Figure 2. Attitudes towards regulation of the hazards in Fig. 1. The larger the point, the greater the desire for strict regulation to reduce risk. From Slovic *et al.* (1985).

tims—deaths, injuries, and damages. The impacts of an unfortunate event, however, sometimes extend far beyond these direct harmful effects, and may include indirect costs to the responsible government agency or private company that far exceed direct costs. In some cases, all companies in an industry are affected, regardless of which company was responsible for the mishap. In extreme cases, the indirect costs of a mishap may even extend past industry boundaries, affecting companies, industries, and agencies whose business is minimally related to the initial event. Thus, an unfortunate event can be thought of as a stone dropped in a pond. The ripples spread outward, encompassing first the directly affected victims, then the responsible company or agency, and, in the extreme, reaching other companies, agencies, and industries.

Some events make only small ripples; others make big ones. Early theories equated the magnitude of impact to the number of people killed or injured, or to the amount of property damaged. Unfortunately, things are not this simple. The accident at the Three Mile Island (TMI) nuclear reactor in 1979 provides a dramatic demonstration that factors besides injury, death, and property damage impose serious costs. Despite the fact that not a single person died at TMI, and few if any latent cancer fatalities are expected, no other accident in our history has produced such costly societal impacts. The accident at TMI devastated the utility that owned and operated the plant. It also imposed enormous costs (estimated at 500 billion dollars by one source) on the nuclear industry and on society, through stricter regulation, reduced operation of reactors worldwide, greater public opposition to nuclear power, reliance on more expensive energy sources, and increased costs of reactor construction and operation. It may even have led to a more hostile view of other large-scale, modern technologies, such as chemical manufacturing and genetic engineering. The point is that traditional economic and risk analyses tend to neglect these higher-order impacts, hence they greatly underestimate the costs associated with certain kinds of mishaps.

An important concept that has emerged from psychometric research is that the seriousness and higher-order impacts of an unfortunate event are determined, in part, by what that event signals or portends (Slovic *et al.*, 1984b). The informativeness or "signal potential" of an event, and thus its potential social impact, appears to be systematically related to the characteristics of the hazard and the location of the event within the factor space (Fig. 3). An accident that takes many lives may produce relatively little social disturbance, beyond that caused the victims' families and friends, if it occurs as part of a familiar and well-understood system (such as a train wreck). However, a small accident in an unfamiliar system (or one perceived as poorly understood), such as a nuclear reactor or

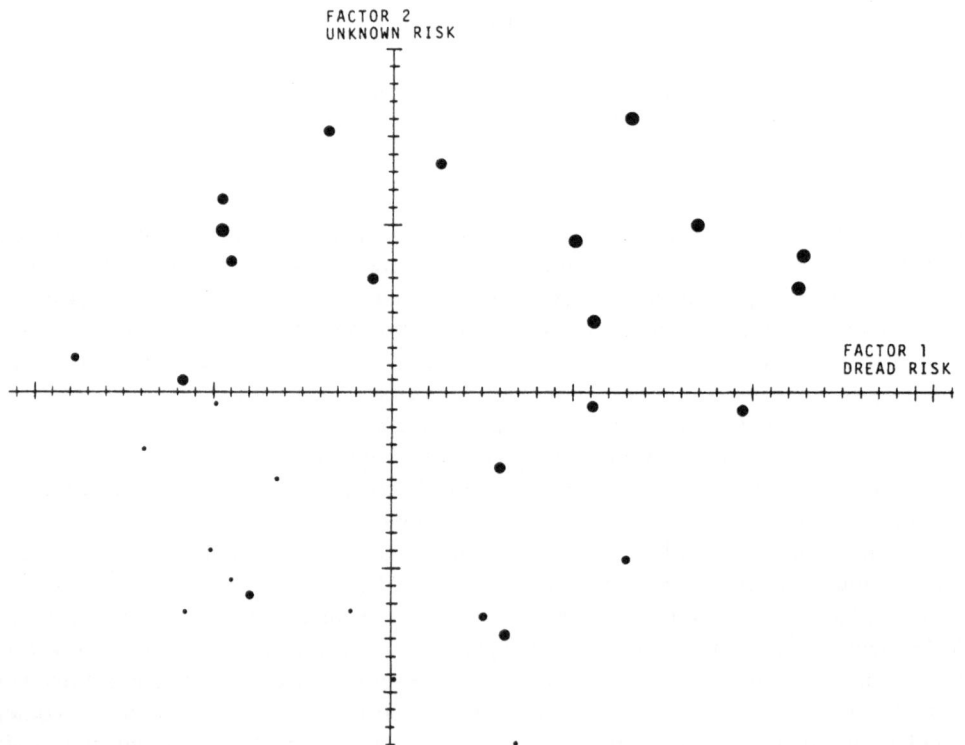

Figure 3. Relation between signal potential and risk characterization for 30 hazards in Fig. 1. The larger the point, the greater the degree to which an accident involving that hazard was judged to "serve as a warning signal for society, providing new information about the probability that similar or even more destructive mishaps might occur within this type of activity." The higher-order costs of a mishap are likely to be correlated with signal potential. From Slovic *et al.* (1984).

a recombinant DNA laboratory, may have immense social consequences if it is perceived as a harbinger of further and possibly catastrophic mishaps.

The concept of accidents as signals was eloquently expressed in an editorial addressing the tragic accident at Bhopal, India: "What truly grips us in these accounts [of disaster] is not so much the numbers as the spectacle of suddenly vanishing competence, of men utterly routed by technology, of fail-safe systems failing with a logic as inexorable as it was once—indeed, right up until that very moment—unforseeable. And the spectacle haunts us because it seems to carry allegorical import, like the whispery omen of a hovering future" (*The New Yorker,* February 18, 1985).

One implication of the signal concept is that effort and expense beyond that indicated by a cost–benefit analysis might be warranted to reduce the possibility of "high-signal accidents." Unfortunate events involving hazards in the upper-right quadrant of Fig. 1 appear particularly likely to have the potential to produce large ripples. As a result, risk analysis of these hazards needs to be sensitive to these possible higher-order impacts.

PLACING RISKS IN PERSPECTIVE

A consequence of the public's concern and opposition to risky technologies has been an increase in attempts to inform and educate people about risk. Risk perception research has a number of implications for such educational efforts (Slovic, 1986).

One frequently advocated approach to broadening people's perspectives is to present quantitative risk estimates for a variety of hazards, expressed in some unidimensional index of death or disability, such as risk per hour of exposure (Sowby, 1965), annual probability of death (Wilson, 1979), or reduction in life expectancy (Cohen and Lee, 1979; Reissland and Harries, 1979). Even though such comparisons have no logically necessary implications for acceptability of risk (Fischhoff *et al.,* 1981), one might still hope that they would help improve the public's intuitions about the magnitude of risks. Risk perception research suggests, however, that these comparisons may not be very satisfactory even for this purpose. Perceptions and attitudes of the public are determined not only by the sort of unidimensional statistics used in such tables but also by the variety of quantitative and qualitative characteristics reflected in Fig. 1. To many people, statements such as "the annual risk from living near a nuclear power plant is equivalent to the risk of riding an extra three miles in an automobile" give inadequate consideration to the important differences in the nature of the risks from these two technologies.

In short, "riskiness" means more to people than "expected number of fatalities." Attempts to characterize, compare, and regulate risks must be sensitive to this broader conception of risk. Fischhoff *et al.* (1984) have made a start in this direction by demonstrating how one might construct a more adequate measure of risk. They show that variations in the scope of one's definition of risk can greatly change the assessment of risk from various energy technologies.

The concept of accidents as signals indicates that, when informed about a particular hazard, people may "read between the lines," generalizing beyond the immediate problem to other related and possibly more ominous hazard. In response to information provided by the Environmental Protection Agency about the small degree of carcinogenicity associated with exposure to the pesticide ethylene dibromide (EDB), one newspaper editor wrote: "The cumulative effect—the 'body burden count' as scientists call it—is especially worrisome considering the number of other pesticides and carcinogens humans are exposed to." (*The Sunday Star-Bulletin and Advertiser,* Honolulu, Feb. 5, 1984)

On the same topic, another editor wrote: "Let's hope there are no cousins of EDB waiting to ambush us in the months ahead." (*San Francisco Examiner,* Feb. 10, 1984)

As a result of this broad (and legitimate) perspective, communications from risk managers pertaining to the risk and control of a single hazard, no matter how carefully presented, may fail to alleviate people's fears, frustrations, and anger. However, if people trust the ability of the risk manager to handle the risk problem, these broader concerns will probably not surface.

Whereas psychometric research implies that risk debates are not merely about risk statistics, some sociological and anthropological research implies that some of these debates may not even be about risk (Douglas and Wildavsky, 1982; Short, 1984). Risk concerns may provide a rationale for actions taken on other grounds or they may be a surrogate for other social or ideological concerns. When this is the case, communication about risk is simply irrelevant to the discussion. Hidden agendas need to be brought to the surface for open discussion, if possible (Edwards and von Winterfeldt, 1987).

Perhaps the most important message from the research done to date is that there is wisdom as well as error in public attitudes and perceptions. Laypeople sometimes lack certain information about hazards. However, their basic conceptualization of risk is much richer than that of the experts and reflects legitimate concerns that are typically omitted from expert risk assessments. As a result, risk communication efforts are destined to fail unless they are structured as a two-way process. Each side, expert and public, has something valid to contribute. Each side must respect the insights and intelligence of the other.

ACKNOWLEDGMENTS. The text of this paper draws heavily upon the author's joint work with Baruch Fischhoff and Sarah Lichtenstein. Support for the writing of this paper was provided by the National Science Foundation under Grant No. SES-8796182 to Decision Research. Portions of this chapter appeared in Slovic (1987).

REFERENCES

Brown, R. A., and Green, C. H., 1980, Precepts of safety assessments, *J. Operat. Res. Soc.* **11**:563–571.
Cohen, B., and Lee, I., 1979, A catalog of risks, *Health Phys.* **36**:707–722.
Douglas, M., and Wildavsky, A., 1982, *Risk and Culture,* University of California Press, Berkeley and Los Angeles.
Edwards, W., and von Winterfeldt, D., 1987, Public values in risk debates, *Risk Anal.* **7**:141–158.
Fischhoff, B., Slovic, P., Lichtenstein, S., Read, S., and Combs, B. 1978, How safe is safe enough? A psychometric study of attitudes towards technological risks and benefits, *Pol. Sci.* **8**:127–152.
Fischhoff, B., Lichtenstein, S., Slovic, P., Derby, S. L., and Keeney, R. L., 1981, *Acceptable Risk,* Cambridge University Press, New York.
Fischhoff, B., Watson, S., and Hope, C., 1984, Defining risk, *Pol. Sci.* **17**:123–139.
Gardner, G. T., Tiemann, A. R., Gould, L. C., DeLuca, D. R., Doob, L. W., and Stolwijk, J. A. J., 1982,

Risk and benefit perceptions, acceptability judgments, and self-reported actions toward nuclear power, *J. Soc. Psychol.* **116**:179–197.

Green, C. H., 1980, Risk: Attitudes and beliefs, in: *Behavior in Fires* (D. V. Canter, ed.), Wiley, Chichester.

Green, C. H., and Brown, R. A., 1980, "Through a Glass Darkly: Perceiving Perceived Risks to Health and Safety," (Research paper). School of Architecture, Duncan of Jordanstone College of Art, University of Dundee, Dundee, Scotland.

Johnson, E. J., and Tversky, A., 1984, Representations of perceptions of risks, *J. Exp. Psychol. [Gen.]* **113**:55–70.

Lindell, M. K., and Earle, T. C., 1983, How close is close enough? Public perceptions of the risks of industrial facilities, *Risk Anal.* **3**:245–254.

MacGill, S. M., 1983, Exploring the similarities of different risks, *Environ. Plan. [B]* **10**:303–329.

Reissland, J., and Harries, V., 1979, A scale for measuring risks, *New Sci.* **83**:809–811.

Renn, O., 1981, *Man, technology and risk: A study on intuitive risk assessment and attitudes towards nuclear power,* Report Jul-Spez 115, Jülich, June, Nuclear Research Center, Federal Republic of Germany.

San Francisco (California) Examiner, 1984 (Feb. 10,1984).

Short, J. F., Jr., 1984, The social fabric at risk: Toward the social transformation of risk analysis, *Am. Sociol. Rev.* **49**:711–725.

Slovic, P., 1986, Informing and educating the public about risk, *Risk Anal.* **6**:403–415.

Slovic, P., 1987, Perceptions of risk, *Science* **236**:280–285.

Slovic, P., Fischoff, B., and Lichtenstein, S., 1974, Rating the risks, *Environment* **21**(3):14–20, 36–39.

Slovic, P., Fischhoff, B., and Lichtenstein, S., 1980, Facts and fears: Understanding perceived risk, in: *Societal Risk Assessment: How Safe Is Safe Enough?* (R. Schwing and W. A. Albers, Jr., eds.), pp. 181–216, Plenum Press, New York.

Slovic, P., Fischhoff, B., and Lichtenstein, S., 1981, Perceived risk: Psychological factors and social implications, in: *The Assessment and Perception of Risk* (F. Warner and D. H. Slater, eds.), The Royal Society, London.

Slovic, P., Fischhoff, B., and Lichtenstein, S., 1984a, Behavioral decision theory perspectives on risk and safety, *Acta Psychol.* **56**:183–203.

Slovic, P., Lichtenstein, S., and Fischhoff, B., 1984b, Modeling the societal impact of fatal accidents, *Manag. Sci.* **30**:464–474.

Slovic, P., Fischhoff, B., and Lichtenstein, S., 1985, Characterizing perceived risk, in: *Perilous Progress: Managing the Hazards of Technology* (R. W. Kates, C. Hohenemser, and J. X. Kasperson, eds.), pp. 91–125, Westview Press, Boulder, Colorado.

Sowby, F. D., 1965, Radiation and other risks, *Health Phys.* **11**:879–887.

Starr, C., 1969, Social benefit versus technological risk, *Science* **165**:1232–1238.

The New Yorker, 1985, Talk of the town, *The New Yorker* **60**(53):29–30 (Feb. 18, 1985).

The Sunday Star-Bulletin and Advertiser, 1984, Honolulu, Hawaii (Feb. 5, 1984).

Vlek, C. A. J., and Stallen, P. J., 1981, Judging risk and benefit in the small and in the large, *Org. Behav. Hum. Perform.* **28**:235–271.

von Winterfeldt, D., John, R. S., and Borcherding, K., 1981, Cognitive components of risk ratings, *Risk Anal.* **1**:277–288.

Wildavsky, A., 1979, No risk is the highest risk of all, *Am. Sci.* **67**:32–37.

Wilson, R., 1979, Analyzing the daily risks of life, *Technol. Rev.* **81**(4):40–46.

14

Risk Assessment and Comparisons
An Introduction

Richard Wilson and E. A. C. Crouch

Every day we take risks and avoid others. It starts as soon as we wake up. One of us lives in an old house that had old wiring. Each time he turned on the light, there was a small risk of electrocution. Every year about 200 people are electrocuted in the United States in accidents involving home wiring or appliances, representing a risk of death of about 10^{-6} per year, or 7×10^{-5} per lifetime. To reduce this risk, he got the wiring replaced. When we walk downstairs, we recall that 7000 people die each year in falls in U.S. homes. But most are over 65, so we pay little attention to this risk since both of us are younger than that.

How should we go to work? Walking is probably safer than using a bicycle, but would take five times as long and provide less healthful exercise. A car or, better, public transport would be both safer and faster. Expediency wins out, and the car comes out of the garage. Fortunately, the choice nowadays is not between horse or canoe—both of which are much more dangerous. The day has just begun, and already we are aware of several risks, and have made decisions about them.

Most of us act semiautomatically to minimize our risks. We also expect society to minimize the risks suffered by its members, subject to overriding moral, economic, or other constraints. In some cases these constraints will dominate, in others there will be trade-offs between the values assigned to risks and the constraints. Risk assessments, except in the simplest of circumstances, are not designed for making judgments, but to illuminate them (Lave, 1987). To effectively illuminate, and then to minimize, risks requires knowing what they are and how big they are. This knowledge usually is gained through experience, and the essence of risk assessment is the application of this knowledge of past mistakes (and deliberate actions) in an attempt to prevent new mistakes in new situations.

Richard Wilson • Department of Physics and the Energy and Environmental Policy Center, Harvard University, Cambridge, Massachusetts 02138   *E. A. C. Crouch* • Energy and Environmental Policy Center, Harvard University, and Metasystems, Cambridge, Massachusetts 02138.

The results of risk assessments will necessarily be in the form of an estimate of probabilities for various events, usually injurious. The goal in performing a risk assessment is to obtain such estimates, although we consider the major value in performing a risk assessment is the exercise itself, in which (ideally) all aspects of some action are explored. The results, goals, and values of performing the risk assessment must be sharply contrasted with the cultural values assigned to the results. Such cultural values will presumably be factors influencing societal decisions and may differ even for risk estimates that are identical in probability.

RISK AND UNCERTAINTY

The concept of risk and the notion of uncertainty are closely related. We may say that the lifetime risk of cancer is 25%, meaning that approximately 25% of all people develop cancer in their lifetimes. Once an individual develops cancer, we can no longer talk about the risk of cancer, for it is a certainty. Similarly if a man lies dying after a car accident, the risk of his dying of cancer drops to near zero. Thus estimates of risks, insofar as they are expressions of uncertainty, will change as knowledge improves.

Different uncertainties appear in risk estimation in different ways (Wilson *et al.*, 1985). There is clearly a risk that an individual will be killed by a car if that person walks blindfolded across a crowded street. One part of this risk is stochastic; it depends on whether the individual steps off the curb at the precise moment that a car arrives. Another part of the risk might be systematic; it will depend on the nature of the fenders and other features of the car. Similarly, if two people are both heavy cigarette smokers, one may die of cancer and the other not; we cannot tell in advance. However, there is a systematic difference in this respect between being, for instance, a heavy smoker and a gluttonous eater of peanut butter, which contains aflatoxin. Although aflatoxin is known to cause cancer (quite likely even in humans), the risk of cancer from eating peanut butter is much lower than that from smoking cigarettes. Exactly how much lower is uncertain, but it is possible to make estimates of how much lower and also to make estimates of how uncertain we are about the difference.

Some estimates of uncertainties are subjective, with differences of opinion arising because there is a disagreement among those assessing the risks. Suppose one wishes to assess the risk (to humans) of some new chemical being introduced into the environment, or of a new technology. Without any further information, all we can say about any measure of the risk is that it lies between zero and unity. Extreme opinions might be voiced; one person might say that we should initially assume a risk of unity, because we do not know that the chemical or technology is safe; another might take the opposite extreme, and argue that we should initially assume that there is zero risk, because nothing has been proven dangerous. Here and elsewhere, we argue that it is the task of the risk assessor to use whatever information is available to obtain a number between zero and one for a risk estimate, with as much precision as possible, together with an estimate of the imprecision. In this context, the statement "I do not know" can be viewed only as procrastination and not responsive to the request for a risk estimate (although this should not be read as condemning procrastination in all circumstances).

The second extreme mentioned, the assumption of zero risk, can arise because people and government agencies have a propensity to ignore anything that is not a proven hazard. We argue that this attitude is inconsistent if the objective is to improve the public health, may also lead to economic inefficiencies, and often leads to unnecessary contention between experts who disagree strongly. Fortunately, if risk assessors have been diligent in searching out hazards to assess, few hazards posing large risks will be missed in this way, so that there may be minor direct danger to human health from a continuation of the attitude.

RISK ESTIMATION BASED ON HISTORICAL DATA

The way in which risks are perceived is strongly correlated with the way in which they are calculated. Risks based on historical data are particularly easy to understand and are often perceived reliably. It is therefore easy to illustrate a risk calculated from historical data to understand some characteristics of risk estimation. There are plenty of data on automobile accidents (although never enough to make risk assessors happy). One thing that these data can tell us is the frequency of such accidents in the past and their trend through time. To make predictions, however, we must use a model. The simplest model is that there will be as many accidents next year as last, to within a statistical error of the square root of the number. A slightly more complicated, but perhaps more accurate, model might be to fit a mathematical function to numbers from previous years and to argue that next year's accidents will follow the trend given by this function. A possibly better and possibly more accurate model still might use all available information that might influence accident trends. For example, an oil embargo with a concomitant rise in oil price and reduction in automobile travel would be likely to reduce the risk of accident. In any event, it becomes clear that it is impossible to calculate any risk without a model of some sort, even the simple one that tomorrow will be like today.

RISKS OF NEW TECHNOLOGIES

We can only use the historical approach to estimating risks when the hazard (for example, technology, chemical, or simply some action) has been present for some time and the risk is large enough to be directly measured (although when it is not large enough to be measured, an upper limit may be calculated, if one assumes some sort of model). If there is no historical database for the hazard (a new power plant or industrial facility, for instance), one approach is to consider it in separate parts, calculating the risks from each part and adding them together to estimate a risk for the whole. For example, all possible chains of events from an initiator to a final accident are followed in an "event tree," with the probabilities of each event in the tree being estimated from historical data in different situations.

A particularly well-known example is the calculation of the probability of a severe accident at a nuclear power plant (Rasmussen *et al.*, 1975). That this procedure has at least a partial validity is due to the fact that the design of nuclear power plants proceeded in approximately this factorable way; attempts were made to imagine all major accident possibilities, "maximum credible accidents" or "design basis accidents," and then to add an independent device to prevent this accident from having severe consequences. To the extent that the added safety device is independent, the failure probability is independent, and the small overall accident probability is the product of individual failure probabilities which are larger.

RISKS BY ANALOGY: CARCINOGENIC RISKS

Some carcinogenic risks may be estimated from historical data. But this is complicated by the time delay between the insult and the final cancer, one reason why causality is hard to prove if the risk is small. This is the difficult field of epidemiology.

Although some of the largest cancer risks have been identified through the use of epidemiology (Doll and Peto, 1984), preventive public health suggests that we endeavor to estimate risks even where no historical data exist and the risk is small. This is often done by analogy with the cancer risks to animals, usually rodents, which are deliberately exposed to large enough quantities of pollutant so that an effect is observed. To use these data to estimate the risk at low doses in people involves (to oversimplify matters) two difficult steps—the comparison of carcinogenic potency in animal and man (Anderson *et al.*, 1983; Crouch and Wilson, 1979; Calabrese, 1983) and the extrapolation from a high dose to a low dose. Because both steps require a certain amount of theory, they are controversial. Indeed, there are those who regard the uncertainty as so great that they prefer not to provide numerical estimates of risk (Peto, 1985; Ames *et al.*, 1987) although they may order materials in carcinogenic potency. The difference between this and providing a numerical estimate is important, but is one of presentation rather than substance.

If there are no animal data, or if in an animal experiment there is no statistically significant effect, it does not necessarily mean that there is no risk. If the experimenters have been diligent, the risk is probably small, although never zero, even though that may be the best estimate. Various attempts are made to use data even less direct than the animal bioassays to estimate risks in such cases. These include simple analogies based on chemical similarity (*Fed. Regist.*, 1968), and comparison with outcomes other than cancer—for example, mutagenesis (Meselson and Russell, 1977) and acute toxicity (Parodi *et al.*, 1982; Zeise *et al.*, 1984). Not surprisingly, these more indirect procedures arouse even more controversy than the animal bioassays.

There have been few attempts to perform risk assessments for biological end points other than cancer. However, it is known that the pollutants in cigarette smoke cause at least as many deaths through heart problems as by cancer (Public Health Service, 1979) and we should not be surprised if other carcinogens were to produce chronic effects other than cancer. For now, the cancer risk assessment has to act as surrogate for these other risks also.

RISK VALUE VERSUS CERTAINTY OF INFORMATION

After risks of a number of situations have been assessed, we often want to order them in order to decide which should command our attention. It is not always the order of increasing risk that is used for such purposes. There have been proposals to order potential carcinogens on other factors (Peto, 1985; Squire, 1981), such as the certainty of information.

Vinyl chloride gas has been found to cause angiosarcomas both in people and in rats. Since an angiosarcoma is a rare tumor, the risk ratio (the ratio of the observed number of cancers in those exposed to the number expected by chance) is of order 100 or more in some cases. If an angiosarcoma is seen in a vinyl chloride worker, the attribution to vinyl chloride exposure is almost certain. On the other hand, the number of persons who have been heavily exposed to vinyl chloride is small, so that only about 125 angiosarcomas have been seen among vinyl chloride workers worldwide in the last 20 years. Now that exposures in the workplace have been greatly reduced, no angiosarcomas attributable to recent occupational exposure have been seen. We do not know the dose–response relation, but it is generally believed that the response falls at least linearly as the exposure is reduced, so that no more than one cancer is expected in several years.

We can compare this with the possible cancer incidence that was predicted by the Food and Drug Administration (FDA) in 1977 from use of saccharin (*Fed. Regist.*, 1977). This was based on experiments with rats, leading to an additional uncertainty. More people ate saccharin than were exposed to vinyl chloride, and nearly 500 cancers per year were estimated for the United States alone. For vinyl chloride we therefore have the situation that the individual risk is now low, yet there is considerable certainty that there is a risk. For saccharin the risk is higher, but there is more uncertainty about the value of the risk. Some persons, in some situations, may demand that more attention be given to the risk from vinyl chloride than to the risk from saccharin; for other persons or situations the reverse may be the case.

COMPARISON OF RISKS

The purpose of risk assessment is to be useful in making decisions about the hazards causing risks, and so it is important to gain some perspective about the meaning of the magnitude of the risk. Comparisons can be useful. We are not born with an instinctive feeling for what a risk of one in a million per lifetime means, although we do learn that some risks are small and others large. It is particularly helpful to compare risks that are calculated in a similar way. For example, the risk of traveling by automobile can be compared to that of traveling by horse with the use of historical data.

Another common procedure is to compare exposures only. Table 1 shows a list of radiation exposures in typical situations (Wilson and Jones, 1974). The dose–response relation for radiations with similar energy deposition per unit track length will be similar, although there may be some correction required for dose–rate effects, so that ordering by exposure should be similar to ordering by risk. In estimating the number of lethal cancers on a linear hypothesis, we have here assumed approximately 8000 man-rems per cancer (at low doses), in itself uncertain by 30% or more.

An example of comparison of risks that are similarly calculated is the comparison of risks of various chlorinated hydrocarbons in drinking water. The risks to humans are estimated from carcinogen bioassays in rodents (rats and mice). Since these are similar materials, we might expect that the dose–response relationships have the same shape.

Table 1. Comparison of Several Common Radiation Risks

Action	Dose (mrem/year)	Cancers if all U S. population exposed (assuming linearity)
Medical x-rays	40	1100
Radon gas (1.5 pCi/liter, equivalent dose)[a]	500	13,500
Potassium in own body	30	1000
Cosmic radiation at sea level	40	1100
Cosmic radiation at Denver	65	1800
Dose to average resident near Chernobyl first year	5000	Not relevant
One transcontinental round trip by air	5	135
Average within 20 miles of nuclear plant	0 02	>1

[a]The radon exposure is to the lungs and cannot be directly compared to whole body external exposure The comparison here is on the basis of the same magnitude of risk The uncertainty of the radon number is at least a factor of 3

Chloroform, which is produced by interaction of chlorine with organic matter during the chlorination of surface waters to kill bacteria, produces cancer in animals 20 times as readily as does trichloroethylene, an industrial solvent that is occasionally found in well waters as a result of accidental pollution. Although neither is known to cause cancer in people, we might expect that chloroform would do so about 20 times as readily.

Table 2 shows a variety of risks calculated in various ways and our estimate of the

Table 2. Some Commonplace Risks (Mean Values with Uncertainty)

Action	Annual risk	Uncertainty
Motor vehicle accident (total)	2.4×10^{-4}	10%
Motor vehicle accident (pedestrian only)	4.2×10^{-5}	10%
Home accidents	1.1×10^{-4}	5%
Electrocution	5.3×10^{-6}	5%
Air pollution, eastern United States	2×10^{-4}	Factor of 20 downward only
Cigarette smoking, one pack per day	3.6×10^{-3}	Factor of 3
Sea-level background radiation (except radon)	2×10^{-5}	Factor of 3
All cancers	2.8×10^{-3}	10%
Four tablespoons peanut butter per day	8×10^{-6}	Factor of 3
Drinking water with EPA limit of chloroform	6×10^{-7}	Factor of 10
Drinking water with EPA limit of trichloroethylene	2×10^{-9}	Factor of 10
Alcohol, light drinker	2×10^{-5}	Factor of 10
Police killed in line of duty (total)	$2 2 \times 10^{-4}$	20%
Police killed in line of duty (by felons)	1.3×10^{-4}	10%
Frequent flying professor	5×10^{-5}	50%
Mountaineering (mountaineers)	6×10^{-4}	50%

uncertainty. They are deliberately jumbled to provoke thought by juxtaposition. [Risk estimates quoted by the Environmental Protection Agency (EPA) for carcinogens tend to be greater than those shown in Table 2 by a factor approximately equal to the uncertainty factor—this is not accidental (Anderson *et al.*, 1983; Russell and Gruber, 1987).]

CONTRASTING RISKS

Objections have been raised to risk comparisons on the ground that they are misleading. This would be true if all risks of the same numerical magnitude were treated in the same way. But they are not. In some cases it is useful to contrast risks to indicate the different ways in which they are treated in society. In Table 3 we give an example by comparing and contrasting the carcinogenic effects of aflatoxin B1 and dioxin, both among the most carcinogenic chemicals known. The difference in treatment of these two materials is perhaps a reflection of different values assigned to various aspects of the problems caused by their presence.

Aflatoxin and dioxin have similar toxicities and carcinogenic potency (perhaps within a factor of 10, although both measures for both chemicals vary substantially with species tested). The certainty of information for aflatoxin is great. There is less information about carcinogenicity of dioxin. Dioxin may be a promoter and pose a minuscule risk at low doses, whereas aflatoxin is almost certainly an initiator also. Nonetheless such standards as there are appear to be more stringent for dioxin, possibly because dioxin is an artificial chemical and possibly because it was a trace component of a chemical mixture (Agent Orange) that was used in warfare.

Table 3. Comparison of Two Very Toxic Chemicals,
Aflatoxin B1[a] and Dioxin[b]

Measure	Aflatoxin B1	Dioxin
Acute toxicity	High	Equal
Carcinogenic potency to people [(kg/day)/mg]	~500	Unknown
Carcinogenic potency to rats [(kg/day)/mg]	~5000	~5000
Mutagenic	Yes	No
Certainty of information on human carcinogenicity	High	Low
Activity (initiator or promoter)	Initiator	Promoter (?)
Possibility of threshold dose–response	Low	High
Source	Natural	Artificial
Common knowledge	Little known	Agent Orange
FDA action level in peanuts (ppb)[c]	20	—
CDC[d] level of concern in soil (ppb)	—	1

[a]From Roberts (1977)
[b]From Kimbrough *et al* (1984)
[c]ppb, part per billion
[d]CDC, Centers for Disease Control

The small risk of a large accident in a nuclear power plant can also be contrasted with the more numerous small accidents or events that occur every day in the mining, transport, and burning of coal. One feature that is brought out clearly here is that we do not always compare the risk averaged over time, but worry more about risks that are sharply peaked in time.

EXPRESSION OF RISKS

Just as a comparison of risks is an aid in understanding them, so is a careful selection of the methods of expression. It is hard to comprehend the statistical (stochastic) nature of risk. There are ways to mitigate this difficulty in comprehension. We are almost all used to one such statistical concept—the expectation of life. When we talk about the expectation of life being 79 years (for a nonsmoking male in the United States) we all know that some die young and that many live to be over 80. Thus the expression of a risk as the reduction of life expectancy caused by the risky action conveys some of the statistical concept essential to its understanding. One particular calculation of this type can be used as an anchor for many people, because it is easy to remember. The reduction of life expectancy by smoking cigarettes can be calculated from the risk, one in 2 million, of smoking one cigarette, multiplied by the difference of the average life-span of a nonsmoker and a lung cancer victim. This turns out to be five minutes, or the time it takes to smoke the one cigarette.

It is important to realize that risks appear to be very different when expressed in different ways (Tversky and Kahneman, 1981). One example of this can be seen if we consider the cancer risk to those persons exposed to radionuclides after the Chernobyl disaster. According to the Soviets (U.S.S.R. Committee for the Utilization of Atomic Energy, 1986) the 24,000 persons between 3 and 15 km from the plant, but excluding the town of Pripyat, received and are expected to receive 1.05 million man-rems total integrated dose, or about 44 rems average. Even if we assume a linear dose–response relation, with 8000 man-rems per cancer, the risk may be expressed in different ways. Dividing 1.05 million man-rems by 8000 gives 131 cancers expected in the lifetimes of that population. This is larger than, and for some people more alarming than, the 31 people within the power plant itself who died within 60 days of acute radiation sickness combined with burns. Dividing the 131 again by the approximately 5000 cancer deaths expected from other causes, the accident caused "only" a 2.6% increase in cancer. This seems small compared to the 30% of cancers attributable to cigarette smoking. The difference is even more striking if we consider the 75 million people in Byelorussia and the Ukraine who received, and will receive, 29 million man-rems over their lifetimes. On the linear dose–response relation this leads to 3500 "extra cancers," surely a large number for one accident. But dividing by the 15 million cancers expected in this population leads to an "insignificant" increase of 0.023%. Of course, none of the methods of expressing the risk can be considered "right" in an absolute sense. Indeed, it is our belief that a full understanding of the risk involves expressing it in as many different ways as possible.

COST OF REDUCING A RISK

Another interesting and instructive way of comparing risks is by comparing the amount people have paid in the past to reduce them. It might be thought that people would try to adjust their activities until the amount spent is roughly the same. Cohen (1980) has shown that the amounts spent vary by a factor of more than a million. He shows that it would be possible even for an American to save lives in Indonesia by aiding in immunization at $100 per life saved. Society is willing to spend more on environmental protection to prevent cancer (over $1 million per life) than on cures (about $50,000 per life with the high value of $200,000 for kidney dialysis raising some objections). This ratio is in rough accord with the maxim "an ounce of protection is better than a pound of cure." People are willing to spend still more on radiation protection at nuclear power plants and on waste disposal. Economists and others often argue that efficiency depends on adjusting society until the amounts spent to save lives in different situations are equalized. It seems to us that society does not work that way. People are aware of the order of magnitude of these differences, and approve of them. Nonetheless, we believe that providing this information to a decision maker is essential for an informed decision.

ACKNOWLEDGMENT. Our work on risk assessment has been supported by donations from Clairol, Inc., the Dow Chemical Company, the Cabot Corporation, the General Electric Foundation, and the Monsanto Corporation.

REFERENCES

Ames, B. N., Magaw, R., and Gold, L. S., 1987, *Science* **236**:271.

Anderson, E. L. *et al.*, 1983, *Risk Anal.* **3**:277.

Calabrese, E. J., 1983, *Principles of Animal Extrapolation*, Wiley, New York.

Cohen, B. L., 1980, *Health Phys.* **38**:33.

"Control of trihalomethanes in drinking water," 1968, proposed rule, *Fed Regist.* **43**:5756; see also the advanced notice [*Fed. Regist.* **41**, 28991 (1976)] and the final rule [*Fed. Regist.* **44**, 68624 (1979)].

Crouch, E. A. C., and Wilson, R., 1979, *J. Toxicol. Environ. Health* **5**:1095.

Doll, R., and Peto, R., 1984, *J. Natl. Cancer Inst.* **66**:1191

Kimbrough, R. D., Falk, H., Stehr, P., and Fries, G., 1984, *J. Toxicol. Environ. Health* **14**:47.

Lave, L. B., 1987, *Science* **236**:291.

Meselson, M., and Russell, K., 1977, in: *Origins of Human Cancer* (H. H. Hiatt, J. D. Watson, J. A. Winsten, eds.), p. 1473, Cold Spring Harbor Laboratory, Cold Spring Harbor, New York.

Parodi, S., Taningher, M., Boero, P., and Santi, L., 1982, *Mutat. Res.* **93**:1.

Peto, R., 1985, in: *Assessment of Risk from Low-Level Exposure to Radiation and Chemicals* (A. D. Woodhead, C. J. Shellabarger, V. Pond, A. Hollaender, eds.), pp. 3–16, Plenum Press, New York.

Rasmussen, N. C. *et al.*, 1975, "Reactor safety study—an assessment of accident risks in U.S. commercial nuclear power plants" (WASH 1400, NUREG 75/014, U.S. Nuclear Regulatory Commission, Washington, DC, 1975); see also D. Okrent, 1987, *Science* **236**:296.

Roberts, H. R., 1977, "The regulatory outlook for nut products," paper presented at the Annual Convention of the Peanut Butter Manufacturers and Nut Salters Association, West Palm Beach, Florida, Nov. 1977.

Russell, M., and Gruber, M., 1987, *Science* **236**:286.

"Saccharin and its salts," proposed rule and hearing, *Fed. Regist.* **42**:19996 (1977).

Smoking and Health, a Report of the Surgeon General, 1975, PHS79-50066, Public Health Service, Washington, D.C.

Squire, R. A., 1981, *Science* **214:**877.

Tversky, A., and Kahneman, D., 1981, *Science* **211:**453; see also P. Slovic, 1987, *Science* **236:**280.

U.S.S.R. State Committee for the Utilization of Atomic Energy, "The accident at the Chernobyl Nuclear Power Plant and its consequences," working document for the Post Accident Review Meeting, 25–29 August 1986, International Atomic Energy Agency, Vienna.

Wilson, R., and Jones, W. J., 1974, *Energy, Ecology and the Environment,* Academic Press, New York, table 9-6. Other entries may be readily calculated from data in the reports of the United Nations scientific committee on the effects of atomic radiation ["Sources and effects of ionizing radiation" (United Nations, New York, 1977)] and the report of the Committee on the Biological Effects of Ionizing Radiations ["The effects on populations of exposure to low levels of ionizing radiations" (National Academy Press, Washington, DC, 1980)].

Wilson, R., Crouch, E. A. C., and Zeise, L., 1985, in: *Risk Quantitation and Regulatory Policy: Banbury Report 19,* pp. 133–147, Cold Spring Harbor Laboratory Press, Cold Spring Harbor, New York.

Zeise, L., Wilson, R., and Crouch, E. A. C., 1984, *Risk Anal.* **4:**187.

15

Risk Communication

Vincent T. Covello, Detlof von Winterfeldt, and Paul Slovic

INTRODUCTION

Risk communication takes place in a variety of forms, ranging from warning labels on consumer products to interactions among governmental officials, industry representatives, the media, and members of the public on such highly charged situations as Love Canal, ethylene dibromide (EDB) contamination of food, Three Mile Island, cigarette smoking, asbestos in school buildings, and Chernobyl. Experience has shown that risk communication efforts are a source of frustration for both risk communicators and for the intended recipients of the information. Government officials, industry representatives, and scientists note that laypeople frequently do not understand highly technical risk information and that individual biases and limitations may lead to distorted and inaccurate perceptions of many risk problems. Representatives of citizen groups and individual citizens are often equally frustrated, perceiving risk communicators and risk assessment experts to be uninterested in their concerns and unwilling to take immediate and direct actions to solve seemingly straightforward health, safety, and environmental problems. In this context, the media often plays the role of transmitter and translator of information between risk communicators and the public. But the media has been criticized for exaggerating risks and for emphasizing drama over scientific facts.

A recent review of the literature (Covello *et al.*, 1986) on efforts to communicate information about health and environmental risks—such as the controversies over the risks of saccharin, the pesticide EDB, dioxin, AIDS, toxic wastes, smoking, driving

Vincent T. Covello • Risk Assessment Program, National Science Foundation, Washington, D.C. 20550. *Detlof von Winterfeldt* • Institute of Safety and System Management, University of Southern California, Los Angeles, California 90089.   *Paul Slovic* • Decision Research, Eugene, Oregon 97401.   The views and conclusions expressed in this paper are solely those of the authors and do not necessarily reflect the views and conclusions of the National Science Foundation.

without seat belts, and nuclear power plant accidents—suggests that risk communication problems arise from (1) message problems (e.g., limitations of scientific risk assessments), (2) source problems (e.g., limitations of risk communicators and risk assessment experts), (3) channel problems (e.g., limitations in the means or media by which scientific information about health or environmental risks is transmitted), and (4) receiver problems (e.g., characteristics of the intended recipients of the communication) (Table 1).

Message problems include:

• Deficiencies in scientific understanding, data, models, and methods resulting in large uncertainties in risk estimates.
• Highly technical analyses that are often unintelligible to laypersons.

Source problems include:

• Lack of trust and credibility.
• Disagreements among scientific experts.
• Limited authority and resources for addressing risk problems.
• Lack of data addressing the specific fears and concerns of individuals and communities.
• Failures to disclose limitations of risk assessments and resulting uncertainties.

Table 1. Problems in Risk Communication

Origin of the problem	Example	Nature of the problem
Message problems	Government or industry data on health risks	High level of scientific complexity Large data uncertainties
Source problems	Government or industry officials	Lack of institutional trust and credibility Expert disagreements Use of technical, bureaucratic language Lack of understanding of public concerns
Channel problems	Media	Selective and biased reporting Focus on sensational or dramatic aspects Premature disclosure of scientific information Inaccuracies and distortions
Receiver problems	Individual citizens	Inaccurate perceptions of risk Overconfidence in ability to avoid harm Unrealistic demands for scientific certainty Reluctance to make tradeoffs

- Limited understanding of the interests, concerns, fears, values, priorities, and preferences of individual citizens and public groups.
- Use of bureaucratic, legalistic, and technical language.

Channel problems include:

- Selective and biased media reporting that emphasizes drama, wrongdoing, disagreements, and conflict.
- Premature disclosures of scientific information.
- Oversimplifications, distortions, and inaccuracies in interpreting technical risk information.

Receiver problems include:

- Inaccurate perceptions of levels of risk.
- Overconfidence in one's ability to avoid harm.
- Strong beliefs and opinions that are resistant to change.
- Exaggerated expectations about the effectiveness of regulatory actions.
- Desire and demands for scientific certainty.
- A reluctance to make trade-offs between different types of risks or between risks, costs, and benefits.
- Difficulties in understanding probabilistic information related to unfamiliar technologies.

Given these problems and the widespread dissatisfaction with the current state of risk communication, increasing numbers of researchers have turned their attention to problems of risk communication. Much of this work has focused on communications between government agencies and the public. Such communications are currently the subject of intense controversy and represent one of the most challenging and difficult aspects of risk management today (Ruckelshaus, 1984; EPA, 1984).

Reflecting the broad scope of risk communication, the literature on risk communication encompasses such diverse fields as cognitive psychology, social psychology, consumer behavior, marketing, advertising, economics, mass communications, linguistics, anthropology, decision science, sociology, political science, health education, behavioral medicine, public health, environmental health, law, and philosophy.

RISK COMMUNICATION TASKS AND PROBLEMS

For purposes of this review, risk communication is defined as any purposeful transfer or exchange of information about health or environmental risks between interested parties. More specifically, risk communication is the act of conveying or transmitting information between interested parties about (1) levels of health or environmental risks, (2) the significance or meaning of health or environmental risks, or (3) decisions, actions, or policies aimed at managing or controlling health or environmental risks. Interested parties include government agencies, corporations and industry groups, unions, the media, scientists, professional organizations, public interest groups, and individual citizens.

As shown in the Table 2, risk communication tasks can be organized into four general types, according to the primary objective or intended effect of the communication:

- Information and education.
- Behavior change and protective action.
- Disaster warnings and emergency information.
- Joint problem solving and conflict resolution.

In the real world, these four types of risk communication tasks overlap substantially, but they still can be conceptually differentiated. The task of informing and educating the public can be considered primarily a nondirective, although purposeful, activity aimed at providing the lay public with useful and enlightening information. In contrast, both the task of encouraging behavior change and personal protective action and that of providing disaster warnings and emergency information can be considered primarily directive activities aimed at motivating people to take specific types of action. These three tasks, in turn, differ from the task of involving individuals and groups in joint problem solving and conflict resolution, in which officials and citizens exchange information and work together to solve health and environmental problems. As shown by the descriptions of the four communication tasks provided below, each task is also associated with a different set of characteristic problems. An extended discussion of recommendations for handling these problems can be found in the recent literature review by Covello *et al.* (1986).

Type 1: Information and Education

Problems.   A variety of problems complicate the task of informing and educating people about risks and risk assessment.

Table 2. A Typology of Risk Communication Objectives

Type 1: Information and education
   Informing and educating people about risks and risk assessment in general.
   Example. Statistical comparisons of the risks of different energy production technologies.

Type 2: Behavior change and protective action
   Encouraging personal risk-reduction behavior.
   Example. Advertisements encouraging people to wear seat belts.

Type 3: Disaster warnings and emergency information
   Providing direction and behavioral guidance in disasters and emergencies.
   Example. Sirens indicating the accidental release of toxic gas from a chemical plant.

Type 4: Joint problem solving and conflict resolution
   Involving the public in risk management decisionmaking and in resolving health, safety, and environmental controversies.
   Example. Public meetings on a possible hazardous waste site.

- Risk information is often highly technical, complex, and uncertain. Because of uncertainties deriving from a lack of scientific data and from deficiencies in available methods and models, it is not uncommon to find substantial variations in risk estimates. For example, a committee of the National Academy of Sciences (1978) estimated that the expected number of bladder cancers resulting from the consumption of saccharin over the next 70 years ranges between 0.22 and 1,144,000 cases, depending on the assumptions that are made.
- Experts often disagree on the assumptions underlying a risk assessment and, as a result, often provide widely differing risk estimates. One result of these disagreements is public confusion about the validity of risk estimates.
- Government agencies often lack public trust and credibility. Trust and credibility are intimately linked and can be undermined by numerous factors, including public perceptions that an agency lacks technical competence, that the agency has withheld critical information or provided misleading information in the past, that agency decisions are overly influenced by special interest groups, or that an agency is inappropriately biased in favor of a particular technology or political strategy.
- Experts and laypeople often define risk differently. Experts typically define risk strictly in terms of expected annual mortalities. Lay people almost always include other factors in their definition of risk, such as catastrophic potential, equity (that is, whether those receiving benefits from the technology bear their share of the risks), effects on future generations, controllability, and involuntariness (Table 3). These differing conceptions often result in laypeople assigning relatively little weight to risk assessments conducted by technical experts and government agencies.
- Government officials often use technical, legalistic, or bureaucratic language. Besides being difficult to comprehend, such language gives the impression that officials are being unresponsive or evasive. For example, an official's statement that "groundwater contamination of 5 parts per billion is within the limits of acceptable safety standards set by the agency" may be technically correct but may also leave individuals suspicious and confused about the meaning and relevance to a particular situation. Government officials may argue that technical language is unavoidable, given the constraints placed on them by the nature of the data, by agency regulations, and by the law.
- People are frequently unwilling to believe government officials who claim that their decisions and actions are constrained by resource, statutory, and other limitations. Individuals who are directly affected by a government decision are especially reluctant to accept such claims and often demand that the risk agent be banned or that the hazardous activity be curtailed.
- People are often not as interested in risk problems as officials in government agencies. Given competing interests and priorities, issues that are high on the agendas of government agencies may be low on the agendas of average citizens. It may thus be difficult to get people to pay attention to risk information. Those that do pay attention may be highly selective and focus on unusual and dramatic aspects of the problem instead of on representative data and statistics.
- Risk information can be frightening. A statement by a government official meant

Table 3. Factors Involved in Public Risk Perception

Factor	Conditions associated with increased public concern	Conditions associated with decreased public concern
Catastrophic potential	Fatalities and injuries grouped in time and space	Fatalities and injuries scattered and random
Familiarity	Unfamiliar	Familiar
Understanding	Mechanisms or process not understood	Mechanisms or process understood
Uncertainty	Risks scientifically unknown or uncertain	Risks known to science
Controllability (personal)	Uncontrollable	Controllable
Voluntariness of exposure	Involuntary	Voluntary
Effects on children	Children specifically at risk	Children not specifically at risk
Effects on future generations	Risk to future generations	No risk to future generations
Victim identity	Identifiable victims	Statistical victims
Dread	Effects dreaded	Effects not dreaded
Trust in institutions	Lack of trust in responsible institutions	Trust in responsible institutions
Media	Much media attention	Little media attention
Accident history	Major and sometimes minor accidents	No major or minor accidents
Equity	Inequitable distribution of risks and benefits	Equitable distribution of risks and benefits
Benefits	Unclear benefits	Clear benefits
Reversibility	Effects irreversible	Effects reversible
Personal involvement	Individual personally at risk	Individual not personally at risk
Scientific evidence	Risk estimates based on human evidence	Risk estimates based on animal evidence

to assure the public that its water is safe to drink, its air is safe to breathe, or its food is safe to eat may have exactly the opposite effect. Instead of alleviating concern, it may increase fear, anxiety, and avoidance of an activity that previously was assumed to be safe. The very fact that an official investigation is under way may be sufficient to create an atmosphere of fear and suspicion.

- People holding strong beliefs are exceedingly resistant to changing such beliefs, even when confronted with substantial and opposing scientific evidence. Motorcyclists, for example, often deny that they engage in a high risk activity, even when presented with statistics on the high incidence of motorcycle accidents. Such persons frequently question the accuracy of the statistics or the relevance of the statistics to their unique situation. For example, they may refer to their superior abilities and experience in handling motorcycles or to their own accident-free records.

- Although strong beliefs are difficult to change, weakly held beliefs can often be manipulated by subtle differences in the presentation of risk information.

- People have difficulty interpreting probabilistic information. Extremely small probabilities, such as a chance of one in a million or smaller, are especially difficult to comprehend.

Relevant Research. Of the various academic disciplines concerned with problems related to information and education, researchers in the fields of cognitive and social psychology have been among the most active. (See, for example, Combs and Slovic, 1979; Slovic *et al.*, 1978, 1979, 1980, 1981, 1982; Green, 1980; Johnson and Tversky, 1983; McNeil *et al.*, 1982; Renn, 1981; Fischhoff *et al.*, 1978, 1979, 1984; Lichtenstein *et al.*, 1978; Otway, 1980; Otway and von Winterfeldt, 1982; Otway *et al.*, 1978; Tversky and Kahneman, 1981; von Winterfeldt *et al.*, 1981; Vlek and Stallen, 1981; Squyres, 1980; Gardner *et al.*, 1982; Lowrance, 1976; Kasperson and Kasperson, 1983; Covello, 1983, 1984.) Cognitive and social psychologists have explored questions such as: How do people define and perceive risks and what determines the risk's acceptability? Does newspaper coverage bias the perception of risks? What are the determinants of attitudes and attitude change? What factors influence the success or failure of educational efforts? How does the presentation of risk information influence the public's perceptions and preferences?

Sociologists, economists, political scientists, anthropologists, health educators, and communications researchers have also been active in the study of problems related to information and education. While psychologists have usually focused on the mental processing and evaluation of risk information, sociologists, economists, political scientists, anthropologists, and health educators have focused on the influence of social, economic, institutional, organizational, or cultural factors as well as the influence of the media on the public's risk perceptions, preferences, and behavioral responses to risk-related information. (See, for example, Conrad, 1980; Mazur, 1973, 1981; Nelkin, 1984; Nelkin and Brown, 1984; Perrow, 1984; Wildavsky and Douglas, 1982; Gross and Rayner, 1983; Twentieth Century Fund, 1984; Mitchell, 1980; Short, 1984; Douglas, 1966; Rothman, 1982; Sharlin, 1985; Levine, 1982; Shelanski *et al.*, 1982; Winsten, 1985; Sandman, 1973, 1975, 1982; Sandman and Paden, 1979; Johnson and Covello, 1986; Morris *et al.*, 1980; Lipset and Schneider, 1983; Barber, 1983; Short, 1984; Burger, 1984; Media Institute, 1985.)

Type 2: Behavior Change and Protective Action

Problems. In addition to problems already noted in relation to other communication tasks, a variety of problems complicate the task of encouraging behavior change and protective action.

- The losses incurred by changing behavior are tangible and immediate, such as the loss of the pleasure of smoking or the taste of a favorite food, while the gains are abstract, intangible, and remote in time.
- People frequently display an "optimism bias." For example, a person may believe that fate or luck is on his or her side and that it "can't happen to me." This is especially true in activities that require skill and involve individual control, such as driving or skiing.
- People often resist government efforts aimed at changing behavior for political or ideological reasons. For many, such efforts represent unacceptable intrusions by government in their personal lives.

- The target audience of a behavior change campaign is often unmotivated and uninvolved, and, consequently, it may ignore the message.
- People rationalize their resistance to behavior change. For example, smokers who need the psychological relief of smoking a cigarette often cite the pressures of modern life as their justification and minimize the risks.
- People seldom respond appropriately to high-threat or fear communications, such as photographs or films graphically depicting the physical symptoms of disease or the results of a disfiguring or fatal accident. Such communications may induce excessive fear and anxiety, which, in turn, may reduce people's attention, induce defensive responses, and evoke hostility toward the source of the communication.

Relevant Research. Of the various academic disciplines concerned with problems of behavior change and protective action, researchers in the fields of consumer behavior, marketing, advertising, social psychology, sociology, health promotion, and disease prevention have been among the most active. (See, for example, McGuire, 1985; Eagly and Chaiken, 1985; Earle and Cvetkovich, 1983; Earle, 1984; Vertinsky and Vertinsky, 1982; Weinstein, 1984; Maccoby *et al.*, Maccoby and Solomon, 1977, 1981; Fishbein and Ajzen, 1975; Kiesler *et al.*, 1968; Gusfield, 1982; Robinson, 1976; Robinson *et al.*, 1974; Sutton, 1982; Alcalay, 1983; Adler and Pittle, 1984; Evans and Clarke, 1983; Rice and Page, 1981.) Researchers in consumer behavior, marketing, and advertising have been concerned primarily with factors that underlie consumer choice. Social psychologists, sociologists, and health promotion specialists have been interested primarily in attitude change and persuasion, as well as in the social and institutional processes that precede behavior change.

Type 3: Disaster Warnings and Emergency Information

Problems. In addition to problems already noted in relation to other communication tasks, a variety of problems complicate the task of providing disaster warnings and emergency information.

- In most disasters and emergencies, the primary objectives of government officials are to minimize loss of life and to minimize property damage. These macroobjectives often come into conflict with the microobjectives of local residents (and sometimes local disaster or emergency workers), who frequently assign highest priority to the protection of their own family members, friends, personal possessions, and property.
- Time pressures often compound an already difficult situation.
- Coordination between agencies and organizations frequently breaks down during disasters; confusion about responsibility and authority often results in multiple and competing sources of information.
- Communication channels frequently break down during disasters and may result in confusion and the spread of rumors.
- Warning systems frequently produce false alarms, which confuse people, generate mistrust in the warning system, and may desensitize people to future warnings.
- People often deny the possibility of a disaster or that it may affect them personally.

Thus, it is often difficult to capture public interest and attention before a disaster occurs. These observations appear, however, to apply more to natural disasters than to technological disasters.

- People are sometimes reluctant to evacuate, especially in natural disasters. Concerns about the loss of personal belongings and of opportunities to save their homes and property often outweigh the motivation to evacuate.
- People usually require confirmation of the original emergency communication through several communication channels before taking action, for example, through telephone calls to the local police or to friends. However, these channels often break down during a disaster or emergency. Without the ability to confirm the original message, people may become confused and not act appropriately.

Relevant Research. Of the various academic disciplines concerned with disaster warnings and emergency information, sociological and social psychological researchers have been among the most active. The literature includes general reviews (see Mileti *et al.*, 1975; Quarantelli and Dynes, 1977; Kreps, 1984; Saarnen, 1982), case studies of risk communication prior to and during disasters and emergencies (see Cutter and Barnes, 1982; Friedman, 1981; Greene *et al.*, 1980; Kunreuther *et al.*, 1978; Lindell *et al.*, 1983; Lagadec, 1982; Shelanski, 1982; Bowonder, 1985), and studies of specific aspects of the disaster process, such as warning systems (see Mileti, 1975; Turner, *et al.*, 1981; Nilson and Nilson, 1981; Hodler, 1982; Pate-Cornell, 1986), media coverage (see Mazur, 1981; Mazur *et al.*, 1982; Rogers and Sood, 1986; Sandman, 1979; Peltu, 1985), and evacuation behavior (see Perry *et al.*, 1980; Lindell *et al.*, 1985; Quarantelli, 1980).

Type 4: Joint Problem Solving and Conflict Resolution

Problems. In addition to problems already noted in relation to other communication tasks, a variety of problems complicate the task of involving the public in joint problem solving and conflict resolution.

- Actions by a government agency aimed at involving the public in the regulatory decisionmaking process may be viewed as an attempt by the agency to abdicate its legal duties and responsibilities. For example, such attempts are sometimes viewed as an attempt by the agency to avoid enforcing health and environmental laws.
- It is difficult to hold public meetings in a highly charged, emotional atmosphere. A common characteristic of joint problem solving exercises is strong involvement by stakeholder groups, with each group bringing its own values and concerns to the arena. Frequently, the initial atmosphere is one of distrust and confrontation, rather than openness and cooperation.
- Officials often do not understand the nature of the conflict or sources of disagreement. Such disagreements can range from factual disputes about levels of risk to fundamental disagreements about values and ethical principles.
- Many communication strategies are inappropriate for specific types of conflict. For example, when conflicts are about facts and statistics, information and education strategies are relevant. However, when conflicts are about the equity (fairness) of risk–benefit distributions or about basic values, education and information strat-

egies are of little value. Such cases require careful diagnosis of the concerns of all interested parties and the design of options (such as safeguards or compensation schemes) that specifically address these concerns.

- The media may aggravate communication problems by highlighting personal fears and anxieties, by focusing only on the dramatic or sensational aspects of a story, and by emphasizing conflict rather than agreement.

- Individuals and groups involved in the process are often unwilling to compromise or accept tradeoffs. For example, local residents may exhibit a "not in my backyard" attitude when exposed to a new risk and frequently demand complete elimination of the risk regardless of costs, resources, or other constraints.

- Individuals and groups are often invited to participate in decision making only after many of the most important decisions have been made.

Relevant Research. Of the various academic disciplines concerned with joint problem solving and conflict resolution, researchers in the fields of decision science, political science, and sociology have been among the most active. Within these disciplines, specialists on public involvement and on social conflict have been especially productive. Public involvement studies have examined numerous examples of interactions between the public and government agencies (see Creighton, 1980; Delli Priscoli *et al.*, 1983; Popper, 1985; Susskind, 1978; Susskind *et al.*, 1978). Researchers have also drawn on the literature on game and decision theory (see Luce and Raiffa, 1957; Keeney and Raiffa, 1976; von Winterfeldt and Edwards, 1985) and on bargaining, negotiation, and mediation (see Raiffa, 1982) to develop tools for diagnosing the nature of conflict among groups and mechanisms for resolving these conflicts. Three additional research traditions have also made substantial contributions: sociological research on the causes and the dynamics of technological controversies (see Tribe *et al.*, 1976; Coser, 1956; Mazur, 1980, 1981; Nelkin, 1978; Perrow, 1984); research on environmental mediation and arbitration (see Busterud, 1980; Bingham, 1984; Cormick, 1980; Wellborn, 1979; O'Hare, 1977, 1984; Susskind and Wheeler, 1983; Bacow *et al.*, 1983; Bacow and Wheeler, 1983; Mernitz, 1980); and research on informed consent and decision making (see Gibson, 1985; MacLean, 1986).

CONCLUSIONS

Several general conclusions can be drawn from the literature on risk communication that cut across all four types of communication tasks.

- The roots of most risk communication problems are deeply embedded in broader social issues. What sometimes appears to be a simple and direct issue often turns out to be an issue of enormous scientific, economic, social, and political complexity.

- Interactive and participatory approaches to risk communication appear to offer the greatest promise of better, less controversial, or less divisive decisions. Even the most directive types of risk communication tasks, such as encouraging personal behavior change and providing disaster warnings, can benefit substantially from public involvement, direct interaction, and exchanges of information. Such interactions are an important source of knowledge of public needs and concerns, without which communication efforts are likely to fail or be ineffective.

- As a target for risk communication, there is no such entity as "the public"; instead, there are many publics, each with its own interests, needs, concerns, priorities, and preferences.
- The choice of one communication strategy over another often requires a complex balancing of multiple, competing objectives, including the community's "right to know," the duty to protect public health, the costs of unnecessarily alarming people, and the possible repercussions of premature or delayed action.
- Government officials and individual citizens often hold different views of risk problems. Most regulatory agencies view risk problems from a societal or macroperspective. As a result, most analyses by government agencies provide only aggregate or population statistics for the community or nation as a whole. Aggregate or population statistics are, however, usually of little interest to individual citizens, who are more likely to view risks from a microperspective and to be concerned about the risks to themselves or to their loved ones than to society or the community as a whole. Given this divergence of viewpoints, government officials are often at a disadvantage, since they often do not have immediate access to information that addresses the highly personalized questions asked by citizens.
- A large amount of research has been conducted that bears on problems of risk communication, but the literature specifically focused on risk communication is relatively small. Substantial progress has been made on some topics, such as psychological research on public perceptions of risk, but large gaps exist in our understanding of virtually every issue relevant to risk communication. Institutional arrangements and financial resources for research on risk communication issues are inadequate.

REFERENCES

Adler, R., and Pittle, R. D., 1984, Cajolery or command: Are education campaigns an adequate substitute for regulation?, *Yale J. Reg.* **1**:159–193.

Alcalay, R., 1983, The impact of mass communication in the health field, *Social Sci. Med.* **17**:87–94.

Barber, B., 1983, *The Logic and Limits of Trust*, Rutgers University Press, New Brunswick, New Jersey.

Bingham, G., 1984, *Resolving Environmental Disputes: A Decade of Experience*, The Conservation Foundation, Washington, D.C.

Bowonder, B., 1985, "Low Probability Event: A Case Study in Risk Assessment," Unpublished paper presented at the workshop *Risk Analysis in Developing Countries*, Hyderabad, India, Oct. 1985.

Burger, E., 1984, *Health Risks: The Challenge of Informing the Public*, The Media Institute, Washington, D.C.

Busterud, J., 1980, Mediation: The state of the art, *Environ. Pro.* **2**:34–39.

Combs, B., and Slovic, P., 1979, Newspaper coverage of causes of death, *Journalism Q.* **56**:837–843.

Covello, V. T., 1983, The perception of technological risks: A literature review, *Technol. Forecast. Social Change*, **23**:285–297.

Covello, V. T., 1984, Uses of social and behavioral research on risk, *Environ. Int.* **10**(June):541–545.

Covello, V., von Winterfeldt, D., and Slovic, P., 1986, Communicating scientific information about health and environmental risks: Problems and opportunities from a social and behavioral perspective, in: *Uncertainties in Risk Assessment and Risk Management* (V. Covello, L. B. Lave, A. Moghissi, and V. R. R. Uppuluri, eds.), pp. 221–239, Plenum Press, New York.

Conrad, J. (ed.), 1980, *Society, Technology, and Risk Assessment,* Academic Press, New York.

Cormick, G. W., 1980, The theory and practice of environmental mediation, *Environ. Pro.* 2:24–33.

Coser, L. A., 1956, *The Functions of Social Conflict.* Free Press, New York.

Creighton, J. L., 1980, *Public Involvement Manual: Involving the Public in Water and Power Resource Discussions.* U.S. Government Printing Office, Washington, D.C.

Cutter, S., and Barnes, K., 1982, Evacuation behavior and Three Mile Island, *Disasters* 6:116–124.

Delli Priscoli, J., Creighton, J., and Dunning, C. M. (eds.), 1983, *Public Involvement Techniques: A Reader of Ten Years Experience of the Institute for Water Resources,* U.S. Army Corps of Engineers, Institute for Water Resources, IWR Research Report 82-R1, May, 1983.

Douglas, M., 1966, *Purity and Danger,* Routledge and Kegan Paul, London.

Douglas, M., and Wildavsky, A., 1982, *Risk and Culture,* University of California Press, Berkeley.

Eagly, A. H., and Chaiken, S., 1985, Psychological theories of persuasion, in: *Advances in Experimental Social Psychology* (L. Berkowitz, ed.), Academic Press, New York.

Earle, T. C., 1984, "Risk Communication: A Marketing Approach," Unpublished paper presented at the National Science Foundation/Environmental Protection Agency Workshop on *Risk Perception and Risk Communication,* Long Beach, California, Dec. 1984.

Earle, T. C., and Cvetkovich, G., 1983, Risk judgment and the communication of hazard information: Toward a new look in the study of risk perception, *BH ARC* (400/83/017), Battelle Human Affairs Research Centers, Seattle, Washington.

Environmental Protection Agency (EPA), 1984, *Risk·Assessment and Risk Management: Framework for Decision Making,* Environmental Protection Agency, Washington, D.C., Dec. 1984.

Evans, S. H., and Clarke, P., 1983, When cancer patients fail to get well: Flaws in health communication, in: *Communication Yearbook 7* (R. N. Bostrom, ed.), Sage, Beverly Hills.

Fischhoff, B., Slovic, P., Lichtenstein, S., Read, S., and Combs, B., 1978, How safe is safe enough? A psychometric study of attitudes towards technological risks and benefits, *Pol. Sci.* 8:127–152.

Fischhoff, B., Slovic, P., and Lichtenstein, S., 1979, Weighing the risks, *Environment* 21:17–20, 32–38.

Fischhoff, B., Watson, S., and Hope, C., 1984, Defining risk, *Pol. Sci.* 17:123–139.

Fishbein, M., and Ajzen, I., 1975, *Belief, Attitude, Intention and Behavior: An Introduction to Theory and Research,* Addison-Wesley, Reading, Massachusetts.

Friedman, S. M., 1981, Blueprint for breakdown: Three Mile Island and the mass media before the accident, *J. Commun.* 31:85–96.

Gibson, M. (ed.), 1985, *To Breathe Freely: Risk, Consent, and Air,* Rowman and Allanheld, Totowa, New Jersey.

Green, C. H., 1980, Risk: Attitudes and beliefs, in: *Behavior in Fires,* (D. V. Canter, ed.), Wiley, Chichester.

Greene, M., Perry, R. W., and Lindell, M. K., 1980, The March 1980 eruptions of Mount St. Helens: Citizens perceptions of volcano hazard, *Disasters* 2:49–66.

Gross, J. L., and Rayner, S., 1983, *Measuring Culture: A Paradigm for the Analysis of Social Organization,* Columbia University Press, New York.

Hodler, T. W., 1982, Residents' preparedness and response to the Kalamazoo tornado, *Disasters* 2:44–49.

Johnson, B., and Covello, V. (eds.), 1987, *The Social and Cultural Construction of Risk,* Reidel, Boston.

Johnson, E. J., and Tversky, A., 1983, Affect, generalization and the perception of risk, *J. Person. Social Psychol.* 45:20–31.

Kasperson, R., and Kasperson, J., 1983, Determining the acceptability of risk: Ethical and policy issues, in: *Risk: A Symposium* (J. Rogers and D. Bates, eds.), pp. 133–155, The Royal Society of Canada, Ottawa.

Keeney, R. L., and Raiffa, H., 1976, *Decisions with Multiple Objectives: Preferences and Value Tradeoffs,* Wiley, New York.

Kiesler, C. A., Collins, B. E., and Miller, N., 1968, *Attitude Change,* Wiley, New York.

Kunreuther, H., Ginsberg, R., Miller, L., Sagi, P., Slovic, P., Borkan, B., and Katz, N., 1978, *Disaster Insurance Protection: Public Policy Lessons,* Wiley, New York.

Lagadec, P., 1982, *Major Technological Disaster,* Pergamon, Oxford.

Levine, A. G., 1982, *Love Canal: Science, Politics, and People,* D. C. Heath, Lexington, Massachusetts.

Lichtenstein, S., Slovic, P., Fischhoff, B., Layman, M., and Coombs, B., 1978, Judged frequency of lethal events, *J. Exp. Psychol. [Hum. Learn.]* 4:551–578.

Lindell, M., Bolton, P. A., Perry, R. W., Stoetzel, G. A., Martin, J. B., and Flynn, C. B., 1985, *Planning Concepts and Decision Criteria for Sheltering and Evacuation in a Nuclear Power Plant Emergency,*

Technical Report No. AIF/NESP-031, Batelle Human Affairs Research Centers, Seattle, Washington, June, 1985.

Lindell, M., Perry, W., and Greene, M., 1983, Individual response to emergency preparedness planning near Mt. St. Helens, *Disast. Man.* (Jan.–March):5–11.

Lipset, S., and Schneider, W., 1983, *The Confidence Gap: Business, Labor and Government in the Public Mind,* The Free Press, New York.

Lowrance, W., 1976, *Of Acceptable Risk: Science and the Determination of Safety,* Kaufman, Los Altos, California.

Luce, D., and Raiffa, H., 1957, *Games and Decisions,* Wiley, New York.

Maccoby, N., Farquhar, J., Wood, P., and Alexander, J., 1977, Reducing the risk of cardiovascular disease: Effects of a community-based campaign on knowledge and behavior, *J. Community Health* 3:100–114.

Maccoby, N., and Solomon, D. S., 1981, Heart disease prevention: Community studies, in: *Public Communication Campaigns,* (R. E. Rice and W. J. Paisley, eds.), Sage, Beverly Hills.

MacLean, D. (ed.), 1986, *Values at Risk,* Rowman and Allanheld, Totowa, New Jersey.

Mazur, A., 1973, Disputes between experts, *Minerva* 11:243–262.

Mazur, A., 1981, *The Dynamics of Technical Controversy,* Communications Press, Washington, D.C.

Mazur, A., 1980, Media coverage and public opinion on scientific controversies, *J. Commun. Res.* 31:106–115.

Media Institute, 1985, *Chemical Risks: Fears, Facts, and the Media,* Media Institute, Washington, D.C.

Mileti, D., 1975, *Natural Hazard Warning Systems in the U.S.: A Research Assessment,* Technical Report, Institute for Behavioral Science, University of Colorado, Boulder, Colorado.

Mileti, D., Drabek, T., and Haas, E., 1975, *Human Behavior in Extreme Environments,* University of Colorado, Boulder.

McGuire, W. J., 1985, Attitudes and attitude change, in: *Handbook of Social Psychology* (G. Lindzey and A. Aronson, eds.), Addison–Wiley, Reading, Massachusetts.

McNeil, B. J., Pauker, S. G., Sox, H. C., Jr., and Tversky, A., 1982, On the elicitation of preferences for alternative therapies, *N. Engl. J. Med.* 306:1259–1262.

Mitchell, R. C., 1980, *Public Opinion on Environmental Issues: Results of a National Public Opinion Survey,* Council on Environmental Quality, Washington, D.C.

Morris, L., Mazis, M., and Barofsky, I. (eds.), 1980, *Product Labeling and Health Risks,* Banbury Report 6, Cold Spring Harbor Laboratory, Cold Spring Harbor, New York.

National Academy of Sciences/National Research Council, 1978, *Saccharin: Technical Assessment of Risks and Benefits. Committee for a Study on Saccharin and Food Safety Policy,* National Academy of Sciences, Washington, D.C. (Second Ed.) Sage: Beverly Hills, 1984.)

Nelkin, D., (ed.), 1978, *Controversy: Politics of Technical Decisions,* Sage, Beverly Hills.

Nilson, L. B., and Nilson, D. C., 1981, Resolving the "sooner vs. later" controversy surrounding the public announcement of earthquake predictions, *Disasters* 5:391–397.

O'Hare, M., 1977, Not on my block you don't: Facility siting and the strategic importance of compensation, *Public Policy* 197:25:407–458.

O'Hare, M., 1987, Bargaining and negotiation for a conflict resolution, in: *Insuring and Managing Hazardous Risks* (P. Kleindorfer and H. Kunreuther, eds.), pp. 178–198, Springer, New York.

Otway, H., Maurer, D., and Thomas, K., 1978, Nuclear power: The question of public acceptance, *Futures* 10:109–118.

Otway, H. J., 1980, Risk perception: A psychological perspective, in: *Technological Risk: Its Perspective and Handling in Europe,* (M. Dierkes, S. Edwards, and R. Coppock, eds.), Oelgeschlager, Gunn and Hain, Boston.

Otway, H. J., and von Winterfeldt, D., 1982, Beyond acceptable risk: On the social acceptability of technologies, *Policy Sci.* 8:127–152.

Pate-Cornell, M. E., Warning systems in risk management, *Risk Anal.* 6(2):223–234.

Peltu, M., 1985, Risk communication: The role of the media, in: *Risk and Regulation,* (H. Otway, ed.), Butterworths, London.

Perrow, C., 1984, *Normal Accidents,* Basic Books, New York.

Perry, R. W., Greene, M. R., and Lindell, M. K., 1980, Enhancing evacuation warning compliance: Suggestions for emergency planning, *Disasters* 4:433–449.

Popper, F., 1985, The Environmentalists and the LULU (Local Unwanted Land Use), *Environment* (March).

Quarantelli, E., and Dynes, R., 1977, Response to social crisis and disaster, *Ann. Rev. Sociol.* **3**:23–49.

Quarantelli, E. L., 1980, *Evacuation Behavior and Problems: Findings and Implications from the Research Literature*, Department of Sociology, Disaster Research Center, Ohio State University, Columbus, Ohio.

Raiffa, H., 1982, *The Art and Science of Negotiation*, Harvard University Press, Cambridge, Massachusetts.

Renn, O., 1981, Man, technology, and risk: A study on intuitive risk assessment and attitudes towards nuclear power, Report Jul-Spez 115, Julich, Nuclear Research Center.

Rice, R. E., and Paisley, W. J. (eds.), 1981, *Public Communication Campaigns*, Sage, Beverly Hills.

Robertson, L., 1976, The great seat belt campaign flop, *J. Commun.* **26**:41–45.

Robertson, L., Kelley, A., O'Neill, B., Wixom, C., Eiswirth, R., and Haddon, W., 1974, A controlled study of the effect of television messages on safety belt use, *Am. J. Public Health* **64**:1071–1081.

Rogers, E. M., and Sood, R., 1981, "Mass media operations in a quick-onset natural disaster: Hurricane David in Dominica," Working paper, Annenberg School of Communications, University of Southern California, Los Angeles.

Rothman, S., 1982, Risk and nuclear power: Scientists, journalists, and the public, *Public Op.* **3**:47–52.

Ruckelshaus, W., 1984, Risk in a free society, *Risk Anal.* **4**(3):157–163.

Saarinen, T. (ed.), 1982, *Perspectives on Increasing Hazard Awareness*, Institute of Behavioral Science, Boulder, Colorado.

Sandman, P. M., and M. Paden, 1979, At Three Mile Island, *Columbia Journalism Rev.* **18**(no. 2, July–Aug.):43–58.

Sandman, P., 1973, Environmental advertising and social responsibility, in : *Mass Media and the Environment* (D. Rubin and D. Sachs, eds.), Praeger, New York.

Sharlin, H. I., 1985, *EDB: A Case Study in the Communication of Health Risk*, Office of Policy Agency, Environmental Protection Agency, Washington, D.C.

Shelanski, V., Sills, D., and Wolf, C., 1982, *The Accident at Three Mile Island*, Westview Press, Boulder, Colorado.

Short, J., 1984, The social fabric of risk, *Am. Sociol. Rev.* (December).

Slovic, P., Lichtenstein, S., and Fischhoff, B., 1979, Images of disaster: Perceptions and acceptance of risks from nuclear power, in: *Energy Risk Management* (G. Goodman and W. Rowe, eds.), Academic Press, London.

Slovic, P., Fischhoff, B., and Lichtenstein, S. 1980, Facts and fears: Understanding perceived risk, in: *Social Risk Assessment: How Safe is Safe Enough?* (R. Schwing and W. A. Albers, eds.), Plenum Press, New York. [Revision in D. Kahneman, P. Slovic, and A. Tversky (eds.), 1982, *Judgement under Uncertainty: Heuristics and Biases*, pp. 464–489, Cambridge University Press, Cambridge.]

Slovic, P., Fischhoff, B., and Lichtenstein, S., 1980, Informing people about risk, in: *Product Labeling and Health Risks* (L. Morris, M. Mazis, and I. Barofsky, eds.), Banbury Report 6, The Banbury Center, Cold Spring Harbor, New York.

Slovic, P., Fischhoff, B., and Lichtenstein, S., 1981, Perceived risk: Psychological factors and social implications, in: *The Assessment and Perception of Risk* (F. Warner and D. H. Slater, eds.), The Royal Society, London.

Squyres, W. D., 1980, *Patient Education*, Springer, New York.

Susskind, L. E., 1978, *The Importance of Citizen Participation and Consensus-Building in the Land Use Planning Process*, Massachusetts Institute of Technology, Laboratory of Architecture and Planning, Cambridge, Massachusetts.

Susskind, L. Richardson, Jr., and Hildebrand, K., 1978, *Resolving Environmental Disputes: Approaches to Intervention, Negotiation, and Conflict Resolution*, Environmental Impact Assessment Project, Massachusetts Institute of Technology, Cambridge, Massachusetts.

Sutton, S. R., 1982, Fear arousing communications: A critical examination of theory and research, in: *Social Psychology and Behavioral Medicine* (J. R. Eiser, ed.), pp. 303–338, Wiley, New York.

Tribe, L. H., Corrine, S., Shelling, T., and Voss, E. (eds.), 1976, *When Values Conflict: Essays on Environmental Analysis. Discourse and Decision*, Ballinger, Cambridge.

Turner, R. H., Nigg, J. M., Paz, D. H., and Young, B. S., 1981, *Community Response to Earthquake Threat in Southern California*, Institute for Social Science Research, University of California at Los Angeles, Los Angeles, California.

Tversky, A., and Kahneman, D., 1981, The framing of decisions and the psychology of choice, *Science* **211**:235–271.

Twentieth Century Fund, 1984, *Science in the Streets*, Priority Press, New York.

Vertinsky, I., and Vertinsky, P., 1982, Communicating environmental health assessment and other risk information: Analysis of strategies, in: *Risk: A Seminar Series* (H. Kunreuther, ed.), pp. 421–482, IIASA-CP-82-S2, International Institute for Applied Systems Analysis, Laxenburg, Austria.

Vlek, C., and Stallen, D. J., 1981, Judging risks and benefits in the small and in the large, *Organ. Behav. Hum. Perform.* **28:**235–271.

von Winterfeldt, D., John, R. S., and Borcherding, K., 1981, Cognitive components of risk ratings, *Risk Anal.* **1:**277–287.

von Winterfeldt, D., and Edwards, W., 1986, *Decision Analysis and Behavioral Research*, Cambridge University Press, New York.

Weinstein, N. D., 1984, Why it won't happen to me: Perceptions of risk factors and susceptibility, *Health Psychol.* **3:**431–457.

Weinstein, N.D., 1979, Seeking reassuring or threatening information about environmental cancer, *J. Behav. Med.* **2:**125–139.

Wellborn, S., 1979, *The Potential of Mediation for Resolving Environmental Disputes Related to Energy Facilities*, American Management Systems, Inc., DOE/EV/10274-1, Dec. 1979.

Index